Clinically Integrated Histology

Clinically Integrated Histology

David H. Cormack, Ph.D.
Professor
Department of Anatomy and Cell Biology
Faculty of Medicine
University of Toronto
Toronto, Canada

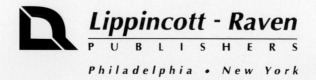

Lippincott - Raven
P U B L I S H E R S
Philadelphia • New York

Acquisitions Editor: Richard Winters
Developmental Editor: Erin O'Connor
Manufacturing Manager: Dennis Teston
Production Manager: Jodi Borgenicht
Assistant Managing Editor: Robert Pancotti
Cover Designer: Kevin Kall
Indexer: Dr. David Cormack
Compositor: Maryland Composition Company
Printer: Toppan Printing Company

Printed and bound in Singapore.

9 8 7 6 5 4 3 2 1

Library of Congress Cataloging-in-Publication Data
Cormack, David H.
   Clinically integrated histology / David H. Cormack.
      p.   cm.
   Includes bibliographical references and index.
   ISBN 0-7817-1211-4
   1. Histology, Pathological—Case studies.   2. Histology.
I. Title.
   [DNLM: 1. Histology—atlases.   2. Histology—case studies.   QS 517 C811c 1997]
   RB25.C67   1997
   611'.018—dc21
   DNLM/DLC
   for Library of Congress

Care has been taken to confirm the accuracy of the information presented and to describe generally accepted practices. However, the author and publisher are not responsible for errors or omissions or for any consequences from application of the information in this book and make no warranty, express or implied, with respect to the contents of the publication.

The author and publisher have exerted every effort to ensure that drug selection and dosage set forth in this text are in accordance with current recommendations and practice at the time of publication. However, in view of ongoing research, changes in government regulations, and the constant flow of information relating to drug therapy and drug reactions, the reader is urged to check the package insert for each drug for any change in indications and dosage and for added warnings and precautions. This is particularly important when the recommended agent is a new or infrequently employed drug.

Some drugs and medical devices presented in this publication have Food and Drug Administration (FDA) clearance for limited use in restricted research settings. It is the responsibility of the health care provider to ascertain the FDA status of each drug or device planned for use in their clinical practice.

Contents

Preface vii
Acknowledgments ix

1. *Introduction to Cell and Tissue Functions* 1
Synopsis of Cell and Tissue Functions 1
Tissue Involvement in Body Processes 4
Functional Units: A Helpful Concept 7
Cell Proliferation and Renewal: Clinical Implications 7
Tissue Identification: Normal and Abnormal Distinguishing Features 8

2. *Skin* 13
Cases 13
Essential Features of Skin 14
Case Discussions 25

3. *Blood, Inflammation, Immunity, and Allergy* 29
Cases 29
Essential Features of Blood Cells 36
Responses to Tissue Injury and Foreign Macromolecules:
    Inflammation, Allergy, and Immune Responses 46
Case Discussions 62

4. *Musculoskeletal and Nervous Systems* 67
Cases 67
Essential Features of Constituent Connective Tissues of
    Joints and Muscles 77
Essential Features of Bone, Cartilage, and Joints 81
Essential Features of Skeletal Muscle 100
Essential Features of Nervous Tissue 105
Case Discussions 111

5. *Cardiovascular and Lymphatic Systems* 119
Cases 119
Essential Features of Cardiac Muscle 122

Essential Features of the Heart 126

Essential Features of Smooth Muscle 129

Essential Features of Blood Vessels and Lymphatics 131

Case Discussions 137

6. *Lungs* 143

Cases 143

Essential Features of the Lungs 148

Case Discussions 158

7. *Kidneys* 163

Cases 163

Essential Features of the Kidneys 167

Case Discussions 181

8. *Gastrointestinal Tract and Liver* 185

Cases 185

Essential Features of the Gastrointestinal Tract 189

Essential Features of the Pancreas 201

Essential Features of the Liver 203

Case Discussions 213

9. *Endocrine and Reproductive Systems* 219

Cases 219

Essential Features of the Endocrine System 237

Essential Features of the Female Reproductive System 251

Essential Features of the Male Reproductive System 264

Case Discussions 275

10. *Eyes* 285

Cases 285

Essential Features of the Eyes 289

Case Discussions 300

Subject Index 303

Preface

A commendable broad objective of the early part of most recently renewed health sciences curricula is to encourage the development of an integrated understanding of the various body tissues, using representative tissue disorders and appropriate patient management as effective sources of motivation. Such an approach acknowledges the fundamental interdependence that exists in tissues between their structure and function. An integrated rendering of histology that brings together basic structural and functional information becomes particularly helpful to students of health science subjects if there is some explanation of how these essentials are involved in actual medical situations. Furthermore, effective organization, consolidation, and application of relevant facts are as essential as their acquisition. Students who are learning their basic science subjects almost entirely in applied clinical contexts obviously need to concentrate on those aspects of histology that are medically applicable. They understandably dislike becoming side-tracked with material that seems irrelevant to their immediate purposes, especially when it is highly detailed. Furthermore, they expect to find histology seamlessly integrated into new curricula, even though the required tailoring may totally destroy the logical progression in complexity that was a hallmark of traditional "Histo Labs." Histology that has been successfully integrated with the allied disciplines, and that is substantially related to actual body functions and their disorders, is not difficult to assimilate, and gradually becomes an integral part of the foundation on which they build.

Many would accept the premise that the inclination to tackle and digest a course in each medical subject requires a certain insight into the potential applicability of the material that is being covered. This book therefore endeavors to present medically relevant histology in a meaningful manner that will enable students to apply it in appropriate clinical situations. The advantage of adopting this approach is that whereas potential health problems need to be addressed, the majority of extraneous details do not need to be included.

A concise and interesting treatment of histology that is clinically integrated and conceptually structured should be of particular interest to students who are participating in problem-based learning (PBL) or other forms of self-directed learning. Key topics are considered in clinical contexts that are compatible with such learning. Case histories and appropriate illustrations of biopsied tissues are presented along with challenging, straightforward basic questions about the tissues and medical conditions that are involved. Students who are given an opportunity to deliberate over such questions (either singly or in groups) will intuitively seek out the histological content that they feel it is appropriate to learn or comprehend at given stages of their training. The various questions posed in each chapter may be used as a means of testing either knowledge or comprehension. Students should endeavor to answer them, at least in part and at appropriate times, before the provided answers are sought.

This book includes a number of specific cross-references to relevant material that is covered in *Essential Histology* by D.H. Cormack, 1993. Hence, it will serve either as a PBL handbook or as an applied supplement to *Essential Histology* that focuses attention on medically important tissues. Some of these references indicate other information that is potentially useful in problem-based learning. Suggested sources for more detailed information on specific topics are given in the bibliographies.

Health professionals familiar with specific tissues generally find pathology reports informative. In cases where the histopathologist or cytopathologist has played a key role in diagnosis, tissue biology can be very relevant. Also, such case histories become an excellent starting point for detailed considerations of pathophysiology and disease management. Adequate advancement of the health practitioner's highly specialized knowledge base requires continuous and diligent self-directed learning. The various facets of histology represented in this book are intended to stimulate and encourage such learning.

Acknowledgments

Restructuring in medical education presents a unique opportunity for realigning conventional textbooks. Problem-based learning (PBL) requires innovative approaches that integrate basic sciences with clinical medicine. Initial consultations with medical students, tutors, and other educators involved with PBL-based curricula at Harvard and McMaster Universities left me with a distinct impression that certain components of histology were useful for PBL, especially in a general sense, whereas others were not really essential. The consensus at that time was that such a textbook should combine carefully selected, interrelated elements of histology, physiology, biochemistry, and pathology, and incorporate them into an accessible framework. My first duty should therefore be to acknowledge the many helpful suggestions that I received from professional colleagues and medical students concerning the content and scope of a book intended for health professionals. R. Butler, D. Carr, and H. Groves, in the Division of Anatomy and Experimental Morphology, Department of Biomedical Sciences, Faculty of Health Sciences, McMaster University, Hamilton, Canada, critiqued my initial proposal and gave me excellent advice about what would be useful. Early contact with D. Goodenough, C. Heth, and a number of their diligent and understanding tutorial students at Harvard Medical School, Boston, reinforced by my further participation in tutorials at McMaster University and our own recently revised curriculum at University of Toronto, helped me to identify and compile a core of basic science content that I consider to be of potential relevance to PBL.

I am also deeply indebted to a substantial number of helpful and supportive individuals at the University of Toronto, McMaster University, and several of the affiliated teaching hospitals, primarily McMaster University Medical Center, St. Joseph's Hospital, and Henderson District Hospital in Hamilton, and Mount Sinai Hospital, Toronto Hospital (General Division), Princess Margaret Hospital, and St. Michael's Hospital in Toronto, for providing most of the source material needed to illustrate and document the case histories. I would particularly like to thank R. Riddell and other assiduous members of various Hospital and University Departments of Pathology, Medicine, and Radiology in the cities of Hamilton and Toronto who, at my request, sought representative histological material for these clinical cases and identified useful medical and radiological records. The many individuals who generously contributed in this manner include I. Alexopoulou, M. Auger, J. Bilbao, V. Chen, A. Daya, A. Gotlieb, W. Hunter, E. Kovacs, J. Meharchand, C. Nahmias, W. Orr, K. Pritzker, R. Riddell, J. Roberts, E. Sevilo, B. Shapiro, M. Silver, I. Teshima, and L. Vincic. Thanks are due to R. Powers for assisting with collection of the material. I would also like to thank all other contributors for use or reuse of their illustrations (see following list). B. Smith deserves due credit and much gratitude for his expertise and painstaking care in obtaining the majority of color photomicrographs in this book. The fine drawings are by B. Vallecoccia and D. Irwin, to whom I am also grateful. Many thanks also to J. Pittman, P. Stewart, and D. Holman for contributing excellent electron micrographs. All these contributors were of great assistance in fulfilling my intended task.

I am particularly obliged to those colleagues who willingly found time to read and offer helpful comments on parts of the manuscript, particularly C. Bayliss, J. Hay, M. Johnson, J. Meharchand, and R. Murray. I would like to thank C. Bayliss, J. Dorrington, S. George, Y. Israel, and R. Murray for advice and critical review during development of the various graphic illustrations in this book. Also, I am grateful to R. Winters of Lippincott–Raven Publishers for patiently allowing enough time for this new project to materialize and for expediting its completion. Illustrations are duly acknowledged from the following sources.

Figure 1-2: Courtesy of L. Arsenault

Figures 2-1, **A** and **B,** 2-2, **A** and **B,** and 2-3, **A** and **B:** Courtesy of J. Roberts

Figure 2-9: Courtesy of V. Kalnins

Figures 3-1, **A** and **B,** 3-2, **A** and **B,** 3-3, **A** and **B,** 3-4, **A** and **B,** 3-5, 3-6, 3-7, 3-8, and 3-9: Courtesy of J. Meharchand

Figure 3-13: Clip art component from Techpool Studios

Figure 3-19: After D. Bainton et al.

Figure 3-21, **B:** Hay JB, Yamashita A, Morris B. Lab Invest 31:276, 1974

Figure 4-1, **A, B, C,** and **D:** Courtesy of W. Orr

Figure 4-2, **A:** Courtesy of B. Shapiro

Figures 4-2, **B, C,** and **D,** and 4-3, **A** and **B:** Courtesy of W. Orr

Figure 4-3, **C:** Courtesy of B. Shapiro

Figures 4-4, **B,** and 4-5, **A** and **B:** Courtesy of K. Pritzker

Figure 4-5, **C** and **D:** Courtesy of D. Holman

Figure 4-6, **A:** Courtesy of W. Orr

Figure 4-6, **B, C,** and **D:** Courtesy of K. Pritzker

Figure 4-7, **A** and **B:** Courtesy of B. Shapiro

Figure 4-8, **A, B,** and **C:** Courtesy of J. Bilbao

Figure 4-9: Courtesy of L. Arsenault

Figure 4-10: Courtesy of P. Lea

Figure 4-15: Courtesy of L. Arsenault

Figure 4-17: Courtesy of D. Holman

Figure 4-21, **A** to **F:** Courtesy of J. Wilson

Figure 4-23: Dale GG, Harris WR. J Bone Joint Surg 40-B:116, 1958

Figure 4-29: Courtesy of J. Pittman

Figure 4-30: Courtesy of P. Stewart

Figure 4-34: Courtesy of J. Wilson

Figure 5-1, **A** to **C:** Courtesy of A. Gotlieb

Figure 5-2, **A:** Courtesy of M. Silver

Figure 5-2, **B** and **C:** Courtesy of A. Gotlieb

Figure 5-3, **D:** Courtesy of M. Silver

Figure 5-8: Courtesy of P. Stewart

Figure 5-8, inset: Courtesy of A. Spiro

Figure 5-9: Courtesy of L. Wilson-Pauwels

Figure 5-12: Courtesy of P. Stewart

Figure 5-16, **A:** Courtesy of H. Movat

Figure 5-17: Courtesy of P. Stewart and M. Wiley

Figure 5-18: After B. Zweifach

Figure 5-19: Uehara Y, Fujiwara T, Kaidoh T. Morphology of vascular smooth muscle fibers and pericytes: scanning electron microscopic studies. In: Motta PM, ed. Ultrastructure of Smooth Muscle. Boston, Kluwer Academic Publishers, 1990, p. 237

Figure 5-20: Courtesy of C. O'Morchoe, P. O'Morchoe, and W. Jones

Figure 6-1, **B:** Courtesy of L. Vincic

Figure 6-2: Courtesy of R. Riddell

Figures 6-3, **B** to **D,** 6-4, 6-5 **A,** and 6-6, **A:** Courtesy of L. Vincic

Figure 6-12: Weibel ER. Physiol Rev 53:419, 1973

Figure 6-13: Courtesy of E. Weibel

Figure 6-14: Weibel ER, Gil J. Structure-function relationships at the alveolar level. In: West JB, ed. Bioengineering Aspects of the Lung. New York, Marcel Dekker, 1977, p. 1

Figure 6-16: Clip art component from Presentation Task Force, Newvision Technologies

Figures 7-1, **A** and **B,** and 7-3, **B** to **D:** Courtesy of I. Alexopoulou

Figure 7-6: Courtesy of J. Wilson

Figures 7-11, 7-12, and 7-13: Courtesy of J. Pittman

Figure 7-16: Tisher CC. Anatomy of the Kidney. In: Brenner BM, Rector FC, eds. The Kidney, vol. 1. Philadelphia, WB Saunders, 1976

Figure 8-1, **A:** Courtesy of R. Riddell

Figure 8-1, **B:** Ottenjann R et al, eds. Atlas of Diseases of the Upper Gastrointestinal Tract, SmithKline Corporation, 1980, p. 292, with permission

Figures 8-2, 8-3 **A** to **C,** and 8-4, **A:** Courtesy of R. Riddell

Figure 8-4, **B** and **C:** Ottenjann R et al, eds. Atlas of Diseases of the Upper Gastrointestinal Tract, SmithKline Corporation, 1980, pp. 103, 105, with permission

Figures 8-5 and 8-6, **B:** Courtesy of R. Riddell

Figure 8-12: Courtesy of S. Ito, R. Winchester, and D. Fawcett

Figure 8-15: Courtesy of C. Leblond

Figure 8-21, **A:** Courtesy of Y. Clermont

Figure 8-22: After J. Grant and J. Basmajian

Figure 9-1, **A:** Courtesy of E. Sevilo

Figure 9-1, **B:** Courtesy of V. Chen

Figure 9-1, **C** and **D:** Courtesy of C. Nahmias

Figures 9-2, 9-3, **A** and **B,** 9-4, 9-5, 9-6, **A** and **B,** and 9-7: Courtesy of V. Chen

Figures 9-8, **A** to **C,** and 9-9, **A** to **C:** Courtesy of E. Kovacs

Figures 9-10, **A** and **B,** and 9-11: Courtesy of I. Teshima

Figure 9-12, **A** and **B:** Courtesy of M. Auger

Figures 9-12, **C** to **E,** 9-13, **A** and **B,** and 9-14, **A** to **D:** Courtesy of A. Daya

Figure 9-15, **A** and **B:** Courtesy of V. Chen

Figure 9-16, **A** to **C:** Courtesy of A. Daya

Figure 9-17: Courtesy of C. Nahmias

Figure 9-23: Courtesy of S. Carmichael

Figure 9-27: Courtesy of K. Kovacs and E. Horvath

Figure 9-29: Courtesy of W. Wilson

Figure 9-30: Courtesy of K. Kovacs and E. Horvath

Figure 9-33: Patten BM. Human Embryology. New York, McGraw-Hill, 1946

Figure 9-40: Modified from Moore KL. The Developing Human: Clinically Oriented Embryology, ed 3. Philadelphia, WB Saunders, 1982

Figure 9-49: Courtesy of J. Sturgess

Figure 9-51: Clermont Y. Am J Anat 112:35, 1963

Figure 9-53: Courtesy of K. Kovacs, E. Horvath, and D. McComb

Figure 10-2, **A** to **D:** Courtesy of W. Hunter

Figures 10-3 and 10-4, **A:** Courtesy of P. Stewart

Figure 10-4, **B:** Courtesy of L. Wilson-Pauwels

Figure 10-4, **C** to **E:** Courtesy of W. Hunter

Figure 10-12: Noback CR, Demarest RJ. The Human Nervous System: Basic Principles of Neurobiology, ed 2. New York, McGraw-Hill, 1975

Figure 10-13: Borwein B. The retinal receptor: a description. In: Enoch JM, Tobey FL, eds. Springer Series in Optical Sciences, vol 23: Vertebrate Photoreceptor Optics. Berlin, Springer-Verlag, 1981, p. 11

Clinically Integrated Histology

CHAPTER I

Introduction to Cell and Tissue Functions

In problem-based learning and other learning that is self-directed, the information sought about cells and tissues often involves facets of *histology* (Gk. *histos,* tissue, *logos,* study of). One of the first steps in gaining a general understanding of the numerous disorders and disease processes that affect the tissues, parts, and systems of the body is to appreciate the underlying cellular and molecular basis of key body processes. The histological basis of some of these processes, therefore, constitutes a useful starting point. Other unifying concepts helpful for building the necessary foundation for self-directed learning will also be considered.

SYNOPSIS OF CELL AND TISSUE FUNCTIONS

The structural and functional characteristics of the many different tissues largely depend on what is occurring within and around their cells. The first part of this chapter, therefore, deals with the principal components, functions, and processes of cells (Fig. 1-1). Some important body processes involving such functions are also discussed.

Organization of the Cell

Almost all nucleated cells share the same basic organization, with a central *nucleus*, surrounding *cytoplasm*, and peripheral *cell membrane (plasmalemma)*. The three basic components of the cell's cytoplasm are (1) the *cytoplasmic organelles*, each kind individually designed to carry out certain functions, (2) the *cytosol (cytoplasmic matrix)*, a macromolecular complex that envelops the various cytoplasmic organelles, and (3) *cytoplasmic inclusions* (eg, stored glycogen, lipid, and pigment) not consistently present in cells.

Specific *cytoplasmic organelles* (a number of which are represented in Fig. 1-2) are required because, in most cases, the enzymes and specific reactants involved in a cellular process or function need to be isolated in a distinct intracellular compartment, separated by an intracellular membrane from all other potentially inappropriate enzymes, substrates, or reactants in the cell. In cells that are highly differentiated (ie, uniquely specialized for particular tasks), the most useful organelles are generally more plentiful and conspicuous than the remainder.

The *nucleus* is the central control compartment where the cell's genetic instructions lie encoded in DNA. It is the site where this DNA becomes transcribed, producing three forms of RNA. Also, it is the site where newly formed RNA is processed. Chromatin granules are attached to the nuclear lamina of the inner nuclear membrane; ribosomes bind to the outer nuclear membrane. These two membranes are fused at the margins of the nuclear pores and constitute the

REVIEW ITEM 1-1
List all the cytoplasmic organelles.

KEY CONCEPT
Distinctiveness of cell structure implies functional specialization.

REVIEW ITEM 1-2
What is the difference between transcription and translation? What makes RNA processing necessary?

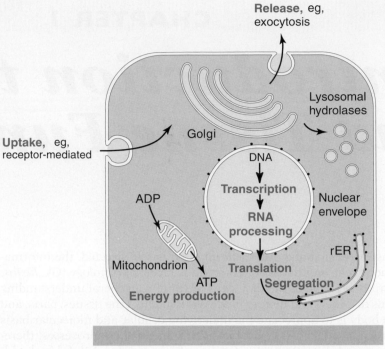

FIGURE 1-1 Key cellular processes.

REVIEW ITEM 1-3

What molecular mechanisms lead to (1) segregation and (2) independent sorting of secretory and lysosomal proteins?

REVIEW ITEM 1-4

List the major intracellular destinations of newly secreted proteins.

nuclear envelope. Inside the nucleus lie one or more rounded, darkly stained masses known as *nucleoli*, which, depending on the nuclear morphology, plane of section, and so on, may or may not be discernible in LM sections. In electron micrographs, nucleoli are electron dense and commonly have a spongelike texture. Nucleoli represent the sites where aggregated *nucleolar genes* coding for *ribosomal RNA* (rRNA) are being transcribed. The newly synthesized rRNA associates with specific proteins and becomes incorporated into ribosomal subunits.

Many cell types possess a spherical-to-ovoid nucleus. In some cell types, however, the nucleus has a distinctive shape that serves as an aid to cell recognition. For example, neutrophils have a nucleus that is segmented. Certain other cells possess more than one nucleus (eg, skeletal muscle fibers, which are multinucleated). The nucleus can also show variation in absolute and relative size and in relative content of extended (transcribed) or condensed (untranscribed) chromatin.

Ribosomes are assembled in the cytoplasm and remain there; hence, protein synthesis occurs only in the cytoplasm. The cell can segregate those proteins that are destined to be secreted, incorporated into the cell membrane, or sequestered in lysosomes, from proteins that are to remain in the cytosol. Segregation from the cytosol occurs when a polypeptide chain passes into the lumen of the *rough-surfaced endoplasmic reticulum* (rER) in the course of being synthesized. Segregated proteins are transferred to the *Golgi apparatus* for posttranslational processing and intracellular sorting. Their eventual intracellular location depends on an elaborate sorting process carried out by the Golgi apparatus. Formation of a secretory product, eg, a peptide hormone, collagen, lipoprotein, or mucus, is an important cellular function that can have clinical implications under certain circumstances.

Organelles With Clinical Relevance

The majority of secretory products are released by exocytosis, but most small molecules and lipid-soluble secretory products can leave the cell by simple dif-

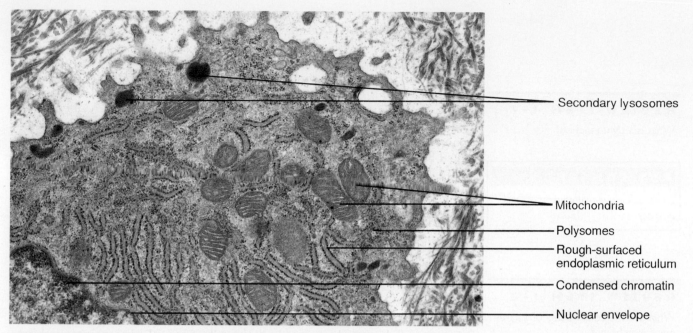

Secondary lysosomes

Mitochondria

Polysomes

Rough-surfaced endoplasmic reticulum

Condensed chromatin

Nuclear envelope

FIGURE 1-2 Several cytoplasmic organelles and an adjacent part of the nucleus (electron micrograph of an osteoblast). Collagen fibrils are present in the surrounding intercellular matrix.

fusion. Extraneous macromolecules are eliminated from the cell's interior through the action of potent lysosomal hydrolases. Such degradation is usually intracellular, and it is carried out in *secondary lysosomes*. In osteoclasts, however, the main site of action of lysosomal enzymes is extracellular (see Fig. 4-16). Sufficient degradation must be achieved, and inherited deficiency of a lysosomal enzyme can cause disease, eg, *Tay-Sach's disease*. Ultimately fatal, this lipid storage disease results from inactivity of hexosaminidase A. A ganglioside known as G_{M2} remains undegraded in neurons, and resulting accumulation of residual material in these cells progressively impairs brain function. At the other extreme, highly destructive lysosomal enzymes liberated by normal neutrophils in intense episodes of *acute inflammation* can cause severe tissue damage.

The *smooth-surfaced endoplasmic reticulum* (sER) is another organelle of major clinical significance. Activity of its *cytochrome P-450* enzymes enables *hepatocytes* to metabolize a large number of drugs, chemical carcinogens, and toxic waste substances that can enter the body from the environment. These sER enzymes represent the body's main *monooxygenases (mixed-function oxidases)*. A complication in polypharmacy (meaning multiple drug prescription) is that almost all the cytochrome P-450 enzymes can become induced by drugs, even to some extent by the excessive consumption of alcohol (see Fig. 8-28). In skeletal and cardiac muscle cells, an elaborate kind of sER called the *sarcoplasmic reticulum* is used to store *calcium ions* withdrawn from myofibrils during relaxation (see Fig. 5-6).

Other Essential Information About the Cell

Uncharged small molecules such as oxygen are able to enter the cell by simple diffusion through the *cell membrane*. However, small molecules do not travel in the opposite direction to their concentration gradient unless they are transported across the cell membrane by transport proteins incorporated into it. Ions can enter the cell by way of gated channels in the cell membrane. Large molecules may be taken into the cell through endocytosis, a special form of which, known as *receptor-mediated endocytosis*, supplies the cell with essential macromolecules.

REVIEW ITEM 1-5

What is a secondary lysosome?

KEY CONCEPT

Lysosomes have key roles in storage diseases and in the acute inflammatory reaction.

KEY CONCEPT

Properties of the cell membrane are an expression of its molecular composition.

REVIEW ITEM 1-6

What is meant by a receptor, and how can it bring a macromolecule into the cell?

The energy needed for the many active processes occurring in the cell comes from the hydrolysis of *adenosine triphosphate* (ATP), which is produced through oxidative phosphorylation in *mitochondria*.

Some cells have to establish and maintain a definite *shape* and structural *polarity* to carry out certain complex functions. Secretory epithelial cells, for example, may require a distinct *apical* or *luminal domain* in the cell membrane to which the Golgi apparatus can send secretory vesicles. *Tight junctions* are needed to delimit this domain from the remainder of the cell membrane and, thus, maintain its distinct composition. The Golgi apparatus in such cells is situated between the rER and the secretory border. Highly asymmetric cells such as multipolar neurons carry out important functions that depend on maintenance of both polarity and shape. The distinctive shapes and other structural features of such cells depend on internal support provided by *microtubules* and *intermediate filaments*, which together with the *microfilaments* found in most cells and the *thin filaments* and *thick filaments* found in muscle cells, comprise the *cytoskeleton*.

In addition to having an internal cytoskeleton, most kinds of cells are externally supported by intercellular matrix. *Epithelial membranes* have a special matrix underlay called a *basement membrane*, which attaches the entire sheet of cells to the adjacent connective tissue. Also, various types of *cell junctions* maintain intercellular attachment and cellular adhesion to the basement membrane. In contrast, *phagocytic cells* such as neutrophils and macrophages have to stay mobile, and long-distance travelers such as *spermatozoa* need to be freely motile. Forward lengthening of microfilaments as a result of actin polymerization at the leading edge of *mobile* or *migrating* cells is used for vigorous crawling over a substrate. Spermatozoa are able to harness a sliding movement generated between neighbouring pairs of microtubules in their flagellum when *dynein*, a microtubule-associated ATPase, hydrolyzes ATP. The body's *ciliated cells* remain stationary; sliding between their microtubule pairs is used to power the bending of cilia and propel fluids, mucus, and small masses in appropriate directions.

The coordination of body functions depends on stringent regulation of all body processes. Cells need to *communicate* with one another and must respond appropriately to specific signal molecules reaching their immediate environment. Electrical excitability of the cell membrane and the presence of hormone receptors on the cell surface or in the cytosol are classic examples of signal response mechanisms. Cells with interiors that are linked by *gap junctions* are able to communicate with each other directly. In recent years, the prevalence of paracrine (local) signaling (eg, short-range interactions based on production of specific growth factors) has also come to light.

Cell *division* is required to compensate for cell depletion. However, the restoration of cell populations that are subject to extensive daily depletion is achieved largely through cell replacement. The necessity for some but not all cells to divide is discussed below in connection with cell renewal. The regulation of cellular proliferation and the inverse relationship that is generally found between marked proliferative capacity and an extreme level of differentiation are matters of considerable relevance to medicine. If proliferation ceases to be regulated in a normal manner, cell production can exceed the level required to compensate for cell depletion and the risk of autonomous growth and cancer development increases.

TISSUE INVOLVEMENT IN BODY PROCESSES

Several of the cell functions reviewed above play key roles in body processes.

REVIEW ITEM 1-7

What is a tight junction?

KEY CONCEPT

Some cell types maintain structural polarity.

REVIEW ITEM 1-8

What are the constituents of a basement membrane?

KEY CONCEPT

Certain cells are motile.

KEY CONCEPT

Cells can communicate with one another.

REVIEW ITEM 1-9

Name some cell types that do not divide.

Individual Compartments Are Involved in Body Processes

As in the cell, certain body processes occur in specific compartments. Digestion, for example, takes place within the gut lumen, a compartment that is external to the body. Gas exchange occurs across the walls of another external compartment—the air space in the lungs—that is invaginated into the pleural cavity. The body's individual internal compartments have to be kept separate, eg, the intravascular compartment has to be partitioned from urinary space. In every case, a continuous sheet of cells called an *epithelial membrane (epithelium)* delimits and maintains the distinctive features of the compartment.

A rapid *exchange* of various constituents (Fig. 1-3A) occurs between different body compartments at such sites as tiny blood vessels, pulmonary alveoli, and the thin-walled portions of kidney tubules. The interface at these sites is *simple squamous epithelium*. This very thin type of epithelium permits effective passive diffusion. In addition, large molecules may be transported across it through a process called *transcytosis*. In this efficient exchange process, vesicles formed by endocytosis at one cell border pass across the cell to the opposite border and discharge their contents. Also, channels open up momentarily through the cytoplasm and create tiny temporary conduits across the epithelium.

Drug Absorption

The various molecules present in each of the body's internal compartments are all derived from substances that are *absorbed* into the body (Fig. 1-3B). Choosing an optimal site for absorption is important when a therapeutic drug has to be given. Lipid-soluble drugs can pass through the lipid bilayer of the cell membrane by passive diffusion. Most water-soluble drugs can diffuse passively through the aqueous channels (ie, the ion channels) in this membrane. However, a few of them are taken up by active transport, and drugs with a high molecular weight are generally taken up by endocytosis. In some cases, the drug interacts with a receptor in the cell membrane.

Therapeutic drugs that are not absorbed efficiently must be injected (usually as a subcutaneous, intramuscular, or intravenous injection) or else infused intravenously. Delivery by such an alternative route is known as *parenteral* (Gk. *para*, beyond, *enteron*, intestine) *administration* of the drug. Sometimes, the only way to ensure that a drug reaches its target in the necessary concentration and with minimal delay is to bypass the absorption process by giving an injection. However, topical application of a drug is the most efficient way of localizing its activity in situations where it is important to minimize systemic activity.

The simple columnar epithelial lining of the intestine is specialized for absorption. Its absorptive cells possess a *brush (striated) border* consisting of absorptive *microvilli*. Many drugs that do not interfere with the digestive process and resist inactivation by it can, therefore, be given by mouth; others are more efficiently delivered from rectal suppositories. Percutaneous (transdermal) absorption is an effective means of continuous administration of drugs such as scopolamine (for those prone to motion sickness) and nicotine (for those seeking relief from tobacco withdrawal). Drugs that can pass through keratinocytes and other cells when placed in contact with undamaged skin are absorbed at a rate that is directly proportional to their lipid solubility.

Filtration

Another important process, *filtration*, plays a key role in the kidneys and also in tissue fluid production. In both instances, fluid filters *between cells* through narrow intercellular slits, and then passes through a basement membrane (Fig. 1-

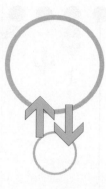

A   Exchange

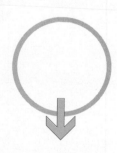

B   Absorption

C   Filtration

FIGURE 1-3 Important tissue-based body processes.

3C). The constituents of basement membranes act as an impediment to the passage of macromolecular substances, particularly those that carry a high net negative charge. Thus, when tissue fluid, a filtrate of blood plasma, is formed, it contains only low concentrations of plasma proteins. Because proteins with molecular weights exceeding 69,000 do not traverse the glomerular basement membrane unless it is damaged, their concentration in the urinary filtrate is normally low. From the water-soluble molecules in plasma that do pass through the glomerular filter, those having potential for re-use by the body are absorbed back into the plasma, ie, *resorbed*.

> **KEY CONCEPT**
>
> Absorption and resorption can bring substances into the body; filtration and secretion can remove them.

> **KEY CONCEPT**
>
> Epithelial damage can result in acute inflammation.

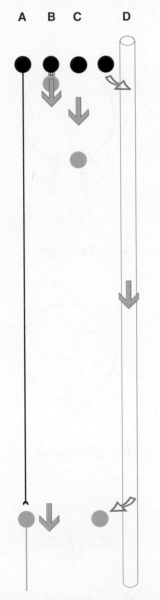

FIGURE 1-4 Principal forms of intercellular communication. (**A**) Synaptic. (**B**) Gap junctional. (**C**) Paracrine. (**D**) Endocrine.

Protection

Cells provide various types of *protection* at body surfaces. The protective epithelium on such surfaces may be made up of many layers, produce mucus as a barrier and lubricant, or undergo keratinization. Insults from the environment that can damage or breach such barriers include inhaled air pollutants, injurious gut contents, wear and tear of body surfaces, and a vast assortment of invading infectious microorganisms. When this happens, the body's first line of defense is the *acute inflammatory reaction*. This is basically a phagocytic response involving neutrophils and macrophages derived from circulating monocytes. The body's second line of defense is the *immune response*, which involves antigen-presenting cells as well as T and B cells, the two essential types of small lymphocytes. Immune responses take a few days to become effective, so acute inflammation serves its useful purpose in the meantime. Damaged epithelia regenerate rapidly, generally through a combination of proliferation and cell migration. The epidermis has the supplementary protective function of producing additional melanin in response to ultraviolet light.

Communication

Sensory input is required to elicit body responses, so certain cells are specialized to detect changes in the body's external and internal environments. Cutaneous tactile receptors, retinal photoreceptors, and hair cells of the inner ear are examples of cells with elaborate arrangements for transducing stimulus energy into electrical signals that contribute valuable information to the central nervous system. The physiological importance of sensory receptors becomes evident when they cease to function, especially if the receptor is a modified neuron that is not replaced if damaged. Synaptic transmission of nerve impulses (Fig. 1-4A) and electrical conduction through gap junctions (Fig. 1-4B) are examples of almost immediate *communication*. The necessity for an extremely rapid exchange of information has long been recognized, eg, between interacting cells, distant interacting parts of the body, sensory receptors and the brain, motor neurons and skeletal muscle fibers, and the numerous muscle cells in the myocardium. Less rapid, short-range *(paracrine)* signaling (Fig. 1-4C), and relatively slow, long-range *(endocrine)* signaling (Fig. 1-4D) are supplementary forms of communication that are widely used to augment and broaden functional responses or fine-tune body processes.

Release of signal molecules into the bloodstream, with feedback inhibition of this release, forms the basis of an important type of homeostatic regulatory mechanism. For homeostasis to be maintained, all the body tissues and organs have to collaborate in the necessary concerted manner. Normal functioning of the kidneys and liver is particularly important for maintenance of this steady state. Patients with end-stage disease of either of these organs, thus, are critically dependent on proper management.

Tissue Repair

A different sort of medical problem is the deterioration of body components as a result of severe wear and tear. Certain constituents of the interstitial matrix (notable those in the skeletal tissues) are susceptible to age-related degeneration or degradation. The cells that might be expected to repair this damage eventually fail to do so. Indeed, there are certain tissues that lack the resources for proper replacement, leaving delay of further deterioration as the best biological option. *Support* and *locomotion* are both highly dependent on adequate tissue maintenance and repair. Many of the limitations imposed by the aging process on daily activity involve degenerative changes in the skeletal tissues.

Tissue maintenance, and also reproduction of the species, are ultimately dependent on properly regulated cell proliferation. Cell division requires the previous error-free replication of DNA and effective repair of any damaged DNA. Although proliferation is strictly regulated in cells that are growth-factor dependent, this regulation is impaired in cells that have lost dependency on external mitogenic growth factors. *Autocrine* (ie, self-stimulating) *production* of mitogenic growth factors by cells that possess their own receptors for these factors is considered ominous. Resulting chronic stimulation of unrestrained proliferation has the potential to contribute to the multistage process of carcinogenesis.

REVIEW ITEM 1-10

Which joints are particularly susceptible to degeneration? Why?

FUNCTIONAL UNITS: A HELPFUL CONCEPT

Many body organs are constructed of units that are distinctively designed to carry out certain functions. In a few instances, these *functional units* correspond to structural units that are recognizable to the unaided eye, but more commonly they are distinguishable only with a microscope. Thus, thyroid follicles are usually discernible with no magnification, whereas renal corpuscles are not. The various parts of the nephron, on the other hand, can readily be recognized in histological sections. A few organs, eg, the liver, have functional units that are morphologically indistinct. The spleen and some other organs that perform a variety of functions have a complicated internal structure that makes definition of their functional unit somewhat difficult.

Organ functions that are being considered in the context of medical conditions often seem more comprehensible, if it is possible to identify the functional units involved. This mechanistic approach encourages analysis of the underlying basis of malfunctions in given clinical situations.

KEY CONCEPT

Functional units are key components of most body organs.

Maintenance

Essential functional units must be kept in good working order. For example, cells that wear out or die may need to be replaced. The main requirement in the kidneys is for the glomerular basement membranes to be kept unobstructed, since macromolecular deposits can occlude them, interfering with the filtration process. Each sort of functional unit is maintained in its own distinctive way, but a basic requirement in all of them, except those that constitute a nonrenewable resource (eg, the myocardium), is cell renewal.

CELL PROLIFERATION AND RENEWAL: CLINICAL IMPLICATIONS

The majority of special functions are carried out by cells that remain in an *extended G_1 phase* of the cell cycle. However, a few specialized cell types, described as *terminally differentiated cells*, have escaped irreversibly from the cell cycle.

REVIEW ITEM 1-11

What is a cell cycle? What is G1?

The term G_0 is applied to cells whose cycling state has gone into an indefinitely prolonged standby mode. The arrest of cycling in G_0 cells, however, is *reversible*. G_0 cells remain *out of cycle* until the cycling state is reestablished.

Those somatic cells that are able to divide must first pass through an S phase, at which time everything needed for the synthesis and repair of DNA has to be available. A shortage of folate or cobalamin (vitamin B_{12}), or inadequacy of DNA repair, eg, because of a defective endonuclease, can have pathological consequences. Such dependency of cells in the S phase is exploitable for effective chemotherapy. For example, agents that impair DNA synthesis are inhibitory to cell proliferation. Therapeutically induced production of fraudulent DNA serves an effective strategy because cells cannot replicate it. Provided the drugs used for cancer chemotherapy are administered under optimally timed and controlled conditions, critical or irreparable concurrent damage to essential normal tissues can be circumvented.

Cell populations typically undergo some form of cell renewal that is either continuous or only meets demands. Certain highly differentiated cells, however, are *not* renewed. Absolute numbers of these cells decrease with age, and no clinically satisfactory replacement occurs when they are destroyed by trauma or disease.

The clinical significance of *continuously renewing populations* is that vast numbers of their cells are in cycle, and many are proliferating at any given moment. These normal cell populations, therefore, are damaged to the greatest extent by chemotherapeutic drugs. To avoid progressive cell depletion of rapidly renewing populations, which include the entire blood cell family and also spermatozoa, their stem cells must be preserved. *Stem cells* are essentially undifferentiated cells with extensive proliferative potential that, in most cases, have gone into G_0. They remain in G_0 until they are triggered back into cycle. In some cases, stem cell proliferation is an emergency amplifying or "boost" response that compensates for severe depletion or catastrophic destruction of differentiated progeny cells. Under less exacting circumstances, the early differentiating progeny of stem cells, still able to divide and known as *progenitors*, can produce enough differentiated non-dividing cells *(end cells)* to meet demands. When a stem cell divides, its two daughter cells have a roughly equal chance of (1) remaining as stem cells or (2) beginning to differentiate (Fig. 1-5). Both daughter cells may even take the same option. Since stem cells possess this unique capacity for *self-renewal*, viable stem cells can repopulate critically depleted continuously renewing populations in emergency and transplant situations.

Hepatocytes and certain hormone-producing cells are noteworthy exceptions to the broad generalization that highly differentiated cells do not divide. Under ordinary circumstances, turnover is minimal in these two kinds of cells. However, a severe loss of either kind of cell due to disease or partial resection causes many of the surviving cells go into cycle. Hepatocyte regeneration continues until the liver regains its former mass.

TISSUE IDENTIFICATION: NORMAL AND ABNORMAL DISTINGUISHING FEATURES

The evidence required to confirm a diagnosis or corroborate a hypothesis may often be found when an affected body part is examined under a microscope. The confirmation generally depends on recognition of a discrepancy between some finding in the tissues sampled and the normal occurrence for this site. An initial rapid identification is made of the tissues in the sample, and then a systematic search is conducted for inconsistencies that are indicative of disease or other abnormality.

> ### KEY CONCEPT
> DNA replication is a prerequisite for mitosis.

> ### KEY CONCEPT
> Various arrangements exist for cell renewal, but some cells are not replaced.

> ### KEY CONCEPT
> Stem cells can (1) self-renew and (2) produce differentiated progeny.

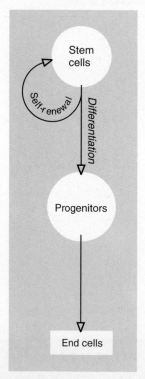

FIGURE 1-5 Self-renewal in cells.

Basic Strategy for Tissue Identification

A number of fairly reliable criteria and a few of the common pitfalls in identifying normal tissues from unknown sources are listed in Table 1-1. An initial scan of the entire slide is necessary for the observer to obtain the "big picture" without missing anything important. It is important to observe not only cells but also any other tissue components that may be present. Also, it is useful to develop an integrated strategy that combines structural recognition with functional knowledge.

Histological Features of Diagnostic Importance

Major or minor tissue malfunctions occur in many disease processes. The finding of disease-related structural changes in histological sections confirms involvement in disease processes and also often facilitates the differential diagno-

TABLE 1-1
HISTOLOGICAL IDENTIFICATION: STRATEGY AND PITFALLS

Basic Questions	Possibilities	Deductions/Explanations
Type of preparation?	Generally a section or film	A film suggests peripheral blood or myeloid tissue
Uniform appearance?	Uniform appearance or dissimilar appearance in different regions	Single component or several different components
Recognizable shapes?	Solid wedge; hollow circular cross sections, holes, etc.	Solid tissue; tubular structures, vessels, ducts, etc.
Dimensions?	Erythrocytes can be used as a handy built-in ruler (diameter = 7 μm).	Sizes may be estimated by comparison with the diameter of erythrocytes in vessels
Do cells or intercellular matrix predominate?	Tissue is mostly cellular, intercellular, or both	Epithelial membranes and glands are essentially cellular, connective tissues are essentially intercellular, etc.
Recognizable components?	Provisional identification of components needs corroboration.	Presence of components serving useful purposes could be expected, and vice versa
Distinctive associations?	Transitional epithelium with urinary tract, mucus-secreting cells + cartilage with upper respiratory tract, megakaryocytes with sinusoids, etc.	Absence of a characteristically associated feature may imply erroneous identification

POTENTIAL DIFFICULTIES

Problem	Basis	Cause/Explanation
Strange color?	A component closely resembles something, but is stained the wrong color	Absolute color is not reliable in H&E sections, but relative color is; also, special stains may impart unfamiliar colors
Strange component?	An unfamiliar component catches the eye	Such components are generally artifacts, but occasionally result from pathological changes
Unrecognizable component?	A structure cannot be identified at all	Tissue may have undergone postmortem degeneration or show some other artifact; unfamiliar plane of section; dead tissue or isolated pathological lesion
Incomplete or incorrect identification?	A familiar component attracts too much attention	Failure to obtain the "big picture" due to haste or anxiety may result in partial or incorrect identification

sis. In diagnostic histopathology, the chief concerns are detection and recognition of changes occurring in tissues because of disease. Generally, it is advantageous to obtain samples of undisrupted tissue using an appropriate biopsy procedure. Such samples disclose the overall architecture of the tissue and yield valuable information as to whether it is normal. In some situations, however, aspiration samples or scrapings are all that is available, giving no information about tissue organization. Evaluation of individual representative cells in cytological preparations is known as diagnostic cytology (cytopathology).

In tissue sections, the pattern of growth can usually be assessed as normal or abnormal. Furthermore, microscopic evidence of cellular responses, such as hypertrophy, hyperplasia, inflammation, or repair may be found. Invasive patterns of growth are regarded as a danger signal. Except for the one non-malignant tissue with invasive activity, placental syncytiotrophoblast, normal tissues have orderly and characteristic growth patterns that are easily recognized. Another danger signal is a local accumulation of mitotic figures that are (1) atypical or (2) more numerous than expected for the tissue, given the prevailing conditions. Increased mitotic activity may indicate disordered growth regulation or the presence of a malignant tumor. An increased incidence of the nuclear changes seen when cells die, on the other hand, commonly indicates *necrosis*, eg, due to acute toxicity or critical ischemia. The alternative possibility, ie, endogenously engendered cell death, is considered in the next section.

PROGRAMMED CELL DEATH

It has been proposed that under certain circumstances, cells may undergo selective elimination through activation of some intrinsic program of self-destruction, as distinct from being killed by some exogenous lethal agent. Nuclear condensation and cell shrinkage are frequently cited as representing the degradation phase of such programmed death, which is alternatively known as *apoptosis* (Gk. *apo*, away from, *ptosis*, fall), but in fact they are nonspecific signs of cell death. Loss of mitochondrial function occurs before postmortem morphological changes in the nucleus are seen. The "self-destruction" program is believed to lead to activation of the cell's Ca^{2+}-Mg^{2+}-dependent endonuclease, with resulting fragmentation of the nuclear DNA, and eventual disintegration of the nucleus. The usual fate of apoptotic cells is for them to become phagocytosed.

Selective elimination of inappropriate (or potentially damaged) cells through a developmentally programmed form of apoptosis is believed to be a necessary part of development of the nervous system. Apoptosis is also thought to be the means through which self-reactive T cells become eradicated in the thymus, and it may account for the depletion of lymphocytes that occurs both during corticosteroid-mediated immunosuppression and after exposure to ionizing radiation. Other suggested examples of programmed cell death are (1) loss of erythroid progenitors that unless "rescued" by the survival-promoting hormone, erythropoietin, seem doomed to apoptosis, and (2) induced apoptosis resulting in the virtual elimination of $CD4^+$ T cells from some patients infected with the human immunodeficiency virus (HIV). It remains difficult to evaluate the importance of extrinsic factors in bringing about such cell death.

This general introduction should provide enough background for an understanding of the interrelated content of subsequent chapters. Each chapter begins with a few case histories that highlight certain aspects of tissue involvement in medical conditions. Tissue involvement is then analyzed, and relevant information is provided about the tissues that may be involved. The Discussion sections address the various questions posed in the Analysis sections.

BIBLIOGRAPHY
General

Damjanov I. Histopathology. A Color Atlas and Textbook. Baltimore, Williams & Wilkins, 1996.

Ganong WF. Review of Medical Physiology, ed 17. Norwalk, Conn., Appleton & Lange, 1995.

Murray RK, Granner DK, Mayes PA, Rodwell VW. Harper's Biochemistry, ed 24. Norwalk, Conn., Appleton & Lange, 1996.

Rubin E, Farber JL, eds. Pathology, ed 2. Philadelphia, J.B. Lippincott, 1994.

Sweeney G. Clinical Pharmacology: A Conceptual Approach. New York, Churchill Livingstone, 1990.

Cell Components, Junctions, Microscopy

Alberts B, Bray D, Lewis J, et al. Molecular Biology of the Cell, ed 3. New York, Garland Publishing, 1994.

Bozzola JJ, Russell LD. Electron Microscopy: Principles and Techniques for Biologists. Boston, Jones and Bartlett, 1991.

Bretscher MS. The molecules of the cell membrane. Sci Am 253(4):100, 1985.

Burgess TL, Kelly RB. Constitutive and regulated secretion of proteins. Annu Rev Cell Biol 3:243, 1987.

Cereijido M, Ponce A, Gonzalez-Mariscal L. Tight junctions and apical/basolateral polarity. J Membr Biol 110:1, 1989.

Cormack DH. Essential Histology. Philadelphia, J.B. Lippincott, 1993.

Darnell JE. RNA. Sci Am 253(4):68, 1985.

Dautry-Varsat A, Lodish HF. How receptors bring proteins and particles into cells. Sci Am 250(5):52, 1984.

Evan G. Regulation of gene expression. Br Med Bull 47:116, 1991.

Felsenfeld G. DNA. Sci Am 253(4):58, 1985.

Goodman SR, ed. Medical Cell Biology. Philadelphia, J.B. Lippincott, 1994.

Gumbiner B. Generation and maintenance of epithelial cell polarity. Curr Opin Cell Biol 2:881, 1990.

Hayat MA. Principles and Techniques of Electron Microscopy: Biological Applications, ed 3. Boca Raton, Fla., CRC Press, 1989.

Hertzberg EL, Lawrence TS, Gilula NB. Gap junctional communication. Annu Rev Physiol 43:479, 1981.

Jackson DA, Cook PR. The structural basis of nuclear function. Int Rev Cytol 162A:125, 1995.

Jasani B, Schmid KW. Immunocytochemistry in Diagnostic Histopathology. Edinburgh, Churchill Livingstone, 1993.

Nickerson JA, Blencowe BJ, Penman S. The architectural organization of nuclear metabolism. Int Rev Cytol 162A:67, 1995.

Osatake H, Tanaka K, Inoué T. An application of rapid freezing, freeze substitution-fixation for scanning electron microscopy. J Electron Microsc Tech 2:201, 1985.

Osborn M, Weber K. Intermediate filaments: Cell type-specific markers in differentiation and pathology. Cell 31:303, 1982.

Panté N, Aebi U. Toward a molecular understanding of the structure and function of the nuclear pore complex. Int Rev Cytol 162B:225, 1995.

Rothman JE. The compartmental organization of the Golgi apparatus. Sci Am 253(3):74, 1985.

Schneeberger EE, Lynch RD. Tight junctions. Their structure, composition, and function. Circ Res 55:723, 1984.

Schwartz AL. Cell biology of intracellular protein trafficking. Annu Rev Immunol 8:195, 1990.

Shaw PJ, Jordan EG. The nucleolus. Annu Rev Cell Biol 11:93, 1995.

Shepherd VL. Intracellular pathways and mechanisms of sorting in receptor-mediated endocytosis. Trends Pharmacol Sci 10:458, 1989.

Singer SJ. The structure and insertion of integral proteins in membranes. Annu Rev Cell Biol 6:247, 1990.

Smith RF. Microscopy and Photomicrography: A Working Manual. Boca Raton, Fla., CRC Press, 1990.

Staehelin LA, Hull BE. Junctions between living cells. Sci Am 238(5):140, 1978.

Steinert PM, Roop DR. Molecular and cellular biology of intermediate filaments. Annu Rev Biochem 57:593, 1988.

Tanaka K, Mitsushima A, Fukodome H, Kashima Y. Three-dimensional architecture of the Golgi complex observed by high resolution scanning electron microscopy. J Submicrosc Cytol 18:1, 1986.

Cell Cycle

Humphrey T, Enoch T. Cell-cycle checkpoints: Keeping mitosis in check. Curr Biol 5:376, 1995.

King KL, Cidlowski JA. Cell cycle and apoptosis: Common pathways to life and death. J Cell Biochem 58:175, 1995.

Kroemer G, Petit P, Zamzami N, Vayssière JL, Mignotte B. The biochemistry of programmed cell death. FASEB J 9:1277, 1995.

Meikrantz W, Schlegel R. Apoptosis and the cell cycle. J Cell Biochem 58:160, 1995.

Murray AW, Kirschner MW. What controls the cell cycle. Sci Am 264:56, 1991.

Norbury C, Nurse P. Animal cell cycles and their control. Annu Rev Biochem 61:441, 1992.

Sanders EJ, Wride MA. Programmed cell death in development. Int Rev Cytol 163:105, 1995.

Schwartz LM, Osborne BA. Programmed cell death, apoptosis and killer genes. Immunol Today 14:582, 1993.

Review Items: Cross References

Information relevant to the Review Items listed in this chapter may be found in the following pages of Cormack, DH. Essential Histology, JB Lippincott, 1993:

REVIEW ITEM	PAGES
1-1	52
1-2	29–33
1-3	62–66
1-4	64–67
1-5	67–68
1-6	55,70
1-7	91
1-8	108–110
1-9	36–37
1-10	185–188
1-11	36
1-12	7-8

CHAPTER 2

Skin

CASE 2-1

Rudy Snyder, aged 42 years, is referred to a dermatologist to investigate a patch of dry non-itching, deep dull red skin that has been present in the sacral region for at least 6 months. Slightly more than 1 cm across, it is now an irregularly shaped plaque with a silvery white, slightly scaly surface and a clearly demarcated margin. Because of its proximity to a pre-existing scar, preliminary evaluation of a punch biopsy seems advisable. The biopsy section submitted for the histopathology report is shown in Fig. 2-1.

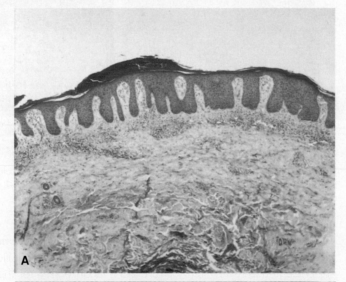

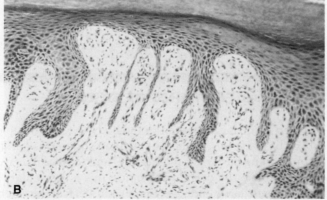

FIGURE 2-1 (**A**) Low-power and (**B**) medium-power views of biopsied tissue in Case 2-1. (The histological findings are considered in part D2-1 of the Discussion section of this chapter.)

ANALYSIS
Case 2-1

A Do you notice anything unusual about the histological appearance of the biopsied skin in Fig. 2-1?

B Is there any evidence in this biopsy that tissue fluid has accumulated in the superficial part of the dermis? If so, where may it have come from?

C What is the pink layer seen along the upper border of Fig. 2-1B?

D How many epidermal cell layers normally contain dividing cells?

E What is the normal turnover time for epidermal keratinocytes?

F Why does the free surface of this patient's skin lesion appear scaly?

(The answers to these questions are considered in the Discussion section of this chapter, under the heading D2-1.)

CASE 2-2

Andrea Hall pays little attention to a mole on her left cheek, but in her 60th year her daughter-in-law advises her to have it examined. A close inspection reveals that it has now become two smaller moles with a tiny reddish area lying between them. During physical examination of her head and neck, an enlarged sub-mandibular node is palpated on the left side. The pathology report returned for an excisional biopsy of the mole confirms the provisional diagnosis. Figure 2-2A shows the mole before excision; Fig. 2-2B shows it in section.

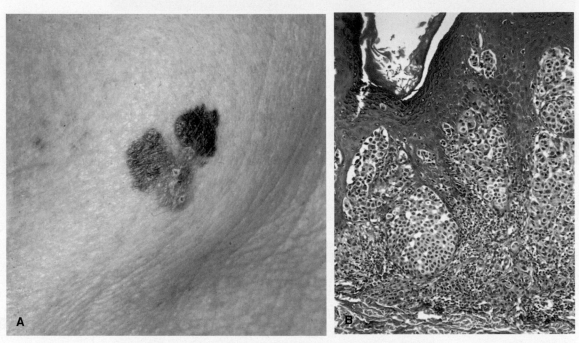

FIGURE 2-2 (A) Photograph of patient's cheek in Case 2-2. **(B)** Histological features of skin biopsy in Case 2-2 (medium power). (The findings are considered in part D2-2 of the Discussion section of this chapter.)

ANALYSIS
Case 2-2

A What is unusual about the area of epidermis seen in Fig. 2-2B?

B What is the prognosis for patients who develop this type of lesion?

C How did such a lesion originate?

D Does its thickness have any clinical significance?

E How common is this type of lesion?

F What precautions decrease the risk of developing this type of lesion?

(The answers are considered in Section D2-2 of the Discussion section of this chapter.

To provide students with a further opportunity to arrive at some of their own conclusions before consulting answers, a number of the component illustrations in this book are presented as review items. Figure 2-3 is incorporated for this purpose.

ESSENTIAL FEATURES OF SKIN

The *skin* is the largest organ in the body. It is made up of (1) an epithelial layer called the *epidermis*, which is stratified squamous keratinizing epithelium with an underlying basement membrane, and (2) a connective tissue layer called the *dermis*. Unlike the dermis, the epidermis is avascular. It nevertheless contains free afferent nerve endings. Epidermal derivatives such as sweat glands, sebaceous glands, hairs and hair follicles, and nails and nail grooves, are classified as *skin (epidermal) appendages*. The epidermis of thick skin has five layers (strata) known as the stratum germinativum (basale), spinosum, granulosum,

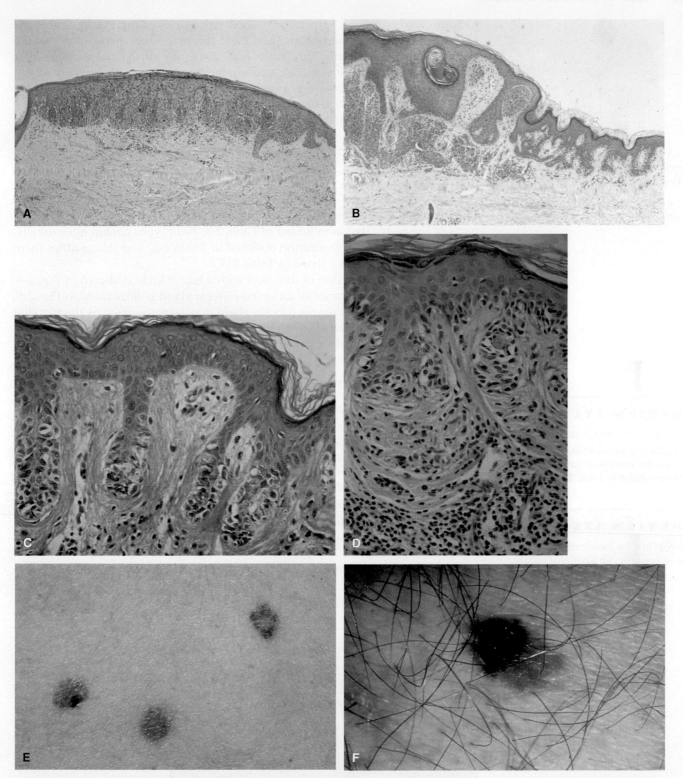

FIGURE 2-3 Evaluation of one of these moles, **A** or **B**, indicates that its histological features are not normal. Is it **A** or is it **B**? In **C** and **D**, parts of section **B** are shown under higher magnification for further information. Would you consider the moles shown in **E** and **F** to be normal? (For answers, see part D2-3 of the Discussion section of this chapter.)

lucidum, and corneum, respectively. Their names reflect increasing degrees of keratinocyte maturation. In thin skin, these layers are less discernible and the stratum lucidum is absent. The *dermis* is made up of a superficial *papillary layer* of loose connective tissue and an underlying *reticular layer* of dense, ordinary connective tissue. The dermis is attached to deeper tissues by an adipocyte-containing layer of connective tissue known as *subcutaneous tissue* or the *hypodermis* because of its position *under* the skin. Hair follicles and the majority of sweat glands, however, extend down into the subcutaneous tissue. Anatomists call this layer the *superficial fascia*.

Thick and Thin Skin

The histological characteristics of *thick skin* and *thin skin*, present on different parts of the body, are summarized in Table 2-1. Both types of skin have the distinctive dual-layered organization outlined in Table 2-2, and this enables them to carry out the functions listed in Table 2-3.

A representative section of thin skin with a hair follicle is shown in Fig. 2-4. The histological appearance of an eccrine sweat gland is illustrated in Fig. 2-5. The duct portion of this simple tubular gland may be recognized by the fact that its walls are two cells thick, which gives it a somewhat darker appearance. Figure 2-6 is a pictorial review item.

Examples of Cutaneous Lesions

Many kinds of skin lesion (Table 2-4) involve particular components of the epidermis or dermis. Burns generally involve a number of components (see below).

Thus, epidermal keratinocytes may undergo excessive proliferation, or their intercellular attachments may be weakened, leading to loss of cohesion and resulting blister formation. A cause of several of these *dyshesive disorders* is autoantibody production to keratinocyte antigens. Such antigens include desmosomal transmembrane linker glycoproteins in patients with *pemphigus vulgaris* and, in patients with *bullous pemphigoid*, a hemidesmosome-associated glycoprotein *(BP antigen)* that is one of the constituents of the epidermal basement membrane (see Fig. 2-10).

Desmosomes and *hemidesmosomes* are cell surface sites that are designed to

REVIEW ITEM 2-1

How does an *apocrine* sweat gland differ from an *eccrine* sweat gland?

REVIEW ITEM 2-2

Using information in this chapter, suggest the skin components that might be involved in formation of the lesions listed in Table 2-4.

REVIEW ITEM 2-3

What are the functions of the other two types of cell junctions?

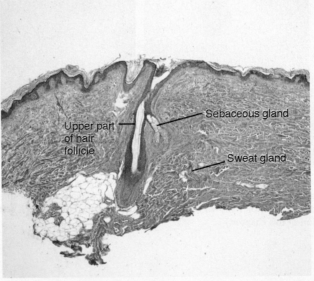

FIGURE 2-4 Thin skin (low power). The small, pale area *(lower left)* is subcutaneous adipose tissue.

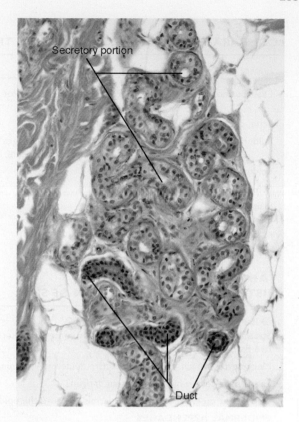

FIGURE 2-5 Sweat gland, eccrine type, in thin skin (medium power). How may the duct be distinguished from the secretory portion? (For details, see text.)

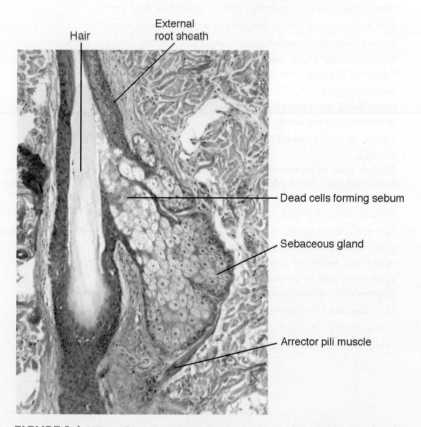

FIGURE 2-6 What effects do androgens have on the processes that are occurring here? (To confirm your answer, see part D2-4 of the Discussion section of this chapter.)

TABLE 2-1
COMPARATIVE FEATURES OF THICK AND THIN SKIN

Feature	Thick Skin	Thin Skin
Distribution	Palmar and plantar, flexor surface of digits	Remainder of body surface
Total thickness (mm)	0.6–4.5	1.0–5.2
Epidermal characteristics	Thick, with friction ridges and a thick stratum corneum	Thin, with no friction ridges and a thin stratum corneum
Epidermal thickness (mm)	0.5–1.5	0.1–0.15
Dermal thickness (mm)	1.0–3.0	0.5–5.0
Hair follicles	Absent	Present
Sebaceous glands	Absent	Present

TABLE 2-2
HISTOLOGICAL ORGANIZATION OF SKIN

EPIDERMIS

Stratified squamous keratinizing epithelium, consisting of keratinocytes, which transform into protective flat scales of soft keratin

Melanocytes, which produce protective epidermal melanin

Langerhans cells, which can present antigens

Dependent on diffusion from the dermis, because the epidermis is avascular

EPIDERMAL APPENDAGES

Hairs in hair follicles, consisting chiefly of protective hard keratin

Nail plates in nail grooves, consisting of protective hard keratin

Eccrine sweat glands, which secrete sweat and, thereby, help to regulate the body temperature

Apocrine sweat glands, which produce an odor-releasing secretion. Bacterial action resulting in release of this body odor is inhibited by deodorants

Sebaceous glands, which produce the sebum that keeps hairs supple

EPIDERMAL BASEMENT MEMBRANE

Attaches epidermis to dermis

Tensile strength provided by type IV collagen

DERMIS

Papillary layer of superficial loose connective tissue, which nourishes the adjacent epidermis: this layer is the main site of inflammatory changes associated with skin infections and cutaneous allergic reactions

Reticular layer of underlying dense ordinary connective tissue, which contributes tensile strength

Numerous blood vessels, mostly in the papillary layer under the epidermis, peripheral nerves, etc.

SUBCUTANEOUS ADIPOSE TISSUE

Adipocytes, which are specialized for lipid storage and lipid metabolism

AFFERENT NERVE ENDINGS

Encapsulated mechanoreceptors responding to compression or tension

Unencapsulated mechanoreceptors responding to compression

Unencapsulated nociceptors responding to injury

Unencapsulated thermoreceptors responding to temperature

KEY CONCEPT

Epidermal layers reflect the maturation of keratinocytes.

TABLE 2-3
SKIN FUNCTIONS

BARRIER
Water loss or gain

Heat loss or gain (regulated)

Ultraviolet light

Microorganisms

DEFENSE
Acute inflammation

Cutaneous immune responses

REPAIR
Self-healing

Promoted by suturing

SENSORY
Touch

Pressure

Temperature

Pain

SYNTHESIS
Melanin

Vitamin D_3

ABSORPTION (LIMITED)
Lipid-soluble drugs

TABLE 2-4
REPRESENTATIVE SKIN LESIONS

INFECTIONS
Bacterial, viral, or fungal

INFLAMMATORY CONDITIONS
Dermatitis (eczema)

Allergic contact dermatitis

Urticaria

Acne vulgaris

EPIDERMAL DISORDERS
Psoriasis vulgaris

Excessive keratinization

Vesicles or bullae (blisters) with loss of adhesion

DERMAL DISORDERS
Connective tissue changes

BENIGN TUMORS
Keratoses

Nevi

MALIGNANT TUMORS
Melanomas

Carcinomas

Kaposi sarcoma

TABLE 2-5
CHARACTERISTICS OF ADHERING (ANCHORING) JUNCTIONS

Junction	Type	Transmembrane and Filament Attachment Proteins	Functions
Desmosome (= macula adherens)	Cell to cell	Desmogleins and desmocollins; desmoplakins, keratocalmin, plakoglobin	Anchors intermediate filaments to cell membrane; bonds to apposed similar membrane site
Adhesion belt (= zonula adherens)	Cell to cell	Cadherin; catenins, vinculin, plakoglobin	Anchors marginal band of microfilaments to cell membrane; bonds to apposed similar membrane site
Hemidesmosome	Cell to extracellular matrix	$\alpha_6\beta_4$ integrin; bullous pemphigoid antigen, HD1	Anchors intermediate filaments to cell membrane; bonds membrane site to basement membrane
Focal contact (= adhesion plaque)	Cell to extracellular matrix	Integrins; α-actinin, vinculin, talin	Anchors microfilament bundle to cell membrane; anchors membrane site to adjacent matrix macromolecules, eg, fibronectin

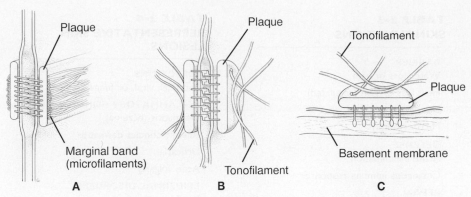

FIGURE 2-7 Adhering (anchoring) junctions. (**A**) Adhesion belt. (**B**) Desmosome. (**C**) Hemidesmosome.

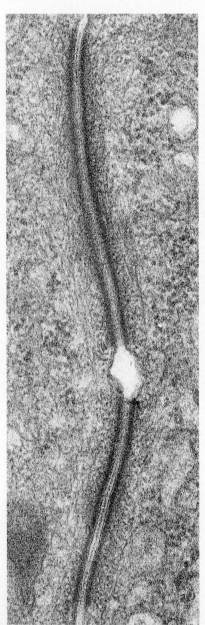

FIGURE 2-9 Can you identify this structure? (To confirm your answer, see Discussion section D2-5 of this chapter.)

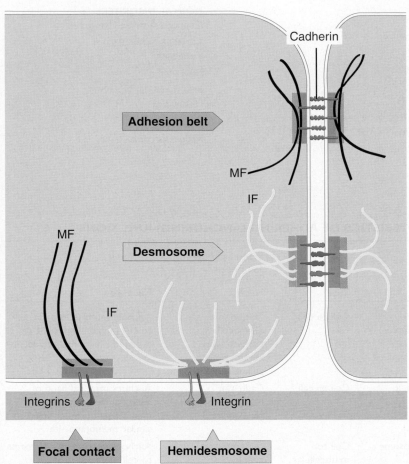

FIGURE 2-8 Epidermal adhering (anchoring) junctions.

hold cells together. They are examples of *adhering (anchoring) junctions*, the various characteristics of which are summarized in Table 2-5 and Figs. 2-7 and 2-8. Figure 2-9 is a Review Item.

Some clinically important features of the epidermis, involving its keratinocytes, Langerhans cells, and melanocytes, are shown in Fig. 2-10.

Several fundamental cutaneous structure-function relationships are summarized in Fig. 2-11.

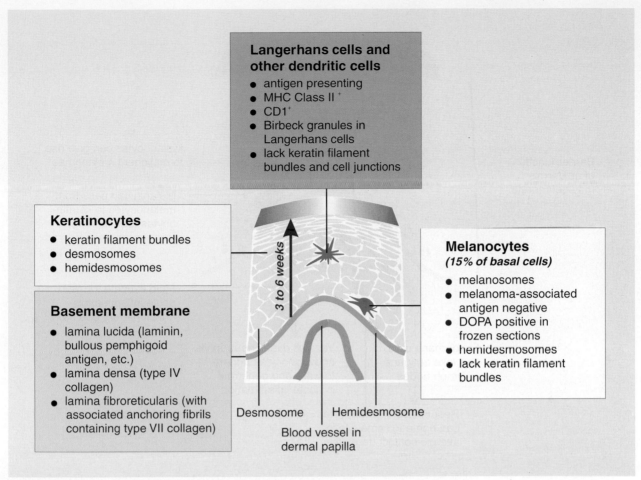

Langerhans cells and other dendritic cells
- antigen presenting
- MHC Class II $^+$
- CD1$^+$
- Birbeck granules in Langerhans cells
- lack keratin filament bundles and cell junctions

Keratinocytes
- keratin filament bundles
- desmosomes
- hemidesmosomes

3 to 6 weeks

Melanocytes
(15% of basal cells)
- melanosomes
- melanoma-associated antigen negative
- DOPA positive in frozen sections
- hemidesmosomes
- lack keratin filament bundles

Basement membrane
- lamina lucida (laminin, bullous pemphigoid antigen, etc.)
- lamina densa (type IV collagen)
- lamina fibroreticularis (with associated anchoring fibrils containing type VII collagen)

Desmosome   Hemidesmosome

Blood vessel in dermal papilla

FIGURE 2-10 Some key components of the skin. Epidermis extends down to the basement membrane, dermis lies below. Living keratinocytes have a mean turnover time of 3.5 weeks. Renewal of the stratum corneum occurs in approximately 2 weeks.

Cutaneous Blood Supply

As indicated in Fig. 2-11, the superficial blood vessels of the dermis play key roles in various skin conditions, especially those with an inflammatory component (see Table 2-4). These vessels also play an essential role in the regulation of body temperature. Figure 2-12 shows the general arrangement of the dermal blood supply. A deep plexus of blood vessels lies at the interface between the fibrous *reticular layer* of dermis and subcutaneous adipose tissue. This *rete cutaneum* or *cutaneous plexus* is supplied by subcutaneous arteries and is drained by small subcutaneous veins. From the cutaneous plexus, vessels extend inward and supply secretory portions of sweat glands, papillae of hair follicles, and the subcutaneous adipose tissue. Vessels extending outward from this plexus supply capillaries in the *papillary layer* of dermis, which is a layer of loose connective tissue. A superficial plexus of arterioles, venules, and capillaries lies at the interface between the reticular and papillary layers of dermis. The epidermis is nourished by diffusion from capillaries that loop up from this *rete subpapillare* or *subpapillary plexus* into the dermal papillae. *Arteriovenous anastomoses (AV shunts)* are present between the deeper arteries and veins, and to an even greater extent interconnect superficial arterioles with venules. These anastomoses enable much of the blood that is delivered to the skin to bypass the cutaneous terminal vascular bed, thereby conserving heat. When blood is permitted to pass through the terminal vascular bed, the skin flushes, ie, it becomes red and hot. Oxyhemoglobin reaching the superficial venules provides the pink color that is

KEY CONCEPT

Epidermal regeneration needs viable stratum germinativum cells, eg, in the surviving parts of epidermal appendages.

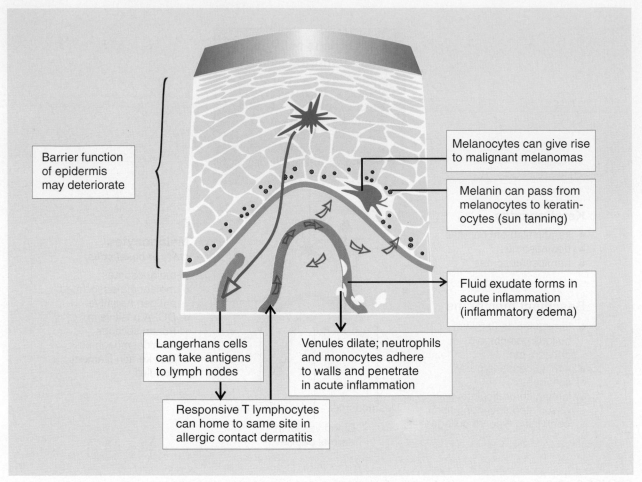

Barrier function
of epidermis
may deteriorate

Melanocytes can give rise
to malignant melanomas

Melanin can pass from
melanocytes to keratin-
ocytes (sun tanning)

Fluid exudate forms in
acute inflammation
(inflammatory edema)

Langerhans cells
can take antigens
to lymph nodes

Venules dilate; neutrophils
and monocytes adhere
to walls and penetrate
in acute inflammation

Responsive T lymphocytes
can home to same site in
allergic contact dermatitis

FIGURE 2-11 Some important structure–function relationships involving the skin.

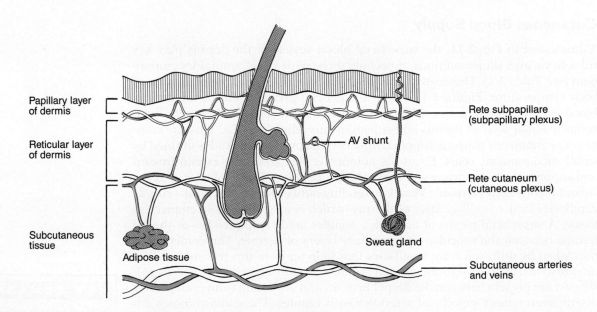

Papillary layer
of dermis

Reticular layer
of dermis

Subcutaneous
tissue

Adipose tissue

Rete subpapillare
(subpapillary plexus)

AV shunt

Rete cutaneum
(cutaneous plexus)

Sweat gland

Subcutaneous arteries
and veins

FIGURE 2-12 Blood supply of the skin.

usually seen, unless it is masked by melanin. For further information on inflammation or the functional role of Langerhans cells, see Fig. 2-10 and Chap. 3.

Cutaneous Burns

Clinical classification of burns and scalds is generally based on their degree of severity. In a *first-degree burn* (or scald), heat coagulation is limited to the superficial part of the epidermis, and the cells in the stratum germinativum remain viable. Destroyed layers of the epidermis are, therefore, subsequently replaced. In a *second-degree burn*, heat damage occurs throughout the epidermis and also in the superficial part of the dermis. However, the lower parts of sweat glands and hair follicles, ie, the deeply situated parts of epidermal appendages, remain undamaged. The surviving stratum germinativum cells of these appendages, therefore, continue to provide the means for epidermal regeneration. Plasma leaks from the venules and capillaries in the damaged papillary layer of dermis, causing edema and often accumulating as pockets of fluid. In thin skin, such fluid-filled blisters *(bullae)* commonly form between the dermis and epidermis. In thick skin, however, intraepidermal blisters may form just above the

TABLE 2-6
EPIDERMAL MELANIN: MAIN STAGES OF FORMATION AND LOSS

In epidermal *melanocytes* (neural crest-derived cells present on the epidermal side of the epidermal basement membrane):

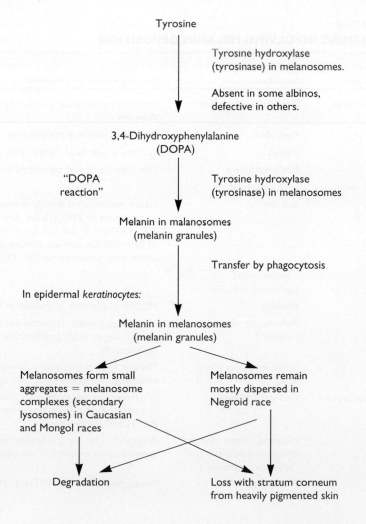

Tyrosine

Tyrosine hydroxylase (tyrosinase) in melanosomes.

Absent in some albinos, defective in others.

3,4-Dihydroxyphenylalanine (DOPA)

"DOPA reaction"

Tyrosine hydroxylase (tyrosinase) in melanosomes

Melanin in malanosomes (melanin granules)

Transfer by phagocytosis

In epidermal *keratinocytes:*

Melanin in melanosomes (melanin granules)

Melanosomes form small aggregates = melanosome complexes (secondary lysosomes) in Caucasian and Mongol races

Melanosomes remain mostly dispersed in Negroid race

Degradation

Loss with stratum corneum from heavily pigmented skin

stratum germinativum as a result of decreased keratinocyte adhesion. Necrotic tissue is sloughed from the burn site following an episode of acute inflammation. Second-degree, deep-dermal thermal burns take more than 3 weeks to heal. For good cosmetic results, skin grafting is sometimes required because the ensuing dermal regeneration can result in scarring. A *third-degree burn* is a full-thickness burn that is severe enough to destroy the entire epidermis and dermis, including all the epidermal appendages. In most cases, a skin autograft is necessary for clinically satisfactory healing because it accelerates the healing process. Without a skin graft, epidermal regeneration can take place only at the perimeter of a third-degree burn site. Loss of blood plasma by exudation from the weeping surface of raw burn sites can lead to development of *hypovolemic shock* if 15% or more of the body surface in adults (or 10% or more in children) is involved.

Epidermal Melanization

The skin color at any given site is only partly determined by the ratio of oxyhemoglobin to reduced hemoglobin. Other contributing factors are the concentration and type of epidermal melanin and the carotene content of the subcutaneous fat. Table 2-6 shows the various stages involved in *epidermal melanization*, which substantially protects the body from penetration by damaging ultraviolet radiation. Some basic examples of melanin production, underproduction *(hypomelanosis)*, and overproduction *(hypermelanosis)* are given in Table 2-7.

The concentration of epidermal melanocytes on different parts of the body

> **KEY CONCEPT**
>
> UV-B, the cause of sunburn, is a risk factor in skin cancer. Epidermal melanization offers partial protection over most of the UV-B range.

TABLE 2-7
CONDITIONS INVOLVING MELANIN DEPOSITION

Extent of Melanization	Condition	Features and Factors Involved
Hypomelanosis	Oculocutaneous albinism	Tyrosine hydroxylase is either absent or else defective
	Piebaldism	Patches of skin lack melanocytes
	Vitiligo	Patches of skin lack melanocytes
	Phenylketonuria	Phenylalanine is not converted into tyrosine
Normal range	Even pigmentation:	
	Sun tan	Heavy melanization greatly reduces transmission of 290–315 nm (UV-B = 290–320 nm). It also decreases transmission of 320–400 nm (UV-A). Preformed melanin darkens on exposure to 320–720 nm
	Circumscribed pigmented macules:	
	Freckles	Macular deposition of melanin in fair skin
	Melanocytic nevi ("moles")	Macular or papular accumulation of nevus cells arising through proliferation of melanocytes
	Senile lentigines ("liver spots")	Macular hyperpigmentation by normal melanocytes that develops with aging
Hypermelanosis	Addison's disease	In adrenocortical insufficiency, the decrease in cortisol output leads to elevation of the ACTH and α-MSH levels
	Melasma, known also as chloasma (circumscribed "mask of pregnancy")	Pregnancy, oral contraceptives; progesterone appears to be involved in the eitology
	Pituitary tumor	Production of excess ACTH or MSH

can vary by a factor of three, but for each body part it is quite similar in light-skinned and dark-skinned races. In infants of the Mongol race, a bluish-gray to brown patch of pigmented skin known as a *mongolian spot* may be present in the sacral area. In this case, the pigmentation results from the presence of melanin-containing cells deep in the dermis. Such spots may vanish spontaneously during childhood.

CASE DISCUSSIONS

D2-1 (CASE 2-1)

At first glance, the section of thin skin seen in Fig. 2-1 may not seem to be atypical. However, dermal papillae are not usually this tall, even in thick skin. Also, the superficial layer of keratin (stratum corneum), where it can be recognized, looks unusually thick (middle of Fig. 2-1A and upper pink border of Fig. 2-1B). Such thickening of the stratum corneum is described as *hyperkeratosis*. Furthermore, nucleated cells are not generally found in the stratum corneum, but here the incorporated keratinocytes have all retained their nucleus. *Parakeratosis*, meaning persistence of the nucleus into the stratum corneum, is in this case regarded as evidence of a maturation defect. No stratum granulosum is recognizable. Because the superficial keratinocytes are defective and unable to form a strongly cohesive layer, the surface of the lesion has a scaly appearance. The deep red color of the lesion is due to the fact that the epidermis overlying its tall, highly vascular dermal papillae is comparatively thin.

In this disorder, which is called *psoriasis vulgaris*, dividing keratinocytes are found in several layers instead of only one or two. The length of the cell cycle in psoriatic keratinocytes is eight times shorter than normal. The turnover time of these cells is under 1 week instead of approximately 5 weeks.

This *epidermal hyperplasia* suggests altered regulation of the cell cycle and defective maturation of the postmitotic keratinocytes. Accelerated production of keratinocytes as a result of excessive proliferation is the probable reason for elongated papillae.

The other main characteristic of psoriasis is accompanying *inflammation* that at times is both chronic and acute. The connective tissue in the affected dermal papillae is edematous, containing fluid exudate from damaged and leaking venules and capillaries. Following early infiltration of the papillary layer of dermis by lymphocytes and macrophages, neutrophils intermittently emerge from the vessels in these papillae. They become attracted to the parakeratotic area, hence, small groups of neutrophils may be found in the epidermis as well as the dermis. Because of this, dermal papillae of psoriatic skin have been appropriately named "squirting papillae."

Implicated in the etiology of this condition are CD4-positive T lymphocytes (helper T cells) that adhere to the endothelium of dermal postcapillary venules, invade the epidermis, and produce various lymphokines. Dermal dendrocytes, which are antigen-presenting phagocytic cells that produce cytokines, also are involved. One of the cytokines that they produce causes keratinocytes to release a cytokine that is capable of attracting T cells and neutrophils.

D2-2 (CASE 2-2)

The irregular borders and variegated colors of the skin lesion shown in Fig. 2-2A, together with the fact that its appearance has changed, suggest that it may be a malignant melanoma. In Fig. 2-2B, it is difficult to identify the epidermal–dermal border because numerous nodules of melanoma cells, which in this case appear amelanotic (melanin-free), have grown down as far as the reticular layer of dermis. The presence of lymphocytes well above this level is evidence that the tumor cells are causing some kind of immune response. This skin cancer, diagnosed as a *malignant melanoma*, has invaded the papillary layer of dermis. There is, therefore, a possibility that the malignant cells, of melanocytic origin, have had an opportunity to enter dermal lymphatics or cutaneous blood vessels and undergo lymphatic or hematogenous dissemination. However, if the melanoma had been diagnosed and excised before it grew into the dermis, at a time when it was <0.75 mm thick, there would have been no significant risk of metastasis. Invasive penetration of the epidermal basement membrane and the basement membrane and endothelium of the superficial plexus of dermal blood vessels and lymphatics sets the stage for ensuing metastasis.

In light-skinned races, an almost certain cause of malignant melanoma is unprotected overexposure to sunlight, particularly for those with a fair complexion who easily become sunburned. General awareness of this hazard and recent availability of effective ultraviolet-blocking sunscreens may help to check the alarming escalation in incidence of this potentially lethal type of skin cancer. Although primary melanomas only constitute 1% or so of all cancers, they metastasize to such an extent that their secondary tumors are the chief lethal outcome of any skin disorder.

D2-3 (FIG. 2-3)

Despite the obvious content of heavily pigmented cells and the raised upper surface of the mole represented in Fig. 2-3A, its histological appearance indicates that it is benign. Described as a *junctional nevus, common (benign) melanocytic nevus,* or *nevocellular nevus,* it contains numerous pigmented basal epidermal melanocytes (*nevus cells*) that in most cases give it a dark brown or light brown uniform color. This mole was considered unsightly and was removed for cosmetic purposes.

In contrast, the moles represented in Fig. 2-3B–F are asymmetric to irregular in outline. Generally, they are larger and more variegated in color. Such moles are also less heavily pigmented, and have somewhat indistinct margins. Their nevus cells extend down into the dermis, and over the course of time, groups of nevus cells possessing an atypical, large nucleus start to appear. This type of mole is accordingly known as a *large atypical mole* or *dysplastic nevus.* Lymphocytes commonly form diffuse aggregates in the papillary layer of dermis beneath nevi of this type (see Fig. 2-3B,D). Any dysplastic nevi that may be present need to be recognized, since their presence can indicate an increased risk of developing malignant melanoma.

D2-4 (FIG. 2-6)

Figure 2-6 shows a *sebaceous gland* with its associated *hair follicle.* Androgens (1) stimulate the growth of terminal hair, (2) augment the autosomal-dominant gene expression in males that results in *male pattern alopecia,* and (3) increase the holocrine secretory activity of sebaceous glands, a response that is excessive in *acne vulgaris.*

D2-5 (FIG. 2-9)

Electron-dense plaque material situated on each side of a cell junction, with associated tonofilaments (intermediate filaments composed of keratins) and an electron-dense line present in the middle of an electron-lucent intercellular space, is characteristic of a *desmosome,* the structure shown in Fig. 2-9.

BIBLIOGRAPHY

Bennett DC. Genetics, development, and malignancy of melanocytes. Int Rev Cytol 146: 191, 1993.

Bos JD, Kapsenberg ML. The skin immune system: Progress in cutaneous biology. Immunol Today 14:75, 1993.

Boyer B, Thiery JP. Epithelial cell adhesion mechanisms. J Membr Biol 112:97, 1989.

Breathnach SM. The Langerhans cell. Br J Dermatol 119:463, 1988.

Eady RAJ. The basement membrane: Interface between the epithelium and the dermis: structural features. Arch Dermatol 124:709, 1988.

Fitzpatrick TB, Szabo G, Wick MM. Biochemistry and physiology of melanin pigmentation. In: Goldsmith LA, ed. Biochemistry and Physiology of the Skin, vol 2. New York, Oxford University Press, 1983, p 687.

Fry L. An Atlas of Psoriasis. Carnforth, Lancs, U.K., Parthenon Publishing Group, 1992.

Fuchs E. Epidermal differentiation. Curr Opin Cell Biol 2:1028, 1990.

Fuchs E. Keratins and the skin. Annu Rev Cell Biol 11:123, 1995.

Garrod DR. Desmosomes and hemidesmosomes. Curr Opin Cell Biol 5:30, 1993.

Green KJ, Jones JCR. Desmosomes and hemidesmosomes: Structure and function of molecular components. FASEB J 10:871, 1996.

Haftek M, Hansen MU, Kaiser HW, Kreysel HW, Schmitt D. Interkeratinocyte adherens junctions: Immunocytochemical visualization of cell-cell junctional structures, distinct from desmosomes, in human epidermis. J Invest Dermatol 106:498, 1996.

Inoué S. Ultrastructure of basement membranes. Int Rev Cytol 117:57, 1989.

Koh HK. Medical progress: Cutaneous melanoma. N Engl J Med 325:171, 1991.

Leffell DJ, Brash DE. Sunlight and skin cancer. Sci Am 275:52, 1996.

Lin AN, Carter DM. Epidermolysis bullosa. Annu Rev Med 44:189, 1993.

Marks R, Christophers E, eds. The Epidermis in Disease. Lancaster, U.K., MTP Press, 1981.

Mehregan AH. Pinkus' Guide to Dermatohistopathology, ed 4. Norwalk, Conn., Appleton-Century-Crofts, 1986.

Millington PF, Wilkinson R. Skin. Cambridge, U.K., Cambridge University Press, 1983.

Nickoloff BJ, ed. Dermal Immune System, Boca Raton, Fla., CRC Press, 1993.

Roenigk HH, Maibach HI, eds. Psoriasis, ed 2. New York, Marcel Dekker, 1991.

Sanchez JA, Robinson WA. Malignant melanoma. Annu Rev Med 44:335, 1993.

Schittney JC, Yurchenco PD. Basement membranes: Molecular organization and function in development and disease. Curr Opin Cell Biol 1:983, 1989.

Schwarz MA, Owaribe K, Kartenbeck J, Franke WW. Desmosomes and hemidesmosomes: Constitutive molecular components. Annu Rev Cell Biol 6:461, 1990.

Slominski A, Ross J, Mihm MC. Cutaneous melanoma: Pathology, relevant prognostic indicators and progression. Br Med Bull 51:548, 1995.

Stevens A, Wheater PR, Lowe JS. Clinical Dermatopathology. A Text and Color Atlas. Edinburgh, Churchill Livingstone, 1989.

Taylor CR, Sober AJ. Sun exposure and skin disease. Annu Rev Med 47:181, 1996.

Tsukita S, Nagafuchi A, Yonemura S. Molecular linkage between cadherins and actin filaments in cell-cell aherens junctions. Curr Opin Cell Biol 4:834, 1992.

Valdimarsson H, Baker BS, Jónsdóttir I, Powles A, Fry L. Psoriasis: A T-cell-mediated autoimmune disease induced by streptococcal superantigens. Immunol Today 16:145, 1995.

Yaar M, Woodley DT, Gilchrest BA. Human nevocellular nevus cells are surrounded by basement membrane components. Immunohistologic studies of human nevus cells and melanocytes in vivo and in vitro. Lab Invest 58:157, 1988.

Review Items: Cross References

Information relevant to the Review Items listed in this chapter may be found in the following pages of Cormack, DH. Essential Histology. Philadelphia, J.B. Lippincott, 1993:

REVIEW ITEM	PAGES
2-1	259, 265
2-3	91–95

CHAPTER 3

Blood, Inflammation, Immunity, and Allergy

CASE 3-1

A recent history of weakness with undue shortness of breath on physical exertion is noted when Mario Dinarello, aged 22 years, presents at the Emergency Service because of severe headaches. Except for finding a mild tachycardia and general pallor, the physical examination is normal. There is no history of poor nutrition, gastrointestinal bleeding, or renal failure. The rectal examination is normal. A test for occult blood in the stools is negative. A peripheral blood film obtained from this patient is shown in Fig. 3-1A. His hemoglobin is 52 g/L.

Persistent questioning eventually establishes that Mario and a few of his friends have been obtaining significant proceeds by diligently marketing their blood. On every second day for the last 3 months, each of them underwent phlebotomy of 40–80 mL of blood and collected $10 for each contribution. This blood was subdivided into smaller samples that were then submitted to local laboratories for routine analyses under fictitious names. Third-party billing for the extraneous analyses is currently under investigation.

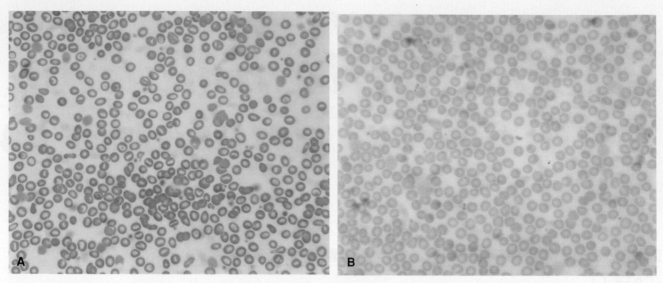

FIGURE 3-1 (**A**) Peripheral blood in Case 3-1. (**B**) Normal peripheral blood.

ANALYSIS
Case 3-1

In how many ways do the blood cells seen in Fig. 3-1A differ from normal? What is the probable diagnosis?

(The answers are discussed in part D3-1 of the Discussion section of this chapter.)

CASE 3-2

Unpleasant tingling sensations with occasional numbness of the feet become yet another source of annoyance for Milt Grover, who at the age of 65 feels unwell or lethargic almost all the time. He blames his ashen appearance, increasing leanness, and chronic tiredness on his poor appetite. It is unusual for him to exert himself, smoke, consume alcoholic drinks, or take medications. He has no history of urinary or bowel symptoms. This patient's peripheral blood film is illustrated in Fig. 3-2. His hemoglobin is 84 g/L. The mean corpuscular volume (MCV) is 120 fL. The reticulocyte count is 3%. The WBC, differential count, and platelet count are all normal. Through a procedure known as the *Schilling test*, the patient's condition is investigated further. In this test, he is given a small oral dose of vitamin B_{12} tagged with ^{57}Co, followed by an intramuscular injection of "cold" vitamin B_{12} within 1 hour. The proportion of the radioactive vitamin that is recovered from urine collected over the next 24 hours is less than 1% of the administered dose. However, when intrinsic factor is given along with the radioactive vitamin, the recovered proportion rises to 18%.

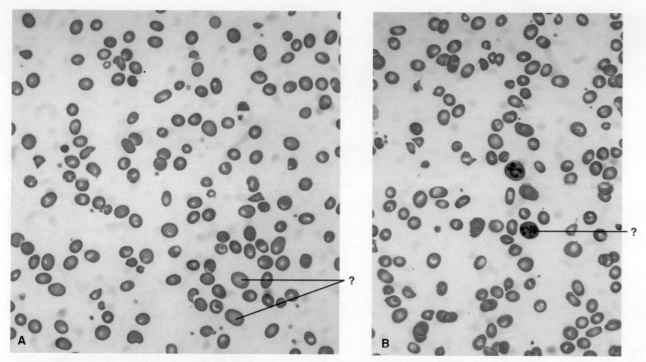

FIGURE 3-2 Peripheral blood in Case 3-2. (**A**) and (**B**) are representative parts of the same blood film. [Features labeled (?) are potentially informative.]

ANALYSIS
Case 3-2

A Do you notice anything unusual about the appearance of this patient's peripheral blood cells (see Fig. 3-2)?

B What does an MCV of 120 fL indicate?

C Do the results of the Schilling test suggest a cause for the low hemoglobin?

(The findings are considered in part D3-2 of the Discussion section of this chapter.)

CASE 3-3

Tony Muffoletto, aged 18 years, is admitted to hospital for investigation of bruising and hematuria (presence of blood in the urine). A complete blood count (CBC) obtained on admission shows hematocrit 23%, MCV 84 fL, WBC 0.5×10^9/L, with 4% segmented neutrophils, 2% eosinophils, and 94% lymphocytes. The platelet count is 15×10^9/L. A biopsy of his bone marrow is seen in Fig. 3-3A. On the basis of these findings, he receives total body irradiation and an allogeneic bone marrow transplant from an HLA-matched brother. Four months after successful engraftment, Tony is doing well. Then his WBC rises to 15.1×10^9/L, with 80% segmented neutrophils, 3% bands, 1% metamyelocytes, and an occasional myelocyte. A peripheral blood film obtained at this time is shown in Fig. 3-4. Tony becomes febrile and has a productive cough with yellow sputum. After treatment with penicillin, the fever and cough subside, and the leukocytosis and neutrophilia resolve. A chest x-ray shows uniform shadowing of the upper lobe of the left lung, consistent with *pneumonitis* (pneumonia), and a sputum sample test positive for Pneumococcus.

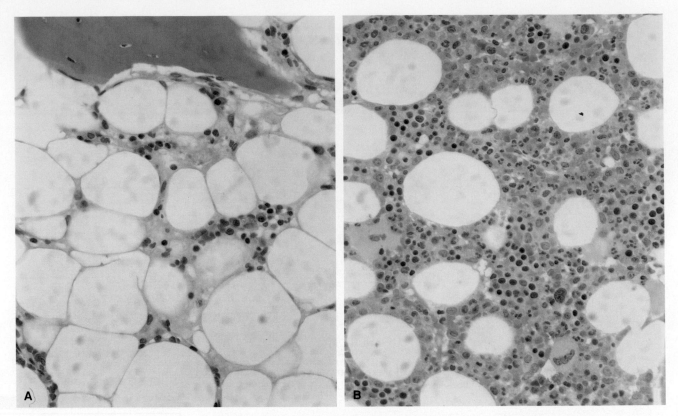

FIGURE 3-3 (**A**) Marrow biopsy in Case 3-3. (**B**) Normal marrow biopsy.

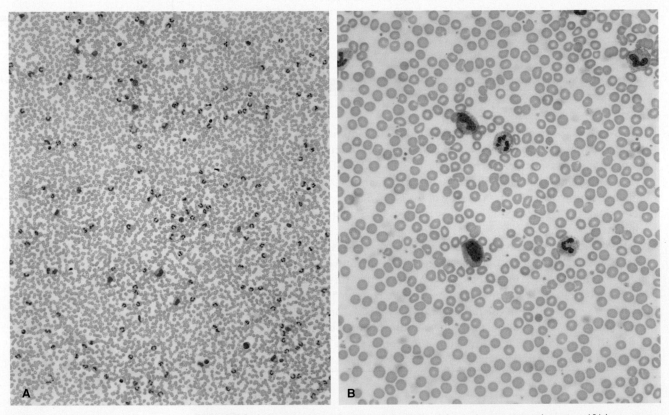

FIGURE 3-4 Peripheral blood in Case 3-3, obtained 4 months post-transplantation. (**A**) Low power. (**B**) Medium power.

CASE 3-4

Toward the end of her second pregnancy, 24-year-old Leslie Bryce notices that she has several bruises on her legs. Three weeks after delivery, the incidence of bruising increases and her gums become puffy and start to bleed easily (Fig. 3-5). Also, Leslie becomes increasingly fatigued, which she attributes to lost sleep due to the baby's night-time crying. Her family physician orders a CBC, and on receiving the report arranges for her hospital admission.

Leslie's physical examination reveals marked swelling of the gums and small ulcers in the mouth and throat. A septic paronychia is found on her left hand. A few recent bruises are also evident on her legs. The blood counts show hemoglobin 79 g/L, WBC 2.3×10^9/L, with 19% neutrophils, 45% monocytes, 25% lymphocytes, and 10% blast cells (Fig. 3-6). The platelet count is 30×10^9/L. For further diagnosis, a bone marrow sample is obtained from the right iliac crest. Representative cells of the aspirate are shown in Fig. 3-7.

Following an intensive course of chemotherapy, the patient goes into complete remission. Her bruises disappear, and the finger infection and gum hypertrophy both resolve. During this remission, her blood values are hemoglobin 120 g/L, WBC 6.5×10^9/L, with 78% neutrophils, 5% monocytes, and 17% lymphocytes. Her platelet count is 151×10^9/L. Her bone marrow regains a normal cellularity, with fewer than 5% blast cells. However, Leslie's condition is characterized by the likelihood of relapse. Arrangements are accordingly made to treat her by more aggressive chemotherapy, followed by total body irradiation. She is then given a bone marrow transplant from Susan, her HLA-matched sister. Donor marrow cells engraft successfully, and when Leslie is discharged home, her blood count is normal. She continues in remission, with a high probability of being cured.

ANALYSIS
Case 3-3

A In what ways does the marrow biopsy obtained from this patient (see Fig. 3-3A) differ from normal (see Fig. 3-3B)?

B From the blood counts obtained on admission, can you identify the blood cell lines that show decreased production?

C Is there any particular constituent in a bone marrow transplant that guarantees successful engraftment? (To confirm your answers, see part D3-3 of the Discussion section of this chapter.)

D What type of leukocyte is prevalent in Fig. 3-4? Is an increased absolute number of such cells in the peripheral blood consistent with pulmonary infection?

(The answer is discussed in part D3-4 of the Discussion section of this chapter.

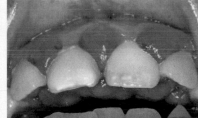

FIGURE 3-5 Appearance of the patient's gums in Case 3-4.

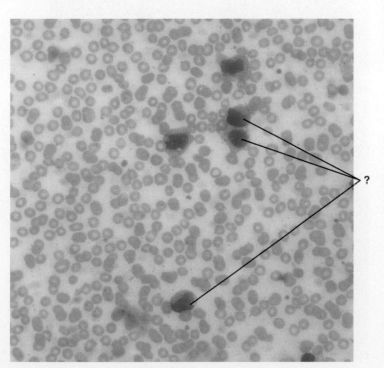

?

FIGURE 3-6 Peripheral blood in Case 3-4 (medium power). [Features labeled (?) are potentially informative.]

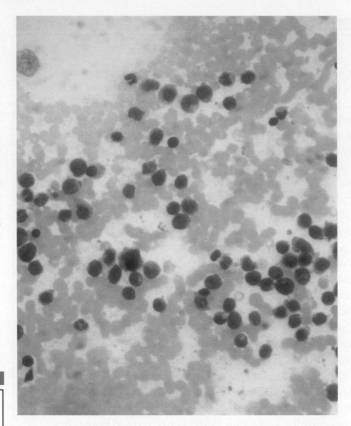

FIGURE 3-7 Marrow aspirate in Case 3-4 (medium power), showing the characteristic blast cells of acute myelomonocytic leukemia. Monoblastic as well as myeloblastic leukemic cells are present in this patient's marrow.

ANALYSIS
Case 3-4

A How does the blood film seen in Fig. 3-6 differ from normal?

B How does the marrow aspirate seen in Fig. 3-7 differ from the normal marrow aspirate shown in Fig. 3-8?

(To check your answers, see part D3-5 of the Discussion section of this chapter.)

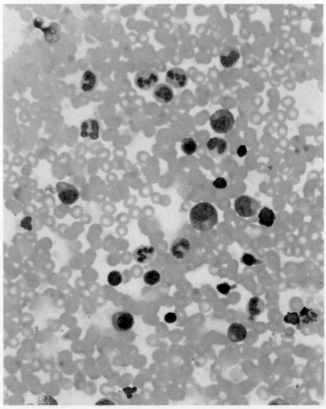

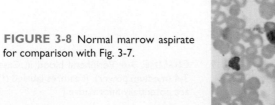

FIGURE 3-8 Normal marrow aspirate for comparison with Fig. 3-7.

OTHER CASES

Figures 3-9 and 3-10 are pictorial review items.

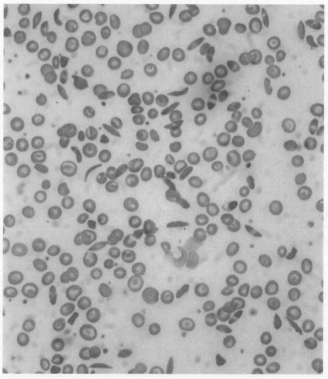

FIGURE 3-9 Peripheral blood obtained from an unrelated case. The oxygen tension of this blood was lowered with sodium metabisulfite before the film was prepared. What is unusual about these blood cells? (For confirmation, see part D3-6 of the Discussion section of this chapter.)

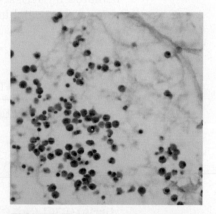

FIGURE 3-10 The cellular infiltrate present in this biopsy supports the clinical diagnosis of nasal polyposis. Which type of inflammatory cell predominates? What other histological sign of inflammation can you find? (For confirmation of your answers, see part D3-7 of the Discussion section of this chapter.)

TABLE 3-1
BLOOD CELLS

ERYTHROCYTES (RED BLOOD CELLS)
Mature

Immature (reticulocytes or polychromatophilic erythrocytes)

PLATELETS (THROMBOCYTES)

LEUKOCYTES (WHITE BLOOD CELLS)
  Granulocytes
    Neutrophils (polymorphs)
    Eosinophils
    Basophils
  Nongranular leukocytes
    Lymphocytes
      B and T cells
    Monocytes

ESSENTIAL FEATURES OF BLOOD CELLS

Oxygen is distributed to the various body tissues by *erythrocytes,* which circulate within blood vessels. If these vessels become damaged, they bleed until circulating *blood platelets* trigger the formation of intravascular or extravascular thrombi (Gk. *thrombus,* clot). The remainder of the blood cells constitute an extremely heterogeneous group called *leukocytes,* which are motile cells that carry out important functions fundamental to the interrelated processes of inflammation, allergy, and immunity.

The blood cells found in peripheral blood are listed in Table 3-1. Figure 3-11 shows their morphological appearance in blood films. In H&E sections, only erythrocytes, neutrophils, and small lymphocytes are easy to recognize in blood vessels or tissues.

Blood cell counts and other clinical laboratory data are expressed in units belonging to the *SI* (Système Internationale) system of measurement. Normal values often required for reference purposes are provided in Table 3-2. (For a concise summary of the main clinical implications of significant deviations from these values and for other useful information, see Fischbach.)

A *complete blood count* (CBC) generally includes determinations of the patient's red blood cell count (RBC), hemoglobin concentration (Hgb or Hb), hematocrit (Hct), several specific erythrocyte indices (eg, the mean corpuscular volume, hemoglobin, and hemoglobin concentration), white blood cell count

TABLE 3-2
NORMAL LABORATORY VALUES* FOR PERIPHERAL BLOOD

RED BLOOD CELL COUNT (RBC)	
Men	$4.8 \times 10^{12}/L$ (4.2–5.4)
Women	$4.3 \times 10^{12}/L$ (3.6–5.0)
HEMOGLOBIN (Hgb or Hb)	
Men	160 g/L (140–180)
Women	140 g/L (120–160)
HEMATOCRIT (Hct) OR PACKED CELL VOLUME (PCV)	
Men	46% (40–54)
Women	43% (37–47)
MEAN CORPUSCULAR VOLUME (MCV)	87 fL–103 fL
RETICULOCYTE COUNT	
Men	0.5%–1.5%
Women	0.5%–2.5%
PLATELET COUNT	150×10^9–$350 \times 10^9/L$
WHITE BLOOD CELL COUNT (WBC)	4.5×10^9–$11.0 \times 10^9/L$
DIFFERENTIAL (DIFF)	
Mature neutrophils (Segs or Polys)	50%–60%
Band neutrophils	0%–5%
Metamyelocytes	0%–1%
Myelocytes	0%
Promyelocytes	0%
Eosinophils	1–4%
Basophils	0.5%–1%
Monocytes	2%–6%
Lymphocytes	20%–40%

* Compiled mostly from Fischbach

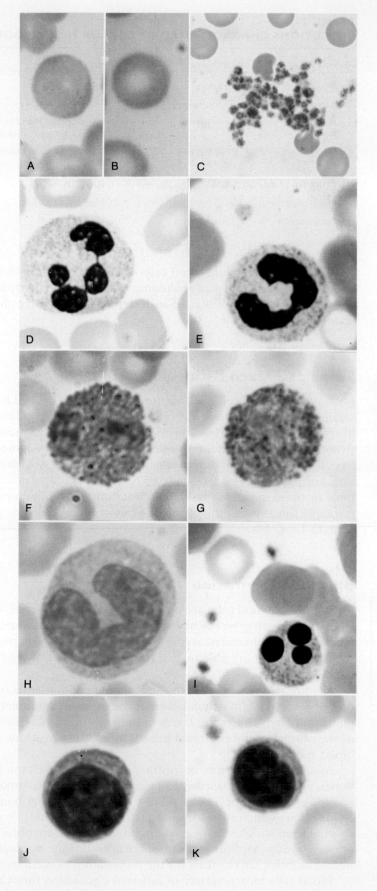

FIGURE 3-11 The cells in peripheral blood films (Wright's blood stain). (**A**) Immature (polychromatophilic) erythrocyte, ie, reticulocyte; (**B**) mature erythrocyte; (**C**) platelets; (**D**) mature neutrophil; (**E**) immature (band) neutrophil; (**F**) eosinophil; (**G**) basophil; (**H**) monocyte; (**I**) degenerating neutrophil; (**J**) large lymphocyte; (**K**) small lymphocyte.

TABLE 3-3
CONDITIONS CHARACTERIZED BY LOW OR HIGH BLOOD CELL COUNTS

Blood Cells	Low Count	High Count
Erythrocytes	Anemias	Polycythemia
Platelets	Thrombocytopenia	Thrombocythemia
Leukocytes:	Leukopenia	Leukocytosis (normal leukocytes); leukemias (neoplastic leukocytes)
Neutrophils	Neutropenia	Neutrophilia (ie, neutrophil leukocytosis)
Eosinophils		Eosinophilia
Basophils		Basophilia
Monocytes		Monocytosis
Lymphocytes	Lymphopenia	Lymphocytosis

(WBC), differential white blood cell count (Diff), and platelet count (Plt), along with routine hematological evaluation of the patient's peripheral blood film.

Some terms frequently used in describing quantitative changes in blood cell counts are listed in Table 3-3.

Specific Characteristics of Blood Cells

Each type of blood cell is characterized by having special functions. Thus, the unique content and shape of *erythrocytes* facilitates uptake, transport, and delivery of oxygen and carbon dioxide. *Platelets* have the capacity to undergo an activation process in which they alter their shape and become more adhesive. As a result of aggregation, they produce *platelet thrombi*, which are essential for the arrest of bleeding. The various types of *leukocytes* carry out a range of key functions involved in inflammation and immunity. The distinguishing features and principal functions of the different types of blood cells are shown in summary form in Table 3-4.

Blood Cell Formation

Most types of blood cells are non-dividing end-cells; hence, continuous replenishment from progenitors in red bone marrow is necessary. Lymphocytes and monocytes are somewhat atypical in that they have the capacity to undergo further division and are able to give rise to other types of cells outside the bloodstream.

As indicated in Fig. 3-12, the site where hematopoiesis begins is the embryonic *yolk sac*. The *liver* then becomes the main hematopoietic organ, with supplementation by the *spleen*. *Red bone marrow* (*myeloid tissue*) ultimately prevails as the normal site of postnatal hematopoiesis and provides a lifelong supply of blood cells.

In adults, red marrow is confined to the axial skeleton (chiefly the cranial bones, vertebrae, pelvis, ribs, and sternum) and the proximal ends of the upper and lower extremities. The medullary cavity of the other bones is filled with *yellow marrow*, which stores fat but is not hematopoietic. Figure 3-13 shows the sources from which marrow aspirates and biopsies are obtained for hematopoietic evaluation. Aspiration biopsies are adequate for cytological evaluation, but needle biopsies are required for the preparation of sections or imprints.

Blood cells have a variety of different circulation times and lifespans, summarized in Table 3-4. The appropriate proportion of each type of blood cell

---

KEY CONCEPT

Hematopoietic populations undergo continuous cell renewal, hence they are easily damaged by chemotherapeutic drugs and ionizing radiation.

TABLE 3-4

MAIN STRUCTURAL AND FUNCTIONAL CHARACTERISTICS OF BLOOD CELLS

Cells	Morphological Features*	Absolute No./L	Estimated Circulation Time or Lifespan	Chief Functions
Erythrocytes	Pink cytoplasm; no nucleus; biconcave disk-shaped; diameter 7 μm	4.3×10^{12} (female) 4.8×10^{12} (male)	Circulate for 100–120 days	Transport O_2 and CO_2
Reticulocytes	Bluish pink cytoplasm (or blue cytoplasmic reticulum if stained with brilliant cresyl blue); no nucleus; biconcave disk-shaped; diameter 7–8 μm	25–85 $\times 10^{12}$	Circulate for 2 days before maturing	Immature cells with the same function as mature erythrocytes
Platelets	Pale blue cytoplasm; purple granules; no nucleus; biconvex disk-shaped; diameter 3 μm	150–350 $\times 10^9$	Circulate for 9–10 days	Arrest bleeding
Neutrophils	Mauve specific granules; purple azurophilic granules; segmented nucleus (2–5 lobes); diameter 13 μm	2.5–7.5 $\times 10^9$	Circulation time 6–10 hours; 2–3 days in tissues	Phagocytose and kill bacteria
Band neutrophils	Granules as in mature neutrophils; band-shaped nucleus, still essentially unsegmented; diameter 14 μm	0–1 $\times 10^9$	Circulation time similar to that of mature neutrophils	Immature cells with the same functions as mature neutrophils
Eosinophils	Large red specific granules; bilobed nucleus; diameter 15 μm	0–0.5 $\times 10^9$	Circulation time 1–10 hours; up to 10 days in tissues	Have antiparasitic and antiallergic capabilities
Basophils	Large blue specific granules; bilobed or segmented nucleus; diameter 11 μm	0–0.2 $\times 10^9$	Circulation time estimated as 1–10 hours; variable time in tissues	Release inflammatory mediators in the course of systemic allergic reactions
Lymphocytes	Blue cytoplasm; spherical nucleus; diameter either 7 μm (small lymphocytes) or 12 μm (large lymphocytes)	1.5–3.5 $\times 10^9$	Mean circulation time 10 hours for majority of cells; variable time in lymphoid organs and tissues; majority of cells are long-lived	Produce the effector cells of immune responses
Monocytes	Pale blue cytoplasm; kidney-shaped nucleus; diameter 12–20 μm	0.2–0.8 $\times 10^9$	Circulate for 1–3 days; variable time in tissues	Phagocytose unwanted material; give rise to macrophages and osteoclasts

*Wright's blood stain, unless otherwise stated

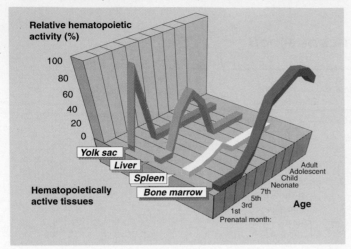

FIGURE 3-12 The sites that participate in prenatal and postnatal hematopoiesis.

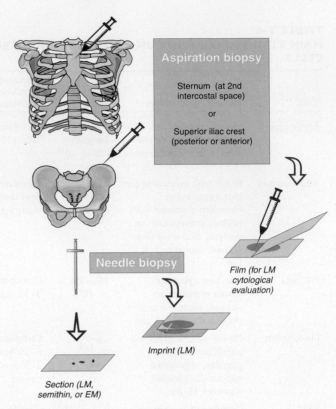

FIGURE 3-13 Standard procedures for cytological and morphological evaluation of bone marrow. Marrow aspirates and biopsies are generally obtainable from the posterior or anterior iliac crests. Alternative sites for sampling are the sternum (adults) or the upper end of the tibia (children).

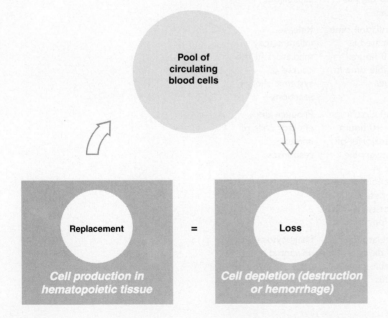

FIGURE 3-14 Blood cell numbers are maintained within normal limits through the production of enough new cells to replace the ones that are lost.

needs to be replaced every day. In each case, the absolute cell number in the peripheral blood stays within normal limits because cell production is consistently commensurate with cell loss (Fig. 3-14).

Marrow Composition

As shown in Fig. 3-15, *red bone marrow* (*myeloid tissue*) is conventionally regarded as being made up of *stromal, myeloid, erythroid,* and *lymphoid* components. Here, the word "myeloid" is highly restricted in meaning. Essentially, it refers only to morphologically recognizable cells of the *neutrophil series*. The *myeloid:erythroid* (M:E) *ratio* is regarded as being diagnostically informative. The normal range for this parameter is 2.5:1 to 5:1.

The various stromal elements of myeloid tissue constitute a special form of connective tissue supported by *reticular fibers* and drained by venous *sinusoids*. Newly formed blood cells leave the marrow by way of these sinusoids. This is because they can squeeze through the attenuated cytoplasm of the endothelial cells that line these vessels. Numerous actively phagocytic *macrophages* lie close to the sinusoids. An important role of many of the stromal cells (notably macrophages, fibroblast-like reticular cells, and endothelial cells) is that they produce hematopoietic growth factors. The levels at which several of these key factors operate are indicated in Fig. 3-16.

Hematopoietic cell populations are made up of (1) *stem cells*, which have the dual capacity of self-renewal and production of differentiating progeny (see Fig. 1-4), (2) *progenitor cells*, which are progeny cells that undergo progressive differentiation, (3) *precursors*, which are progeny cells that have become committed to a specific lineage but are not yet fully functional, and (4) functional *blood cells* (or derivatives, such as platelets), each type of which is highly specialized for certain tasks and, except in the case of lymphocytes or monocytes, is an *end cell* incapable of division. Cells such as *CFU-GEMMs, pluripotential hematopoietic stem cells* (which are the ancestral cells), and the bipotential stem cells that give rise to B and T cells, are classified as *stem cells*. Such cells occupy upper levels in the hierarchical scheme of hematopoietic differentiation (see Fig. 3-16). Below them are a variety of *progenitors*, eg, *BFU-E, CFU-Meg,* and *CFU-GM*, each having substantial proliferative potential but only a limited or negligible capacity for self-renewal. The strange names given to these cells are acronyms denoting their individual or multiple potentialities. The stated potentiality of each progenitor is deduced from the combination of cell types found in the colonies that it produces in vitro. These progenitors, in turn, give rise to morphologically recognizable blood cell *precursors*.

The various erythroid and granulocytic precursors in marrow films are illustrated in Fig. 3-17.

Erythroid Series

Table 3-5 shows the alternative standard terminologies that exist for the morphologically recognizable stages of erythroid differentiation and maturation (Fig. 3-17A through 3-17F). The early cells are large, with a proportionally large, spherical nucleus and discernible nucleoli. As soon as active synthesis of globin chains begins, the cytoplasm becomes intensely basophilic, reflecting its ample content of polysomes. The nucleus then becomes small and tightly packed with condensed chromatin. It is extruded at the *normoblast* stage. Because newly formed erythrocytes still have residual ribosomes that contain rRNA, they stain bluish pink to muddy gray with polychromed blood stains. They are accordingly termed *polychromatophilic* (meaning: love many colors) *erythrocytes*. Such immature erythrocytes are recognized more readily if they have been stained with

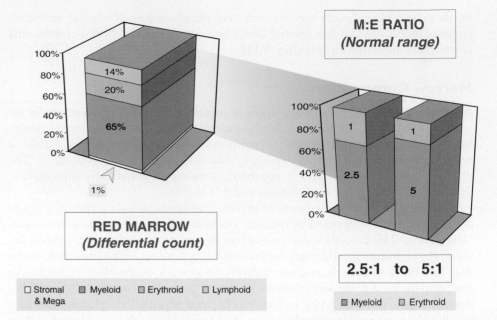

M:E RATIO
(Normal range)

2.5:1   to   5:1

☐ Myeloid   ☐ Erythroid

RED MARROW
(Differential count)

☐ Stromal & Mega   ☐ Myeloid   ☐ Erythroid   ☐ Lymphoid

FIGURE 3-15 The normal cellular composition of red bone marrow, showing its myeloid:erythroid ratio.

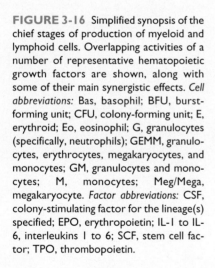

FIGURE 3-16 Simplified synopsis of the chief stages of production of myeloid and lymphoid cells. Overlapping activities of a number of representative hematopoietic growth factors are shown, along with some of their main synergistic effects. *Cell abbreviations:* Bas, basophil; BFU, burst-forming unit; CFU, colony-forming unit; E, erythroid; Eo, eosinophil; G, granulocytes (specifically, neutrophils); GEMM, granulocytes, erythrocytes, megakaryocytes, and monocytes; GM, granulocytes and monocytes; M, monocytes; Meg/Mega, megakaryocyte. *Factor abbreviations:* CSF, colony-stimulating factor for the lineage(s) specified; EPO, erythropoietin; IL-1 to IL-6, interleukins 1 to 6; SCF, stem cell factor; TPO, thrombopoietin.

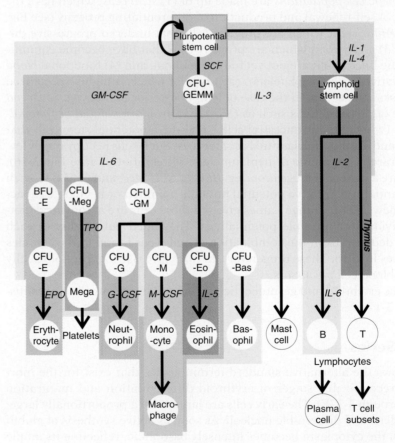

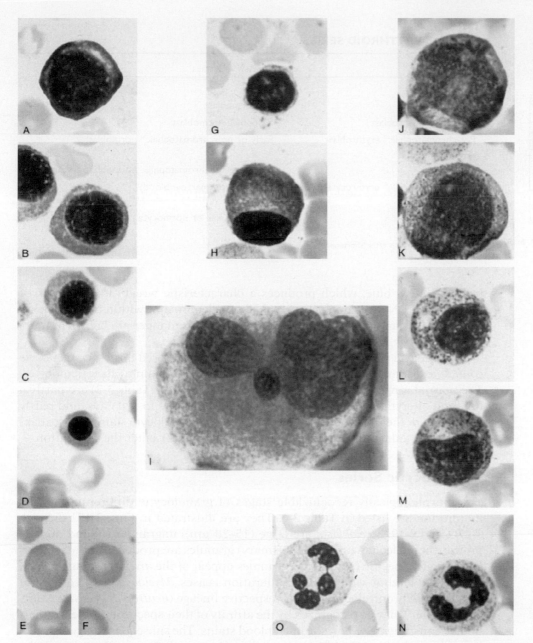

FIGURE 3-17 Morphologically recognizable myeloid cells, at different stages of differentiation and maturation, in marrow films (Wright's blood stain). *Left panel* (**A–F**), erythroid series. *Right panel* (**J–O**), granulocytic series. (**A**) Proerythroblast; (**B**) basophilic erythroblast; (**C**) polychromatophilic erythroblast; (**D**) normoblast; (**E**) polychromatophilic erythrocyte (reticulocyte); (**F**) mature erythrocyte; (**G**) small lymphocyte; (**H**) plasma cell; (**I**) megakaryocyte; (**J**) myeloblast; (**K**) promyelocyte; (**L**) neutrophilic myelocyte; (**M**) neutrophilic metamyelocyte; (**N**) band neutrophil; (**O**) mature neutrophil.

REVIEW ITEM

Can you identify each of these cells before you need to refer to the list provided at left?

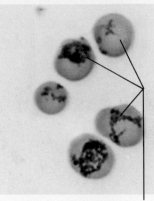

Reticulocytes

FIGURE 3-18 Reticulocytes in a peripheral blood film (high power).

TABLE 3-5
NORMAL ERYTHROID SERIES

Stage	Alternative Names
DIVIDING	
Proerythroblast	Pronormoblast
Basophilic erythroblast	Basophilic normoblast
Polychromatophilic* erythroblast	Early or polychromatophilic* normoblast
MATURING	
Normoblast	Late or orthochromatophilic normoblast/erythroblast
Polychromatophilic* erythrocyte	Reticulocyte (marrow/blood)
MATURE	
Erythrocyte	Red blood cell or normocyte

*Polychromatophilic is often shortened to polychromatic

brilliant cresyl blue, which produces a characteristic wreath-like network of blue-stained RNA (residual ribosomal ribonucleoprotein) within the cytoplasm (Fig. 3-18). Immature erythrocytes identified in this manner are known as *reticulocytes* (L. *rete*, net).

Erythrocyte production may be conveniently monitored through *reticulocyte counts*, ie, estimates of the percentage of erythrocytes staining as reticulocytes. The normal ranges accepted for reticulocyte counts (see Table 3-2) are partly a function of erythrocyte lifespan, which is normally 100 to 120 days, and partly a function of the rate of loss of detectable RNA. Reticulocyte staining is lost approximately 2 days after the newly formed erythrocytes enter the circulation.

Granulocytic Series

The morphologically recognizable stages of granulocytic differentiation and maturation are listed in Table 3-6. They are illustrated in Figs. 3-17J through 3-17O and 3-19. *Myeloblasts* are large (15–20 μm), ungranulated, and possess prominent nucleoli. Azurophilic (primary) granules are produced at the *promyelocyte* stage. Specific (secondary) granules appear at the *myelocyte* stage, which is also the level at which cell proliferation ceases. *Myelocytes* are somewhat smaller than promyelocytes. Their respective lineage (*neutrophilic, eosinophilic,* or *basophilic*) may be recognized by the affinity of their specific granules for particular constituents of polychromed blood stains. The subsequent stages of each lineage may be identified from (1) nuclear shape and (2) the color taken up by their specific granules. In *metamyelocytes* (Gk. *meta*, beyond) the nucleus is kidney-shaped, whereas in *band* forms, it has the shape of a horseshoe. In *maturing granulocytes*, the nucleus becomes segmented, producing three to five lobes in neutrophils or two lobes in eosinophils and most basophils.

The majority of the precursor cells in bone marrow films belong to the myeloid (ie, granulocytic) series (M:E ratio is 2.5:1 to 5.0:1). Neutrophil precursors predominate because neutrophils represent 50–65% of the peripheral blood leukocytes. This large proportion of myeloid precursors is consistent with the brief lifespan of neutrophils (10 hours in the circulation and 1 to 2 days after they have left it). In contrast, erythrocytes last for approximately 4 months, and are then withdrawn from circulation.

Platelet Formation

Platelets are produced through progressive subdivision of the cytoplasm of polyploid *megakaryocytes*. These cells must first become polyploid by undergoing

---

KEY CONCEPT

The fact that cells of the neutrophil series outnumber the other hematopoietic cells helps to explain why myelosuppression increases a patient's susceptibility to bacterial infections.

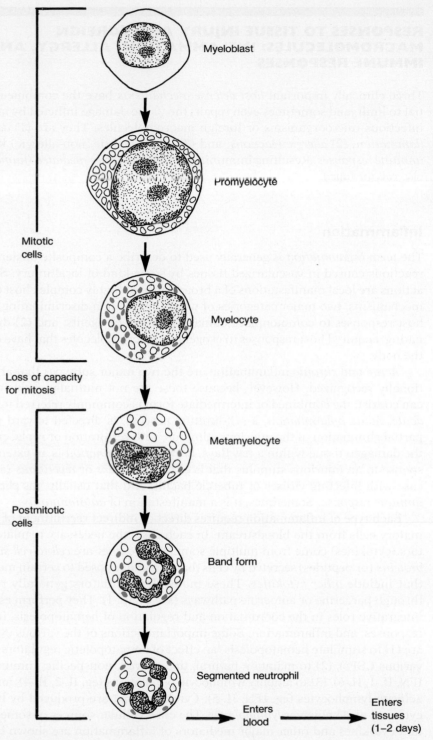

Mitotic cells

Loss of capacity for mitosis

Postmitotic cells

Myeloblast

Promyelocyte

Myelocyte

Metamyelocyte

Band form

Segmented neutrophil

Enters blood

Enters tissues (1–2 days)

FIGURE 3-19 Maturation stages in the neutrophil series. Specific granules are shown in blue.

TABLE 3-6
NORMAL GRANULOCYTIC SERIES

DIVIDING
Myeloblast
Promyelocyte
Myelocyte
MATURING
Metamyelocyte
Band neutrophil
MATURE
Segmented neutrophil (mature neutrophil, Seg or Poly)

endoreduplication, meaning the repetitive replication of their nuclear DNA without its undergoing segregation into separate daughter nuclei. The resulting polyploid complement of chromosomes is confined to a single large *multilobed nucleus* (see Fig. 3-17I). A distinctive hematopoietic growth factor called *thrombopoietin* (TPO) stimulates megakaryocyte maturation and resulting platelet formation (see Fig. 3-16).

RESPONSES TO TISSUE INJURY AND FOREIGN MACROMOLECULES: INFLAMMATION, ALLERGY, AND IMMUNE RESPONSES

Three clinically important *host defense mechanisms* have the combined potential to limit, and sometimes even repair, the tissue damage inflicted by invading infectious microorganisms or foreign macromolecules. They are (1) *acute inflammation*, (2) *allergic reactions*, and (3) additional (ie, non-allergic) kinds of *immune responses*. Resulting immunity is either *antibody-mediated* (*humoral*) or else *cell-mediated*.

Inflammation

The term *inflammation* is generally used to describe a composite of stereotypic reactions caused in vascularized tissues by some kind of local injury. Such reactions are local manifestations of a broad range of highly complex host defense mechanisms, two major categories of which are (1) non-discriminating, innate host responses to commonplace damaging events or agents, and (2) discriminating, acquired host responses to exogenous macromolecules that have entered the body.

Acute and *chronic* inflammation are the two major subtypes that are traditionally recognized. However, because these are not mutually exclusive, they can coexist; the combined or intermediate form is commonly referred to as *subacute*. Acute inflammation, a self-limiting process, is directed toward total or partial elimination of the injurious stimulus, with restoration or replacement of the damaged tissue within a few days. *Chronic inflammation* is an extended response to an injurious stimulus that is either *persistent* or *repetitious* (as is the case with infecting viruses or tubercle bacilli) and that usually has elicited an *immune response*. Sometimes, it is a manifestation of *autoimmunity*.

Each type of inflammation requires direct or indirect recruitment of inflammatory cells from the bloodstream. In each case, the necessary regulatory factors (cytokines) come from multiple sources. *Cytokines* are *cell-to-cell signaling proteins* (or peptides) secreted by cells that become exposed to certain molecules that include *other cytokines*. These molecular mediators generally regulate through paracrine or autocrine pathways (see Chap. 1). They perform essential, integrative roles in the coordination and regulation of hematopoiesis, immune responses, and inflammation. Some important actions of the various cytokines are (1) to stimulate hematopoiesis (an effect of hematopoietic regulators, eg, the various CSFs), (2) to maintain natural, unacquired, nonspecific immunity (eg, IFN, IL-1, IL-6), (3) to amplify lymphocyte populations (eg, IL-2, IL-4), and (4) to activate lymphocytes (eg, IFN, IL-5). Cytokines that are produced by lymphocytes are also known as *lymphokines*. The chief cellular sources of some important cytokines and other major mediators of inflammation are shown in Table 3-7. Detailed studies of inflammation and immunity are virtually inseparable, partly because the acute inflammatory reaction is enhanced by prior formation of specific antibodies, and partly because the two processes are closely interlinked by cytokines. The supply of inflammatory cells depends on rates of cell production in the various blood cell lineages, which in turn is driven by rates of production of hematopoietic growth factors, eg, by T lymphocytes and macrophages. Hence, cytokines (many of which are lymphokines) constitute an integral part of the elaborate regulatory network that coordinates hematopoiesis with (1) natural and acquired immunity and (2) a broad spectrum of inflammatory manifestations.

KEY CONCEPT

Chronic inflammation can be an indication of persistent antigenic stimulation.

TABLE 3-7
MAJOR CELLULAR SOURCES OF SOME REPRESENTATIVE INFLAMMATORY MEDIATORS

Neutrophil	Eosinophil	Mast Cell & Basophil	Macrophage	Endothelial Cell	T Lymphocyte
		Histamine			
Peptides	Peptides	Peptides (some are chemotaxins)	Peptides	Peptides, eg, endothelin	
Enzymes (proteases and hydrolases)	Enzymes, eg, histaminase	Enzymes (proteases and hydrolases)	Enzymes (proteases and hydrolases)	Enzymes	
Lipoxygenase and cyclooxygenase products	Lipoxygenase and cyclooxygenase products	Lipoxygenase and cyclooxygenase products (some are chemotaxins)	Lipoxygenase and cyclooxygenase products	Lipoxygenase and cyclooxygenase products	
PAF	PAF	PAF	PAF	PAF	
Reactive oxygen metabolites	Reactive oxygen metabolites		Reactive oxygen metabolites		
	Major basic protein (MBP)				
			IL-1, IL-6, TNF, and other cytokines	IL-1, Endothelium-derived relaxing factor (nitric oxide radical)	Lymphokines, eg, IL-2, -3, -4, -5, -6, IFN, TNF. Many of these *activate* or *regulate* the activities of inflammaotry cells

PAF = platelet activating factor; TNF = tumor necrosis factor; IL = interleukin

Table 3-8 identifies the cell types involved in simple and composite forms of inflammation. It also indicates that a degree of overlap exists between (1) constitutive, nonspecific defense mechanisms and (2) defense mechanisms that involve induction of specific immunity. Under most circumstances, a suitable combination of these two kinds of host defenses has the potential to eliminate the source of injury, or at least render it harmless.

TABLE 3-8
CELLULAR INVOLVEMENT IN MAJOR TYPES OF INFLAMMATION

Type	Chief Cells Involved
1. *Acute inflammation*	*Neutrophils* and *monocytes/macrophages*—expression of cell adhesion molecules; phagocytosis
	Endothelial cells—expression of cell adhesion molecules; contraction
	Fibroblasts—ECM production; fibrosis
2. *Subacute inflammation*	Intermediate between types (1) and (3)
3. *Chronic inflammation* (persisting cell-mediated immune response, or prolonged response to persisting nonantigenic stimulus)	The features described for (1) but less evident, together with the following additional features:
	Small lymphocytes (chiefly regulatory and effector T cells)—cell-mediated immune responses
	Plasma cells—antibody secretion
	Monocytes/macrophages—immunoregulatory; may become flat, weakly phagocytic "epithelioid cells" or fuse as "giant cells"
4. *Allergic inflammation* (acute reaction, or chronic perpetuating mucosal inflammation)	*Mast cells/basophils*—anaphylactic degranulation with release of inflammatory mediators from IgE-sensitized cells by antigen (type I or immediate-type hypersensitivity, atopy)
	Eosinophils—additional source of inflammatory mediators; weakly phagocytic and regulatory

Acute Inflammation

In some clinical situations, acute inflammation can be so severe that it becomes debilitating or life-threatening. However, the essential contribution of the *acute inflammatory reaction* in combatting and overcoming many kinds of infection should not be underestimated. It is a nonspecific immediate vascular and cellular response to injury characterized by (1) local participation of certain vessels, (2) plasma leakage from small blood vessels into the tissues, often described as formation of *fluid exudate*, (3) migration of *neutrophils* and *monocytes* into the tissues, (4) intense phagocytic activity of leukocytes, and (5) ensuing resolution and revascularization of the site, with repair that may lead to residual scarring (*fibrosis*). Acute inflammation is generally also accompanied by a variable degree of local tissue destruction by toxic products released from neutrophils. If postinflammatory scarring becomes excessive, fibrous adhesions may form and become a cause of progressive immobilization.

Vascular Responses Precede and Facilitate Leukocyte Emigration

The local flow of blood through sites of acute inflammation becomes adjusted in two appropriate ways: (1) *arterioles* dilate, permitting more blood cells to enter the terminal vascular bed, and (2) *postcapillary venules* begin to leak plasma, with resulting internal congestion that slows down the flow of blood. At inflammatory sites, circulating neutrophils begin to round up, roll along the endothelium, and flatten out, becoming stationary (Fig. 3-20). Many of the leukocytes that adhere to the endothelium subsequently become motile. They pass between endothelial cells and migrate into the neighboring tissues. Attracted toward inflammatory sites by chemotactic gradients, migrating *neutrophils* accumulate in large numbers. *Monocytes* migrate in a similar manner, but in smaller numbers. A few recirculating *lymphocytes* may accompany them.

Leukocyte emigration is heralded by a transient increase in *endothelial cell adhesiveness*. Certain adhesion molecules on the endothelial cells of venules are

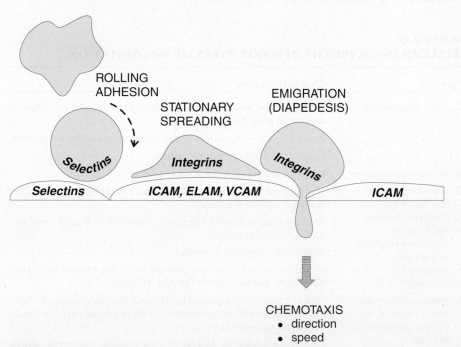

FIGURE 3-20 Cell adhesion molecules that promote the emigration of inflammatory leukocytes.

temporarily up-regulated, and some supplementary adhesion molecules, eg, *endothelial leukocyte adhesion molecule-1* (*ELAM-1*), are induced. Intercellular adhesion molecules (eg, *ICAM-1*), vascular cell adhesion molecules (eg, *VCAM-1*), and leukocyte surface receptors (chicfly *integrins* and *selectins*) also play important roles in the process of leukocyte recruitment through trapping and emigration (see Fig. 3-20). Sequential cytokine-mediated expression of adhesion molecules results in the concomitant or consecutive emigration of different types of leukocytes. Neutrophils recruited early in the reaction are accompanied by monocytes and, in inflammation that becomes subacute or chronic, lymphocytes as well.

Phagocytosis

Once microorganisms have become coated with specific antibody and have bound complement-derived products, known as *opsonins* (ie, become *opsonized*), their capture by means of phagocytosis is greatly facilitated. The main reason for this is that neutrophils possess individual surface receptors for (1) the complement fragment *C3b*, (2) its derivative *iC3b*, and (3) *IgG*. However, elimination of microorganisms through phagocytosis is not particularly effective in situations where these have a means of evading opsonization.

> **KEY CONCEPT**
>
> An important role of acute inflammation is to defend the body from bacterial infections.

Neutrophils are able to destroy their ingested bacteria through two distinct mechanisms. The basis of the first, an *oxygen-dependent* mechanism, is that neutrophils experience a sudden increase in oxygen consumption when their phagocytic activity is enhanced. Primarily a manifestation of activation of their NADPH oxidase, this *"respiratory burst"* produces relatively large quantities of certain reactive oxygen metabolites. *Superoxide radicals* (O_2^-) generated by this augmented enzyme activity become converted into H_2O_2, HOCl, and other potent microbicidal products. A similar kind of "respiratory burst" accompanied by the release of superoxide radicals occurs when eosinophils become activated.

The second mechanism that neutrophils employ for microbial elimination is essentially *nonoxidative*. It depends on the destructive action of lysosomal enzymes and other antimicrobial proteins that enter phagosomes from the primary and secondary granules that fuse with them (Table 3-9).

Neutrophil granules are of two distinct types, *azurophilic* (lysosomal) and *specific*. The chief contents of each granule type are listed in Table 3-9. Some of their active constituents are as follows. *Myeloperoxidase*, present in the azurophilic granules, produces bactericidal hypochlorite (OCl$^-$) ions from H_2O_2. The characteristic greenish color of pus is the natural color of myeloperoxidase. Also present in the same granules are *lysozyme* (muramidase), capable of hydrolyzing peptidoglycans in the cell wall of gram-positive bacteria, and a number of *cationic proteins* and *peptides* with antimicrobial activity. These include a *bactericidal/permeability-increasing protein* (B/PI), a *chymotrypsin-like cationic protein* (CLCP, also known as *cathepsin G*), and bactericidal peptides known as the *defensins*. *Lactoferrin* (apolactoferrin), an active constituent of the specific granules, is a glycoprotein that chelates ferric iron and, therefore, inhibits growth of iron-requiring bacteria. It also promotes neutrophil adhesion to endothelium.

Other functionally important constituents are present in *eosinophil*, *basophil*, and *mast cell granules*. These are included in Table 3-9.

Allergic Reactions

Clinical manifestations of *allergic reactions* may be *immediate* in onset, as in systemic hypersensitivity reactions to allergens (*type I hypersensitivity*), or they may be *delayed*, as in tuberculin-type hypersensitivity (*type IV hypersensitivity*). Examples of immediate-type hypersensitivities, which develop in a matter of min-

TABLE 3-9
FUNCTIONALLY IMPORTANT CONSTITUENTS OF THE GRANULES IN LEUKOCYTES AND MAST CELLS

Cell	Activity of Constituent	Azurophilic (Primary) Granules	Specific (Secondary) Granules	Additional Granules
Neutrophil	Bactericidal	Myeloperoxidase	Lactoferrin (apolactoferrin)	
		Lysozyme	Lysozyme	
		Bactericidal/permeability increasing protein (B/PI)	Phospholipase A_2	
		Cationic proteins and peptides, eg, defensins		
		Phospholipase A_2		
	Acid hydrolase	Acid phosphatases		Cathepsins
		Cathepsin D		
		Sulfatases		
		Lipases		
	Neutral protease	Collagenase	Type IV collagenase	Gelatinase
		Elastase		
		Cathepsin G (CLCP)		
	Other	Glycosaminoglycans	Flavoproteins	
			Vitamin B_{12}-binding R protein	
Eosinophil		Charcot-Leyden crystal protein (lysophospholipase)		Acid phosphatase
				Aryl sulfatase B
	Antiparasitic		Major basic protein (MBP) in dense core	
			Eosinophil cationic protein (ECP)	
	Other		Eosinophil peroxidase (EPO)	
			Eosinophil-derived neurotoxin (EDN)	
			Cathepsin D	
			Catalase	
			β-Glucuronidase	
			Lysozyme	
			Collagenase	
			Alkaline phosphatase	
Basophil			Histamine	
			Chondroitin sulfate A	
			Acid hydrolases	
			Major basic protein (MBP)	
			Charcot-Leyden crystal protein (lysophospholipase)	
Mast cell			Histamine	
			Heparin	
			Chondroitin sulfate E	
	Neutral protease		Tryptase	
			Chymase	
			Carboxypeptidase	

utes or hours as distinct from days, are allergic reactions to bee venom, wasp venom, penicillin, certain foods (eg, some shellfish), and many types of pollen. In generalized, systemic immediate reactions (*systemic anaphylaxis*), eg, to bee venom, wasp venom, or penicillin, massive release of inflammatory mediators from *basophils* as well as *mast cells* can lead to severe, potentially fatal respiratory and cardiovascular complications. Delayed-type hypersensitivities to food antigens may be manifested in a variety of body parts and systems, with resulting composite or diffuse symptoms.

Cellular Involvement

Mast cells play a key role in immediate-type and certain delayed-type hypersensitivities. *Basophils* participate to a variable extent. *Eosinophils* become attracted by chemotaxis to sites where allergic reactions are occurring, particularly during later stages of the response. Their presence in nasal mucus supports a diagnosis of *allergic rhinitis*, eg, in association with hay fever. Eosinophils can also be found in the lamina propria of bronchi of patients with *asthma*.

Some actions of eosinophils can be considered regulatory. Thus, eosinophils phagocytose IgE-allergen complexes and mast cell granules, and produce histaminase and aryl sulfatase, two mediator-counteracting enzymes. A local concentration of eosinophils, however, can contribute significantly to tissue damage. This is because eosinophils possess a surface receptor for IgE, in addition to surface receptors for IgG and IgA. As in mast cells and basophils, when allergen bridging occurs between preformed IgE molecules that have become bound to their receptor, inflammatory mediators are immediately released.

Major basic protein liberated from eosinophils damages bronchial epithelial cells, eg, in asthmatic patients; it also exerts a variety of activating effects. Eosinophil cationic protein and eosinophil-derived neurotoxin are both toxic to neurons, and eosinophil-derived neurotoxin has ribonuclease activity. Eosinophil peroxidase has a similar damaging effect on bronchial epithelial cells. Hence, eosinophils, like neutrophils, have the potential to cause considerable tissue destruction.

In patients with *cutaneous contact hypersensitivity* (*allergic contact dermatitis*), IgE becomes similarly bound to epidermal *Langerhans cells*, which are antigen-presenting cells, and this can result in allergen-induced eczematous skin lesions.

In addition to IgE-mediated hypersensitivity, there are IgG- and IgM-mediated hypersensitivities, hypersensitivity-related diseases caused by persisting antigens and deposition of antigen-antibody complexes, and delayed-type hypersensitivities (DTH) that are mediated by the T_D subset of lymphocytes (Table 3-10).

Immune Responses

Immune responses (L. *immunitas*, freedom from) generate specific, acquired immunity. They are of two general types. (1) The *humoral antibody response* involves production of antigen-specific immunoglobulin (*antibody*). It provides the host with protective specific immunity to a variety of bacterial infections. (2) The *cell-mediated immune response* involves production of *cytolytic* (*killer*) *cells* that can destroy antigenically altered or dissimilar cells and eliminate fungal infections. *Delayed hypersensitivity* (DTH) effects are additionally manifested in some cell-mediated responses. Delayed hypersensitivity responses can provide some measure of protection in protracted infectious diseases (eg, tuberculosis, leprosy, and syphilis).

Cell Types Involved in Immune Responses

The effector cells of immune responses are derived from (1) B lymphocytes in the humoral response and (2) T lymphocytes and monocytes in the cell-mediated response. Antigen-presenting cells are also necessary for successful activation.

TABLE 3-10
T LYMPHOCYTE SUBSETS: CHIEF FUNCTIONAL ACTIVITIES

Subset	Designation	Characteristics
Helper T cells	T_H	CD4+.
		Recognize antigen presented in association with MHC Class II surface glycoprotein.
		When activated by antigen, produce lymphokines that:
		(1) stimulate proliferation of B cells and antibody production in their progeny,
		(2) stimulate proliferation and maturation of T cells,
		(3) regulate hematopoiesis, and
		(4) activate macrophages.
		Lymphokines produced by antigen-activated T_H1 cells upregulate cell-mediated immunity and delayed-type hypersensitivity.
		Lymphokines produced by antigen-activated T_H2 cells upregulate the humoral antibody response and immediate-type hypersensitivity.
Suppressor-inducer T cells		CD4+
		Induce suppressor/cytolytic function in CD8+ T cells.
Delayed hypersensitivity T cells	T_D	The majority are CD4+, antigen-sensitized T_H1 cells.
		When activated by antigen, produce several lymphokines with actions that include:
		(1) recruitment and activation of macrophages, and
		(2) inhibition of their migration.
		Activated macrophages then become the effector cells.
Suppressor T cells	T_S	CD8+.
		Down-regulate specific immune responses.
		Rather than being a distinct subset, T_s cells may be heterogeneous, eg, share overlapping activities with T_c (as CD8+ $T_{s/c}$ cells).
Cytolytic (cytotoxic) T cells	CTL or T_c	CD8+.
		Recognize antigen presented with MHC Class I surface glycoprotein.
		Kill allogeneic cells (eg, in transplanted organs), virus-infected cells, and fungi.
		On contacting the target cell, release granules containing cytolytic molecules, notably perforin, a polymerizing protein that produces pores through which degradative enzymes and lymphokines can enter the target cell. Target cell killing is the result of (1) osmotic lysis and (2) induced endonuclease activation, with resulting apoptosis.
Memory T cells		These clonal progeny of activated T cells in each subset remain undifferentiated.
		Long-lived, and (together with memory B cells) collectively responsible for immunological memory.

Cell Markers Provide a Means of Cell Recognition

Different cell types possess distinctive assortments of surface molecules, known as *cell markers,* by which their presence may be demonstrated. Detection of these markers has been helpful in elucidating which cell types are involved in interdependent complex processes, eg, immune responses and inflammation. Most cell markers are cell-specific membrane glycoproteins that are recognized specifically by monoclonal antibodies produced in other species. Many of them bear a "CD" designation. The generic term *CD* was derived from the fact that the differentiation of individual cell types along their respective pathways leaves them with a distinctive "*cluster of differentiation*" combination of antigenic markers. For example, helper T cells are primarily CD3$^+$, CD4$^+$, CD8$^-$; cytolytic T cells are primarily CD3$^+$, CD4$^-$, CD8$^+$; and suppressor T cells are primarily CD4$^-$, CD8$^+$. The detection of specific CD markers by monoclonal antibodies is diagnostically useful in recognizing blood cells, hematopoietic cells, leukemic cells, and other cells that express these markers either permanently or at particular stages in their differentiation.

B Lymphocytes

B cells, which represent approximately 20% of the peripheral blood lymphocytes, are so called because their production from precursors occurs in the *bone marrow*, the functional equivalent of the *b*ursa of Fabricius in birds. A unique feature of each B cell is that its cell membrane contains *immunoglobulin* molecules of a single antigenic specificity. The *surface membrane immunoglobulin* (SmIg) molecule, which represents the *B cell antigen receptor*, is an unequivocal B cell marker. B cells also express HLA Class I and Class II antigens on their surface; hence, they can function as antigen-presenting cells (see below). Their microscopic appearance is that of small lymphocytes. When clonal expansion of B cells occurs as a response to activation by antigen, some of their progeny cells usually differentiate and mature as immunoglobulin-secreting *plasma cells*. These rounded, basophilic secretory cells are readily recognized by the fact that they have an eccentric nucleus with chromatin that commonly has a cartwheel or "clock face" appearance (Fig. 3-21). Their Golgi region generally looks pale in comparison with the remainder of the cytoplasm. Slightly larger than small lymphocytes, these are short-lived, non-dividing cells that tend to stay where they are produced. They are only occasionally found in the peripheral blood.

T Lymphocytes

T cells are so called because they are produced in the *thymic cortex* from immature T cell precursors that enter by way of the bloodstream. Their precursors originate in the bone marrow.

All T cells possess a surface *T cell antigen receptor* (TCR) capable of recognizing a specific foreign antigen. In addition, either CD4 or CD8 is expressed on their surface. Unlike B cells, T cells are able to recognize a foreign antigen only if it is presented as a *peptide fragment* in association with a *self-MHC molecule* (Class I or II). In other words, antigen recognition by T cells is MHC-restricted. Furthermore, the peptide-MHC complex must lie on the surface of an *antigen-presenting cell* (see below).

A number of different *functional subsets* of T cells have been described. Their essential characteristics are given in Table 3-10.

Primate CD4$^+$ cells (which are mostly helper T (T$_H$) cells but also include macrophages, the follicular dendritic cells in lymphoid follicles, 40% of peripheral blood monocytes, and 5% of B cells) are highly susceptible to infection by *human immunodeficiency virus* (HIV), the RNA virus (*retrovirus*) that causes the *acquired immunodeficiency syndrome* (AIDS). High affinity binding occurs between *gp120*, an envelope glycoprotein on the free viral particles, and *CD4* molecules on the uninfected cells. Furthermore, direct binding of gp120 on HIV-infected cells to CD4 on uninfected cells can lead to cell fusion and direct transmission of the virus from cell to cell. Chiefly as a consequence of functional impairment and progressive depletion of T$_H$ cells, humoral and cell-mediated

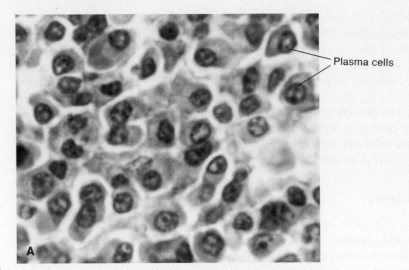

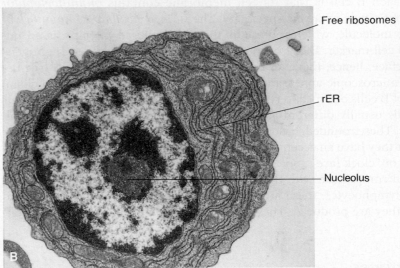

FIGURE 3-21 Plasma cells. **(A)** Medium power. **(B)** Electron micrograph.

immune responses become irreparably impaired, paving the way for opportunistic infections.

T cells, which constitute 65–80% of the peripheral blood lymphocytes, can have two different microscopic appearances. The majority are typical *small lymphocytes*, 6–9 μm in diameter. The remainder are larger (12 μm in diameter), with fine purple-staining (azurophilic) granules representing primary lysosomes. Described as *large granular lymphocytes* (LGLs), they constitute up to 20% of T_H cells and up to 35% of $T_{S/C}$ cells (see Table 3-10).

Lifespan of Lymphocytes

The lifespan of approximately 15–35% of the peripheral blood lymphocytes is 1 week or less. The other 65–85% have a long lifetime. There is controversial evidence suggesting that these cells can remain in G_0 for many years. The majority of long-lived lymphocytes are T cells in G_0.

Natural Killer Cells Represent a Null Cell Population

Alternatively known as *third population cells* (TPCs), the *null cell population* of lymphocytes is negative for both TCR (the T cell receptor that distinguishes T cells) and SmIg (the surface membrane immunoglobulin that distinguishes

B cells). It is accordingly impossible to assign null cells to either of these categories. They represent up to 20% of the peripheral blood lymphocytes.

The most important type of null cell is the *natural killer* (NK) *cell*, which is morphologically similar to the large granular T cell. NK cells have broad-acting cytolytic activity, and they can be induced to secrete cytokines. They are considered a key component of the unacquired, nonspecific immune system. Their main clinical importance is that they are able to lyse certain kinds of cancer cells and virus-infected cells, provided they have free access to them. As in cytolytic T (T_C) cells, actual contact with the target cells is necessary for killing. The dual fatal blow that both NK cells and T_C cells can inflict involves (1) release and polymerization of *perforin* (*cytolysin*), a monomeric protein that rapidly polymerizes into open channels across the target cell membrane, with resulting faulty exclusion of ions and water in the target cell, and (2) accompanying induction of endonuclease-mediated digestion of the target cell's nuclear DNA. Cell death resulting from induced endonuclease-mediated nuclear fragmentation is often described as *programmed cell death* or *apoptosis*.

Antigen-Presenting Cells

Widely recognized antigen-presenting cells for helper T cells include mononuclear phagocytes (eg, macrophages), B cells, activated T cells, dendritic reticular cells, Langerhans cells, and venular endothelial cells. The general term *histiocyte* is now often used to denote not only antigen-presenting cells of the monocyte-macrophage lineage but also dendritic reticular cells and Langerhans cells. Antigens processed by such cells are presented to helper T cells as *peptide fragments* intimately associated with *self-MHC Class II molecules* on the presenting cell surface. An additional population of *follicular dendritic cells* present in lymphoid follicles (including those of lymph nodes and the spleen) plays a supplementary but separate role. Follicular dendritic cells bind antigen–antibody complexes to their cell membrane and hold them there for prolonged periods. Because this increases the chances of exposure of antigen-presenting cells to trapped antigen, it indirectly boosts antigen presentation as peptide fragments.

B Cell Activation

Specific interaction of antigen with the B cell surface membrane immunoglobulin (its receptor) is sufficient to trigger re-entry into the cell cycle. However, with only a few exceptions (notably, bacterial lipopolysaccharides), antigens elicit effective humoral responses only when antigen-specific T_H cells produce the required supporting lymphokines as part of their response to the same antigen. This T cell response requires presentation of the processed antigen as a peptide in intimate association with an MHC Class II molecule on the surface of an antigen-presenting cell. Lymphokine-mediated large-scale B cell responses result in substantial clonal expansion and the production of (1) short-lived, immunoglobulin-secreting *plasma cells* and (2) long-lived *memory B cells*.

T Cell Activation

inactivated T cells (ie, resting or *"naive"* T cells) are activated by complexing of their *TCR* with specific antigen presented as a *peptide* in association with an *MHC Class II molecule* on the surface of an *antigen-presenting cell*. The essential co-stimulator in the dual recognition process appears to be either *IL-1* or *B7*, which is another surface molecule on the antigen-presenting cell. If the second signal (the co-stimulator) is missing, T cells remain unresponsive to the processed antigen and a state of *tolerance* toward that antigen may develop. Activation of T cells in each functional subset induces clonal expansion, producing

(1) *effector cells* representative of the subset, eg, T$_{S/C}$, and (2) long-lived *memory T cells*.

Lymphoid Organs

Lymphoid tissue is diffusely distributed in association with mucosal surfaces throughout the body. However, a substantial part of it lies in the lymphoid organs, which are the thymus, lymph nodes, and spleen. Table 3-11 summarizes the chief distinguishing features of lymphoid tissues and organs.

Thymus

The *thymus* is one of two *primary lymphoid organs*, meaning sites where lymphocytes are produced and differentiate. The *bone marrow* (ie, *bursa* equivalent) is the other primary source of lymphocytes. The thymus is made up of an outer region called its cortex and an inner medulla (Fig. 3-22). The key components of the *thymic cortex* are (1) a loose network of *epithelial reticular cells*, which develop chiefly from third and fourth pharyngeal pouch endoderm and produce *thymic hormones*, and (2) an expanding and differentiating population of *T cell progenitors and T cell progeny* derived from the lymphoid stem cells in bone marrow. Progeny T cells produced in the thymic cortex are subject to two kinds of selection. First, a compounded, antigen-independent *positive selection* process selects only cells that (1) can recognize *self-MHC molecules* on the surface of thymic epithelial reticular cells, and accordingly have become *MHC-restricted*, (2) are *TCR$^+$*, and (3) are either *CD4$^+$* or *CD8$^+$*. *Thymic hormones* (chiefly thymosin, thymulin, and thymopoietin) bring about the expression of CD2, CD3, TCR, and either CD4 or CD8 on the surface of these cells. The second kind of selection that occurs in the thymic cortex is an antigen-dependent *negative selection* process that results in self-destruction (through apoptosis) of any cells that have a TCR capable of recognizing a *self-antigen*. The term *clonal deletion* is often employed in describing the elimination of T cells with such autoimmune potential. The outcome of the dual selection process is that fewer than 10% of the T cells produced in the thymus are permitted to leave. In general, the only T cells that survive and enter the circulation are *self-MHC-restricted T cells* that are *unable to recognize self-antigens*.

Because the thymus is not supplied with afferent lymphatics, its differentiating T cells remain unexposed to lymph-borne antigens. Furthermore, throughout the thymic cortex, a closely arranged combination of vascular endothelium, other components of the vessel wall, and perivascular connective tissue, with an investing contiguous layer of epithelial cells, make up a *blood–thymus barrier*. This arrangement largely excludes circulating antigens from the thymic cortex, where T cells are produced, and also helps to conserve its distinctive internal environment. Cell junctions (1) between adjacent vascular endothelial cells and (2) between contiguous investing epithelial cells are believed to play key roles in providing this degree of antigen shielding.

The main *exit routes* for T cells leaving the thymus are (1) *postcapillary venules* at the corticomedullary border and (2) *efferent lymphatics* draining the medulla. The epithelial component of the thymic medulla is partly arranged as keratinizing concentric whorls of cells known as *thymic (Hassal's) corpuscles* (see Fig. 3-22). Although their significance is obscure, these corpuscles provide a reliable means of identification of thymus sections. The mature T cells found in the thymic medulla generally include some recirculating T cells.

The thymus begins to involute at about the time of puberty and progressively atrophies. Persisting T cell maturation in adult life is widely attributed to residual thymic activity or extrathymic maturation.

TABLE 3-11
DISTINCTIVE FEATURES OF THE LYMPHOID ORGANS AND TISSUES

Lymphoid Tissue or Organ	Structural Characteristics	Functional Features
Thymus	Encapsulated and lobulated; consists of a cortex and medulla	Thymic cortex is the site of T cell production
	Epithelial reticular cells	Source of the thymic hormones produced in the cortex
	Efferent lymphatics only; blood–thymus barrier; lymphoid follicles not present in thymic cortex	Thymic cortex is shielded from high concentrations of circulating and lymph-borne antigens
	Keratinizing thymic (Hassal's) corpuscles present in thymic medulla	Medullary epithelial cells do not produce hormones
Diffusely distributed lymphoid tissue, eg, MALT	Unencapsulated; present as aggregates (lymphoid follicles) or scattered infiltrate	Chiefly B cells; manifestation of immune responses to antigens in tissue fluid
	High endothelial venules (HEVs) in established lymphoid follicles	Site of preferential emigration of circulating T cells
	Generates plasmablasts and plasma cells	These effector cells produce mostly IgA (+ IgE in allergic patients)
Lymph node	Encapsulated; afferent and efferent lymphatics; permeated by lymph sinuses	Major site of immune responses to antigens in lymph
	Lymphoid follicles present in cortex	Sites where B cells are responding to antigens carried by lymph
	T cells present in paracortex (parafollicular region or deep cortex)	Site where T cells respond to antigens carried by lymph
	HEVs present in paracortex	Site of preferential emigration of circulating T cells
	Generates plasmablasts and plasma cells (present in medulla)	These effector cells produce mostly IgG
	Generates cytolytic (cytotoxic) T cells (present in paracortex)	These effector cells destroy allogeneic cells and virus-infected cells
Spleen	Encapsulated; characteristic stromal vessels; large vessels in trabeculae; efferent lymphatics only	Major site of immune responses to circulating antigens
	HEVs absent	T cells pass into the white pulp from the arteriolar supply to the marginal zone
	White pulp is intimately associated with small branches of the splenic artery	Splenic lymphocytes are freely exposed to antigens in plasma
	Splenic arterioles are invested by lymphoid sheaths	Sheaths contain regulatory T cells + any effector T cells generated
	Each splenic lymphoid follicle is supplied by a follicular arteriole	B cells of splenic follicles respond to circulating antigens
	White pulp generates plasmablasts and plasma cells (present in marginal zone)	These effector cells produce mostly IgG
	Red pulp is intimately associated with (and includes) the splenic sinusoids	Temporary extravascular reservoir for erythrocytes, leukocytes, and one-third of the body's total number of platelets
	Endothelial cells of splenic sinusoids are arranged like staves of a leaky barrel	Blood cells and platelets must squeeze through this filter to pass back into circulation from the extravascular compartment of the red pulp; returning erythrocytes are cleared of superfluous nuclear remnants ("pitting")
	Extravascular macrophages are closely associated with splenic sinusoids	Responsible for quality control; scavenge worn-out blood cells before these pass back into circulation

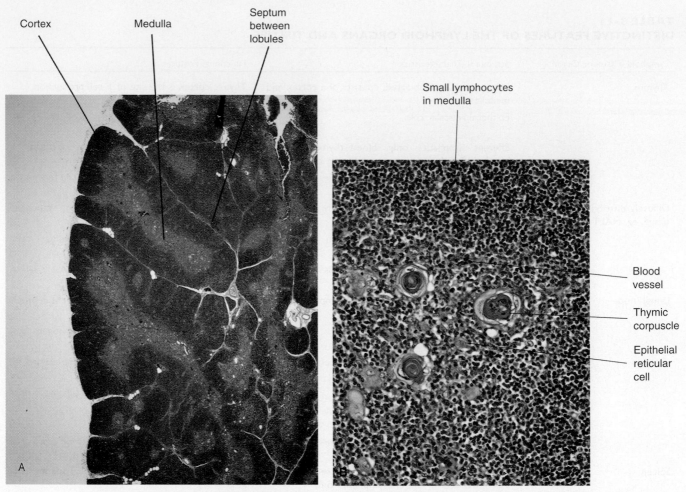

FIGURE 3-22 (**A**) Thymus (low power). (**B**) Thymic (Hassal's) corpuscles of the thymic medulla (medium power).

Mucosa-Associated Lymphoid Tissue

Mucosa-associated lymphoid tissue (MALT), includes *intraepithelial lymphocytes* (which are predominantly CD8$^+$ T cells), the *tonsils*, *Peyer's patches*, and lymphoid follicles of the *appendix*. Some of the recirculating lymphocytes in the lamina propria of mucous membranes become aggregated as unencapsulated *lymphoid follicles* (*nodules*). *B cells* predominate in the central region of these follicles. The chief class of Ig produced by the B cells in MALT is *IgA*, which can be secreted through surface epithelia. Large numbers of lymphocytes and IgA-secreting plasma cells lie diffusely distributed in the lamina propria of the digestive tract (as *GALT*) and respiratory tract (as *BALT*). IgE-secreting plasma cells may also be present, particularly when people have allergies. As in lymph nodes (see below), the *high endothelial venules* (HEVs) in permanent, organized lymphoid follicles such as Peyer's patches can preferentially bind circulating lymphocytes, eg, memory T cells, enabling these cells to "home" to particular sites. Such lymphocytes possess a *MALT homing receptor* with affinity for a complementary *MALT vascular addressin* on the HEV endothelium. Lymphocytes that possess this receptor tend to accumulate in the vicinity of mucosal surfaces.

Lymph Nodes

MALT, lymph nodes, and the spleen are *secondary lymphoid organs*, a term meaning diffuse or enclosed locations where large numbers of lymphocytes respond to foreign antigens. *Lymph nodes* consist of (1) a *cortex* that is a major site of lymphocyte activation by lymph-borne foreign antigens and (2) a *medulla* that, in antigen-stimulated nodes, becomes increasingly packed with plasma cells and their precursors and represents a site of active immunoglobulin secretion. The outer cortex contains *lymphoid follicles* (*nodules*) consisting mostly of B cells. Recirculating T cells are the predominant cell type in the deeper part of the cortex (the *paracortex*).

Lymph enters the node by way of *afferent lymphatics* and passes through a system of intercommunicating sinuses before leaving the medulla by way of *efferent lymphatics* that open onto the concave border of the node (Fig. 3-23). Any excess of *foreign antigen* in the lymph reaching the node is, for the most part, eliminated by macrophages capable of degrading it along with extraneous particulate material. However, lymph nodes also contain (1) antigen-trapping *follicular dendritic cells* and (2) several populations of *antigen-presenting cells* with the capacity to process antigen and subsequently display it as antigenically representative peptides on their surface. Any residual antigen in the efferent lymph reaches the next node. As a result of B cell proliferation that is greatly enhanced by lymphokines from T_H cells, the responding B cells generate additional lymphoid follicles in the outer cortex. Intense proliferation of activated B cells may lead to the formation of a paler-staining *germinal center* in these follicles, which prior to antigenic stimulation are described as *primary follicles* (*nodules*) and following stimulation are known as *secondary follicles* (*nodules*). *Follicular dendritic cells* (the antigen-trapping cells in these follicles) appear large and pale-staining, in contrast to *activated lymphocytes* which, although large, are intensely basophilic. Continuing proliferation of activated B cells leads to progressive displacement of their differentiating progeny (*plasmablasts*) toward the medulla.

Entry of huge numbers of potentially responsive lymphocytes into the interior of lymph nodes is facilitated by their having two different access routes. First, recirculating lymphocytes continue to arrive in the afferent lymph. Sec-

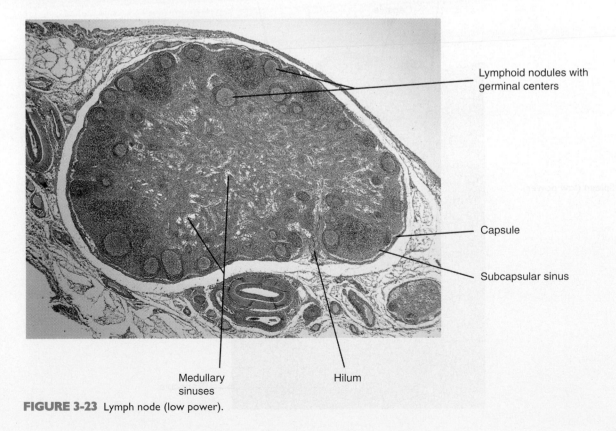

Lymphoid nodules with germinal centers

Capsule

Subcapsular sinus

Medullary sinuses

Hilum

FIGURE 3-23 Lymph node (low power).

ondly, *HEVs* in the deep cortex preferentially bind circulating lymphocytes that then migrate through the vessel wall. As in MALT, a *homing receptor* (eg, *L-selectin*) on these lymphocytes recognizes a specific *vascular addressin* (its complementary binding protein or *ligand*) on the deep cortical HEV endothelium.

Lymph nodes represent a major site of activation in cell-mediated immune responses. They also represent the chief site of IgG production in response to lymph-borne foreign antigens, eg, following local injection of an immunizing antigen. In cancer patients, regional lymph nodes are a common site of metastasis, particularly if tumor cells have disseminated by entering the lymph. Local lymph nodes obtained during the surgical resection of malignant growths are, therefore, screened to assess the probability that malignant cells may have spread.

Spleen

The substantial lymphoid content of the *spleen* is known as its *white pulp*. The extensive interposed regions that contain wide, blood-filled sinusoids and substantial pools of extravasated blood cells are termed its *red pulp* (Fig. 3-24). Splenic white pulp is intimately associated with the arterial blood vessels supplying the spleen (Fig. 3-25). It is made up of (1) *periarterial* and *periarteriolar lymphoid sheaths*, which contain T cells, and (2) *lymphoid follicles* (*nodules*), which consist chiefly of B cells, and are equivalent to the lymphoid follicles in other secondary lymphoid organs. These follicles can become secondary follicles by developing germinal centers in response to antigen. HEVs are not present in the spleen. Most of the Ig-secreting plasmablasts and plasma cells in the

> **KEY CONCEPT**
>
> The histological organization of the lymph nodes and spleen increases the likelihood that immune responses will occur in response to foreign antigens.

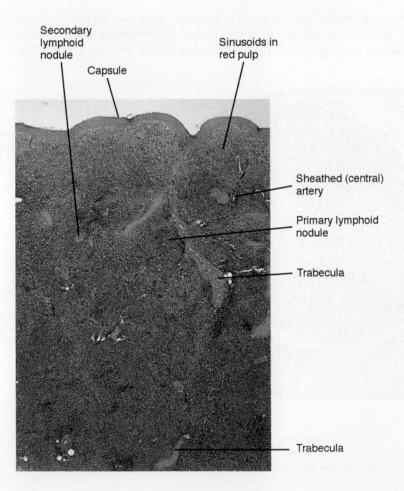

FIGURE 3-24 Spleen (low power).

Secondary lymphoid nodule

Capsule

Sinusoids in red pulp

Sheathed (central) artery

Primary lymphoid nodule

Trabecula

Trabecula

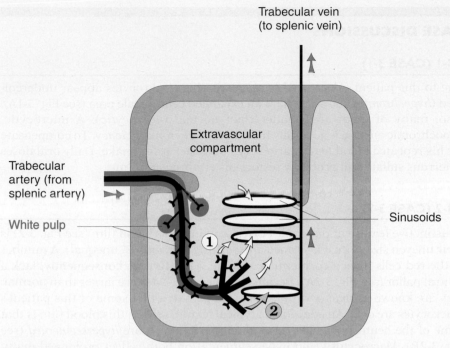

FIGURE 3-25 Essential organization of the spleen vasculature (simplified). Trabecular arteries supply blood to the red pulp through brush-like terminal arrangements of penicillar arteries. (1) Blood from arteriolar branches of penicillar arteries passes into the extravascular compartment of the red pulp. (2) A few arteriolar branches of these arteries deliver blood directly to sinusoids. Pathway (1) is termed the *open circulation*; pathway (2) is termed the *closed circulation* of the spleen.

spleen lie at the interface between the white pulp and red pulp, which is known as the *marginal zone*.

In general, the terminal arteriolar branches of the splenic artery deliver blood to an *extravascular compartment* that is supported by a meshwork of fine reticular fibers. However, a few of these arterial branches open directly into venous sinusoids, providing a *closed* (ie, *bypass*) *circulation* that parallels the generally *open* (ie, *extravasating*) *circulation* that constitutes a unique feature of the spleen (see Fig. 3-25). The majority of venous sinusoids delivering blood to the splenic vein, nevertheless, end blindly in the red pulp. Hence, to leave the spleen, blood cells delivered to its extravascular compartment from the splenic artery must squeeze their way into sinusoids in the red pulp. To facilitate this, the elongated endothelial lining cells of splenic sinusoids are widely separated by slit-like intercellular gaps through which blood cells are able to pass. Macrophages closely associated with these "leaky barrel" sinusoids are able to recognize and phagocytose extravasated blood cells that are damaged or worn out. The spleen, accordingly, serves as an efficient filter for withdrawing old or damaged blood cells. It is also (1) a major site of removal of extraneous particulate matter from the bloodstream and (2) an important site of *platelet storage*. Although under normal circumstances the spleen becomes non-hematopoietic at the end of fetal life, its hematopoietic activity may resume in adult life under conditions of extreme blood cell depletion, eg, in patients with a severe hemolytic anemia. Such supplemental blood cell production is described as *extramedullary hematopoiesis*.

Because the spleen produces antibodies to circulating foreign antigens, it is one of the chief sites of IgG production. The other major site of IgG production is myeloid tissue, which may come to contain vast numbers of plasma cells. As might be expected, splenectomy is associated with an increased susceptibility to bacterial infections, notably *Streptococcus pneumoniae*.

CASE DISCUSSIONS

D3-1 (CASE 3-1)

Due to this patient's decreased hemoglobin, his erythrocytes appear undercolored (*hypochromic*) and some have an expanded central pale area (see Fig. 3-1A). Also, many of them are smaller than normal (*microcytic*). A microcytic, hypochromic anemia is generally indicative of an *iron deficiency*. To compensate for his repeated blood loss, Mario needs a greater iron uptake. Daily oral doses of ferrous sulfate will probably restore his erythrocyte count.

D3-2 (CASE 3-2)

A distinctive feature of the erythrocytes seen in Milt's blood film (see Fig. 3-2) is their uneven size, which is termed *anisocytosis* (Gk. *anisos*, unequal). A number of the red cells have a corpuscular volume >103 fL and, consequently, lack a central pallor (see Fig. 3-2A). Because such erythrocytes are larger than normal, they are known as *macrocytes*. It may also be noted that some of this patient's macrocytes are oval. An additional atypical feature seen in this blood film is that some of the neutrophils have more than five lobes, ie, are *hypersegmented* (see Fig. 3-2B). Macrocytosis and hypersegmentation both reflect prolonged maturation of the precursor cells and, generally, they indicate a deficiency of either vitamin B_{12} or folate.

If the patient's small bowel had been able to absorb the normal amount of vitamin B_{12}, he would have excreted in his urine more than 7% of the radioactive dose administered in the course of the Schilling test. Subsequent investigations showed that this patient is positive for serum antibody to an essential absorption factor called *intrinsic factor* that is secreted by the *parietal cells* of the stomach. Vitamin B_{12} cannot be absorbed in the distal part of the ileum unless it first becomes complexed with intrinsic factor.

This patient's sensory neuropathy substantiates a diagnosis of *pernicious anemia*. Whereas the anemia is chiefly a result of decreased DNA synthesis, it is likely that the neurological symptoms reflect impairment of methylcobalamin-dependent methionine synthesis. The production of myelin basic protein and the methylation of myelin lipids both require S-adenosylmethionine, which is underproduced in patients with pernicious anemia. Furthermore, synthesis of the fatty acids in myelin lipids involves some enzymes that are adenosylcobalamin-dependent.

Inadequate absorption of vitamin B_{12} from the small bowel results in chronically low plasma levels of this vitamin. In this case, absorption is severely restricted by the production and binding of an autoantibody to intrinsic factor. Patients with pernicious anemia, a form of megaloblastic anemia, usually show a favorable response to a 2-week course of six intramuscular or deep subcutaneous injections of vitamin B_{12}. To sustain normal levels of erythropoiesis, however, lifelong monthly injections of this vitamin must be given.

D3-3 (CASE 3-3)

When this patient was admitted, his red cell mass, MCV, WBC, and platelet count were all low. This condition is known as *pancytopenia*, which denotes a deficiency of all the cellular elements of the blood (Gk. *pan*, all). The pancytopenia and marked hypocellularity of the marrow are indicative of *aplastic anemia*. An important feature of this type of anemia is that cell production is greatly impaired along the erythroid, granulocytic, and megakaryocytic lineages; hence, three essential blood cell lines become under-represented. Apart from fat-storing cells, all that can be recognized in Tony's bone marrow is a few lymphocytes and an occasional plasma cell. Normally, there are enough myeloid cells in a marrow biopsy for their total volume to be roughly comparable with that of its fat-storing cells.

The differentiation and maturation pathway that maintains the population size of each blood cell lineage is outlined in Fig. 3-16. From an appreciation of the distinctive mechanism of cell renewal that characterizes continuously renewing cell populations (see Chap. 1) and from Fig. 3-16, it could be correctly surmised that the critical constituent of a bone marrow transplant is the donor's self-renewing *stem cells*. These cells are frequently referred to as *pluripotential hematopoietic stem cells* or *myeloid* (and *lymphoid*) *repopulating cells*. Hematopoietic stem cells seem to be the essential engrafted component. The recipient's stromal cells are able to furnish a microenvironment (hematopoietic growth factors, etc.) that maintains viability of the engrafted stem cells, supporting their continuing proliferation and differentiation. The levels at which the various hematopoietic growth factors act are indicated in Fig. 3-16.

A more recent and successful approach for reconstituting myeloid tissue is *autologous transplantation* using the patient's own *peripheral blood hematopoietic stem cells*. This approach is particularly appropriate in cases where no HLA-matched relative can be found to serve as a donor. These stem cells (which are sometimes referred to as *peripheral blood progenitor cells*) circulate in the peripheral blood of patients during early post-suppressive or post-ablative recovery of the bone marrow. At that time, or prior to therapy, nucleated peripheral blood cells are harvested by *leukapheresis* (Gr. *aphairesis*, a taking away), meaning removal of leukocytes from withdrawn blood and transfusion of the remainder back to the donor. Once harvested, the nucleated cells are submitted to a positive selection procedure for *CD34* antigen, an integral membrane phosphoglycoprotein detectable with monoclonal antibody, which is expressed on pluripotential hematopoietic stem cells, hematopoietic progenitors, and, unfortunately, certain leukemic and other neoplastic cells. The CD34$^+$ cells separated from the withdrawn blood are then transfused back to the patient. Data on respective yields of CD34$^+$ cells indicate that the number of circulating pluripotential hematopoietic stem cells, and also the number of these cells mobilized following myeloablative therapy, are increased by prior administration of the hematopoietic growth factors *GM-CSF* and *G-CSF*. Normal donors manifest the same kind of augmented mobilization response to GM-CSF and G-CSF, making it feasible to collect enough peripheral blood hematopoietic stem cells from normal donors to be able to use them for allogeneic transplants.

D3-4 (CASE 3-3 AND FIG. 3-4)

The proportion and absolute number of neutrophils in this patient's peripheral blood (80%, corresponding to an absolute number of 12.1×10^9/L) are elevated. Such an increase is called a *neutrophilic leukocytosis* or *neutrophilia*. In addition, numerous *immature granulocytes* are present in the peripheral blood. They represent ongoing stages of maturation that precede segmentation of the nucleus and often include *myelocytes* and *metamyelocytes*, as well as *band neutrophils*. At one time, it was conventional to record counts of immature cells to the left of counts of mature forms. An increase in the number of neutrophil precursors seen in a peripheral blood film has, therefore, come to be known as a *shift to the left*. It indicates that many of the cells of the neutrophil series are leaving the bone marrow at an immature stage.

In bacterial infections that result in an acute neutrophilia, a shift to the left can reflect an increased requirement for neutrophils. It can also indicate an effect of *endotoxin*, a lipopolysaccharide in the outer membrane of the cell wall of gram-negative bacteria that stimulates a premature release of immature neu-

> **KEY CONCEPT**
>
> Changes in the proportion of immature blood cells in the peripheral blood can have clinical significance.

trophils from the bone marrow. Thus, endotoxin has the effect of mobilizing maturing neutrophil precursors, as well as functional end cells of the marrow storage pool.

D3-5 (CASE 3-4)

Abundant *monoblastic leukemic cells*, intermixed with *myeloblastic leukemic cells*, are evident in this patient's peripheral blood film (Fig. 3-6). The symptoms and presence of these abnormal cells in her peripheral blood and bone marrow are consistent with the diagnosis of *acute myelomonocytic leukemia*. The case represents a further example of successful engraftment with HLA-compatible hematopoietic stem cells.

D3-6 (FIG. 3-9)

Some of the erythrocytes in Fig. 3-9 are shaped like sickles, which is indicative of *sickle cell disease* or a *sickle cell trait* disorder.

A point mutation in the codon specifying the sixth position from the N-terminal end of the β-globin chain of hemoglobin leads to incorporation of valine in place of glutamic acid at this position. This substitution produces an atypical hemoglobin named *hemoglobin S* (Hb S) that is insoluble at low oxygen tensions. When Hb S becomes deoxygenated, it polymerizes and forms rigid fiber-like aggregates that on lengthening cause erythrocytes to sickle. Sickling becomes irreversible once an erythrocyte's membrane has been damaged. Erythrocytes that have sickled tend to occlude tiny blood vessels. Also, sickle cells are prevented from gaining access to the venous sinusoids of the spleen from the reticular meshwork of the splenic red pulp, an extravascular compartment into which erythrocytes can pass. Hence, a hallmark of the *sickle cell anemia* that characterizes the homozygous Hb S condition is chronic hemolysis within the spleen.

D3-7 (FIG. 3-10)

Nasal polyps are an annoying complication of persistent allergic rhinitis generally caused by inhaled allergens. The presence of *eosinophils* in the lamina propria of the nasal mucosa is considered a reliable indication of *allergic inflammation*. In Fig. 3-10, eosinophils may be recognized from their size, red staining, or bilobed nucleus. They are accompanied by a number of small *lymphocytes* and *plasma cells*. An additional sign of mucosal inflammation is the presence of pale-staining rounded spaces containing *edema fluid* (see Fig. 3-10).

BIBLIOGRAPHY

Blood Cells and Inflammation

Abramson JS, Wheeler JG, eds. The Neutrophil. Oxford, IRL Press at Oxford University Press, 1993.

Adolphson CR, Gleich GJ. Eosinophils. In: Holgate ST, Church MK, eds. Allergy. London, Gower Medical Publishing, 1993, p 6.1.

Beck WS, ed. Hematology, ed 5. Cambridge, Mass., MIT Press, 1991.

Bevilacqua MP, Nelson RM, Mannori G, Cecconi O. Endothelial-leukocyte adhesion molecules in human disease. Annu Rev Med 45:361, 1994.

Chapman PT, Haskard DO. Leukocyte adhesion molecules. Br Med Bull 51:296, 1995.

Dvorak AM. Ultrastructural morphology of basophils and mast cells. In: Blood Cell Biochemistry, vol 4, Basophil and Mast Cell Degranulation and Recovery. New York, Plenum Press, 1991, p 67.

Dvorak AM. Similarities in the ultrastructural morphology and developmental and secretory mechanisms of human basophils and eosinophils. J Allergy Clin Immunol 94 (suppl):1103, 1994.

Erb KJ, Holloway JW, Le Gros G. Innate immunity: Mast cells in the front line. Curr Biol 6:941, 1996.

Esmon CT. Cell mediated events that control blood coagulation and vascular injury. Annu Rev Cell Biol 9:1, 1993.

Fischbach FT. A Manual of Laboratory and Diagnostic Tests, ed 4. Philadelphia, J.B. Lippincott, 1992.

Fuller RW. Macrophages. Br Med Bull 48:65, 1992.

Gleich GJ. Current understanding of eosinophil function. Hosp Pract 23:137, 1988.

Gleich GJ, Adolphson CR, Leiferman KM. The biology of the eosinophilic leukocyte. Annu Rev Med 44:85, 1993.

Górski A. The role of cell adhesion molecules in immunopathology. Immunol Today 15:251, 1994.

Granger DN, Kubes P. The microcirculation and inflammation: Modulation of leukocyte-endothelial cell adhesion. J Leukoc Biol 55:662, 1994.

Harlan JM, Liu DY, eds. Adhesion: Its Role in Inflammatory Disease. New York, W.H.Freeman & Company, 1992.

Harmening D. Clinical Hematology and Fundamentals of Hemostasis, ed 2. Philadelphia, F.A. Davis, 1992.

Henriques GMO, Miotla JM, Cordeiro RSB, Wolitzky BA, Woolley ST, Hellewell PG. Selectins mediate eosinophil recruitment in vivo: A comparison with their role in neutrophil influx. Blood 87:5297, 1996.

Hoffbrand AV, Pettit JE. Color Atlas of Clinical Hematology, ed 2. London, Mosby-Wolfe, 1994.

Hoffman R, Benz EJ, Shattil SJ, et al., eds. Hematology. Basic Principles and Practice. New York, Churchill Livingstone, 1991.

Holgate ST, Church MK. The mast cell. Br Med Bull 48:40, 1992.

Jandl, JH. Blood. Textbook of Hematology, ed 2. Boston, Little, Brown and Company, 1996.

Kaliner MA, Metcalfe DD, eds. The Mast Cell in Health and Disease. New York, Marcel Dekker, Inc., 1993.

Kay AB, Corrigan CJ. Eosinophils and neutrophils. Br Med Bull 48:51, 1992.

Luscinskas FW, Gimbrone MA Jr. Endothelial-dependent mechanisms in chronic inflammatory leukocyte recruitment. Annu Rev Med 47:413, 1996.

Rietschel ET, Brade H. Bacterial endotoxins. Sci Am 267:54, 1992.

Roth GJ. Platelets and blood vessels: The adhesion event. Immunol Today 13:100, 1992.

Spry CJF, Kay AB, Gleich GJ. Eosinophils 1992. Immunol Today 13:384, 1992.

Tracey KJ, Cerami A. Tumor necrosis factor, other cytokines and disease. Annu Rev Cell Biol 9:317, 1993.

Wardlaw AJ. Eosinophils in the 1990s: New perspectives on their role in health and disease. Postgrad Med J 70:536, 1994.

Weissmann G, ed. The Cell Biology of Inflammation. Handbook of Inflammation, vol 2. Amsterdam, Elsevier/North Holland Biomedical Press, 1980.

Zucker MB. The functioning of blood platelets. Sci Am 242(6):86, 1980.

Myeloid Tissue and Hematopoiesis

Atkinson K, ed. Clinical Bone Marrow Transplantation: A Reference Textbook. Cambridge, Cambridge University Press, 1994.

Beck WS. Diagnosis of megaloblastic anemia. Annu Rev Med 42:311, 1991.

Burke F, Naylor MS, Davies B, Balkwill F. The cytokine wall chart. Immunol Today 14:165, 1993.

Erickson N, Quesenberry PJ. Regulation of erythropoiesis. The role of growth factors. Med Clin North Am 76(3):745, 1992.

Geller RB. Use of cytokines in the treatment of acute myelocytic leukemia: A critical review. J Clin Oncol 14:1371, 1996.

Heyworth CM, Vallance SJ, Whetton AD, Dexter TM. The biochemistry and biology of the myeloid hemopoietic cell growth factors. J Cell Sci Suppl 13:57, 1990.

Johnson GR: Erythropoietin. Br Med Bull 45:506, 1989.

Lane TA, Law P, Maruyama M, et al. Harvesting and enrichment of hematopoietic progenitor cells mobilized into the peripheral blood of normal donors by granulocyte-macrophage stimulating-factor (GM-CSF) or G-CSF: Potential role in allogeneic marrow transplantation. Blood 85:275, 1995.

Mayani H, Guilbert MH, Janowska-Wieczorek A. Biology of the hemopoietic microenvironment. Eur J Haematol 49:225, 1992.

Mertelsmann R, Herrman F, eds. Hematopoietic Growth Factors in Clinical Applications, ed 2. New York, Marcel Dekker, Inc., 1995.

Metcalf D. Hemopoietic regulators. Trends Biochem Sci 17:286, 1992.

Metcalf D. Thrombopoietin—At last. Nature 369:519, 1994.

Sims RB, Gewirtz AM. Human megakaryocytopoiesis. Annu Rev Med 40:213, 1989.

Spangrude GJ. Biological and clinical aspects of hematopoietic stem cells. Annu Rev Med 45:93, 1994.

Weiss L. The haemopoietic microenvironment of bone marrow: An ultrastructural study of the interactions of blood cells, stroma, and blood vessels. Ciba Found Symp 71:13, 1980.

Lymphoid Tissue, Immunity and Allergy

Abbas AK, Lichtman AH, Pober JS. Cellular and Molecular Immunology, ed 2. Philadelphia, W.B. Saunders, 1994.

Bochner BS, Schleimer RP. The role of adhesion molecules in human eosinophil and basophil recruitment. J Allergy Clin Immunol 94:427, 1994.

Boyd RL, Tucek CL, Godfrey DI, Izon DJ, Wilson TJ, Davidson NJ, Bean AGD, Ladyman HM, Ritter MA, et al. The thymic microenvironment. Immunol Today 14:445, 1993.

Brostoff J, Scadding GK, Male DK, Roitt IM. Clinical Immunology. London, Gower Medical Publishing, 1991.

Church MK, Caulfield JP. Mast cell and basophil functions. In: Holgate ST, Church MK, eds. Allergy. London, Gower Medical Publishing, 1993.

Church MK, Okayama Y, Bradding P. The role of the mast cell in acute and chronic allergic inflammation. Ann N Y Acad Sci 725:13, 1994.

Davis MM. Molecular genetics of T-cell antigen receptors. Hosp Pract 23:157, 1988.

Dinome MA, Young JD. How lymphocytes kill tumor and other cellular targets. Hosp Pract 22:59, 1987.

Engelhard VH. How cells present antigens. Sci Am 271:54, 1994.

Ferguson A. Mucosal immunology. Immunol Today 11:1, 1990.

Girard JP, Springer TA. High endothelial venules (HEVs): Specialized endothelium for lymphocyte migration. Immunol Today 16:449, 1995.

Gowans JL. The lymphocyte—A disgraceful gap in medical knowledge. Immunol Today 17:288, 1996.

Grey HM, Sette A, Buus S. How T cells see antigen. Sci Am 261:56, 1989.

Holgate ST, ed. Mast Cells, Mediators, and Disease. Dordrecht, Kluwer Academic Publishers, 1988.

Holgate ST, Church MK. Allergy. London, Gower Medical Publishing, 1993.

Kendall MD. Functional anatomy of the thymic microenvironment. J Anat 177:1, 1991.

King PD, Katz DR. Mechanisms of dendritic cell function. Immunol Today 11:206, 1990.

Lichtenstein LM. Allergy and the immune system. Sci Am 269:116, 1993.

Liu YJ, Grouard G, De Bouteiller O, Banchereau J. Follicular dendritic cells and germinal centers. Int Rev Cytol 166:139, 1996.

Marrack P, Kappler J. The T cell and its receptor. Sci Am 254(2):36, 1986.

Massey WA, Lichtenstein LM. Role of basophils in human allergic disease. Int Arch Allergy Immunol 99:184, 1992.

Moqbel R. Eosinophils, cytokines, and allergic inflammation. Ann N Y Acad Sci 725:223, 1994.

Nowak MA, McMichael AJ. How HIV defeats the immune system. Sci Am 273:58, 1995.

Parker DC. T cell-dependent B cell activation. Annu Rev Immunol 11:331, 1993.

Podack ER, Kupfer A. T-cell effector functions: Mechanisms for delivery of cytotoxicity and help. Annu Rev Cell Biol 7:479, 1991.

Roitt IM. Essential Immunology, ed 8. Oxford, Blackwell Scientific Publications, 1994.

Sedlacek HH, Möröy T. Immune Reactions: Headlines, Overviews, Tables, and Graphics. Berlin, Springer-Verlag, 1995.

Smith KA. Interleukin-2. Sci Am 262(3):50, 1990.

Stingl G, Bergstresser PR. Dendritic cells: A major story unfolds. Immunol Today 16:330, 1995.

Szakal AK, Kosco MH, Tew JG. Microanatomy of lymphoid tissue during humoral immune responses: Structure function relationships. Annu Rev Immunol 7:91, 1989.

Williams LA, Egner W, Hart DNJ. Isolation and function of human dendritic cells. Int Rev Cytol 153:41, 1994.

Wolf PR, Ploegh HL. How MHC class II molecules acquire peptide cargo: Biosynthesis and trafficking through the endocytic pathway. Annu Rev Cell Biol 11:267, 1995.

Young JD, Cohn ZA. How killer cells kill. Sci Am 258(1):38, 1988.

Young LHY, Liu C-C, Joag S, Rafii S, Young JD. How lymphocytes kill. Annu Rev Med 41:45, 1990.

CHAPTER 4

Musculoskeletal and Nervous Systems

CASE 4-1

Recurring bouts of painful swelling begin in Jody Smith's right knee when she is 12 years old. An x-ray of her right tibia shows an irregular radiolucent lesion in the upper metaphysis. This lesion appears highly vascular on a bone scan, but no evidence of neovascularization is found on the angiograms. Jody's CBC and levels of plasma calcium, phosphorus, and alkaline phosphatase are all normal. There is no other joint involvement and no indication that she has rheumatic disease.

The tibial lesion is biopsied 2 years later (Fig. 4-1). Rigorous microbiological testing of the biopsied tissue does not reveal any infectious microorganisms but some clinical improvement is noted after several courses of antibiotics.

Almost 18 months elapse before Jody experiences a recurrence of painful swelling in the same knee. Microbiological cultures are started from small samples of the 70 mL of straw-colored fluid that is aspirated from the joint cavity, but again nothing grows from them. The patient still has a normal CBC and remains afebrile. A healed lesion with adjacent sclerosis is observed in an x-ray of the affected knee. However, the right leg is now 1 cm shorter than the left leg, and the right proximal tibial growth plate has gone. A synovial biopsy shows some neutrophils, synovial macrophages containing small numbers of gram-negative bacteria, and a mildly hyperplastic synovium covered by a fibrinous exudate.

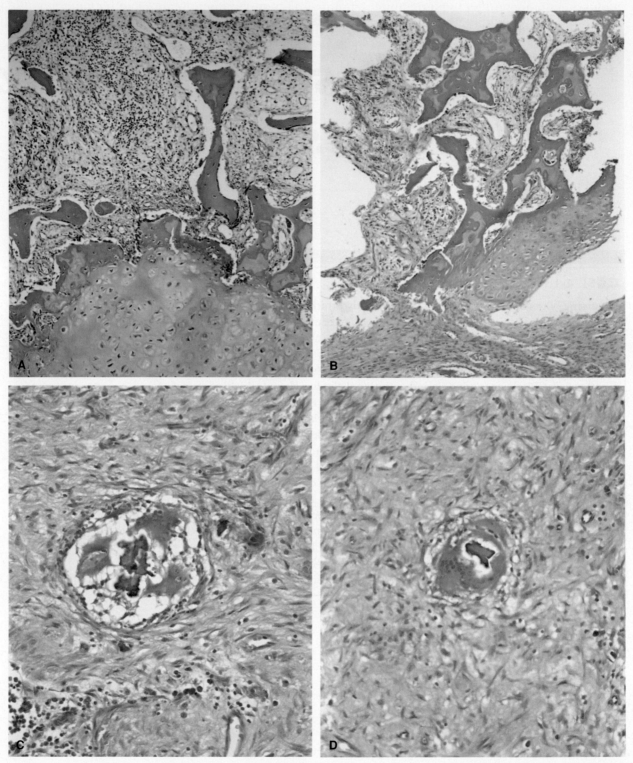

FIGURE 4-1 (**A,B**) Tibial biopsy in Case 4-1 (low power). (**C,D**) Representative parts of this biopsy (medium power).

ANALYSIS
Case 4-1

A Which histological features appearing in parts A and B of Fig. 4-1 enable you to recognize the level from which the biopsy section was obtained?

B Would an abscess cavity be expected in this case?

C How much fluid is normally present in a knee joint cavity?

D What is meant by the synovium?

E Can you interpret what you see in parts C and D of Fig. 4-1?

F Why does the length of this patient's legs become unequal?

G What is the long-term prognosis for Jody's condition?

(The answers are considered in part D4-1 of the Discussion section of this chapter.)

CASE 4-2

Definitive surgery for Jeff Sparling, aged 19 years, is scheduled in 4 month's time. He has a 6-month history of increasingly frequent left knee pain, which generally becomes severe after physical activity. This knee also often gives way when it is put under strain. Jeff now needs to limp rather heavily to reduce the pain. Physical examination shows a diffusely swollen left proximal tibia that is tender and warm to the touch. Flexion and extension are reduced in the left knee, but ligaments are still stable and there is no joint effusion. The serum alkaline phosphatase concentration is increased. The CBC is normal.

A lytic radiolucent lesion is found below the medial condyle of the left tibia in an x-ray of the proximal tibia (Fig. 4-2A). There is evidence of bony destruction and superimposed foci of newly formed matrix. A CT scan confirms the finding. Angiograms indicate the presence of irregular neoplastic blood vessels and a tumor blush. Posterior displacement of the left popliteal artery suggests proximal spread of a soft tissue mass. Jeff's chest x-ray and chest CT scan show no abnormalities. An incisional biopsy (Fig. 4-2B through 4-2D) taken under general anesthesia confirms the provisional diagnosis, so a course of preoperative chemotherapy is begun. Based on the definitive diagnosis returned for the biopsy, the decision must be made whether to (1) replace the left knee joint with a prosthetic implant or (2) proceed with surgical amputation.

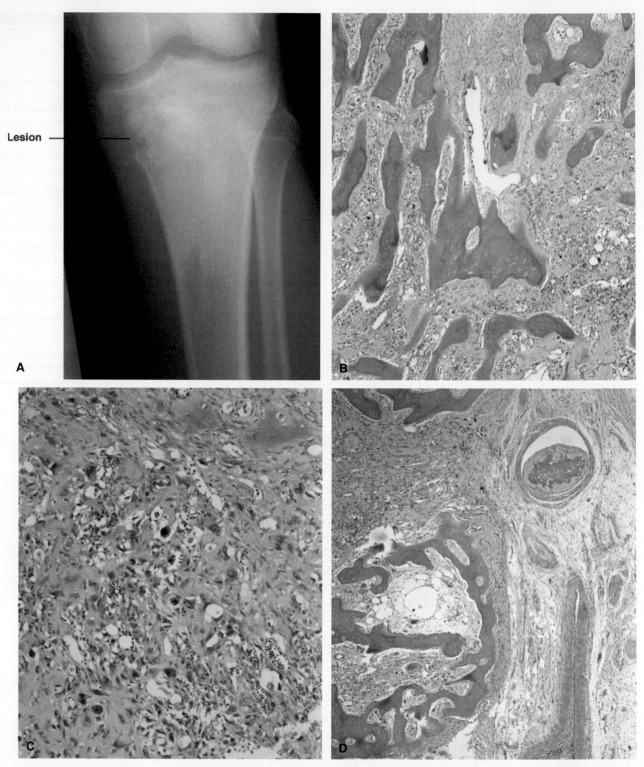

Lesion

A

B

C

D

FIGURE 4-2 (**A**) A x-ray (anteroposterior projection radiograph) of the left proximal tibia in Case 4-2. (**B–D**) Tibial biopsy in Case 4-2 (medium power).

OTHER CASES

Figure 4-3 is an additional pictorial item for analysis.

ANALYSIS
Case 4-2

A Is it significant that many dividing cells are seen in Fig. 4-2C?

B Can you explain the atypical luminal appearance of the vein in Fig. 4-2D?

C Identify as precisely as possible the component tissues of the trabeculae shown in Fig. 4-2B and 4-2D.

D From this patient's medical history and the histological appearance of the biopsy, can you suggest a likely diagnosis?

E Why are a preoperative chest x-ray and CT scan critical to the investigation?

(To confirm your answers, see part D4-2 of the Discussion section of this chapter.)

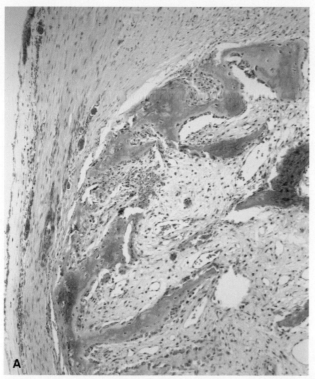

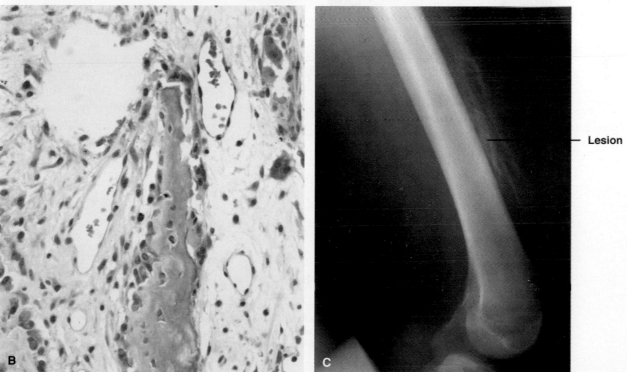

FIGURE 4-3 A rigid, non-painful mass is present in the vastus lateralis (chief component of quadriceps femoris) in the left leg of an athletic 15-year-old boy. Previous history indicates injury of this thigh. The resected mass is seen here under (**A**) low power and (**B**) high power. (**C**) An x-ray (lateral projection radiograph) shows that some calcification has occurred at the site.

Figures 4-4 through 4-7 are additional pictorial items for analysis (see the captions for these figures).

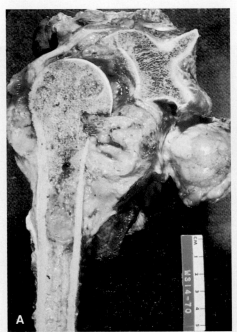

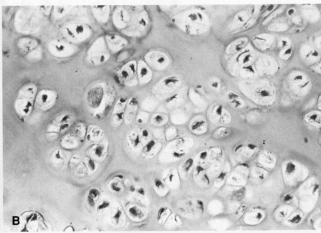

FIGURE 4-4 (**A**) This malignant tumor was resected from the shoulder of a 34-year-old man who experienced shoulder pain that radiated to the wrist when he used his left arm. From its location, general appearance, and histological characteristics, can you tell what type of tissue it is likely to be? (**B**) Resected tumor tissue seen under medium power. (To check your answer, see part D4-4 of the Discussion section of this chapter.)

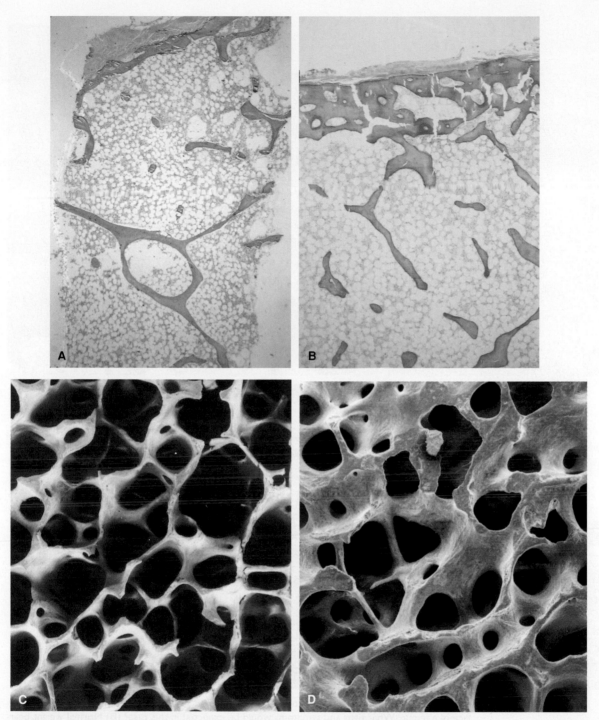

FIGURE 4-5 (A) Iliac crest biopsy from a 90-year-old woman who has severe kyphosis (low power).
(B) Comparable biopsy from a healthy person of similar age (low power). **(C,D)** Scanning electron micrographs of the biopsies shown in **A** and **B**, respectively. (The findings are discussed in section D4-5 of the Discussion section of this chapter.)

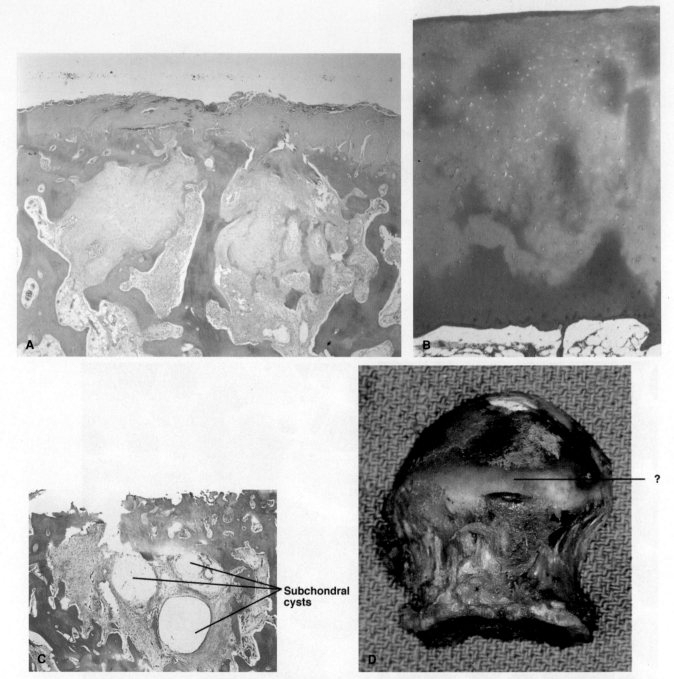

FIGURE 4-6 (**A**) What unusual feature may be discerned at low power in this weight-bearing surface of a femur? What signs and symptoms would be expected in this case? (**B**) Normal weight-bearing surface of a femur (low power). (**C**) These fluid-filled subchondral cysts are also seen in the femoral head shown in **A** (low power). (**D**) Femoral head shown in **A** (surgical specimen). What has happened to it? [In **D, E,** and **F,** the features labeled (?) are all potentially informative.] (**E**) Preoperative x-ray (anteroposterior projection radiograph) of the hip joint containing the femoral head shown in **A** and **D**. (**F**) Comparable radiograph of a normal hip joint. (To confirm your answers, see part D4-6 of the Discussion section of this chapter.)

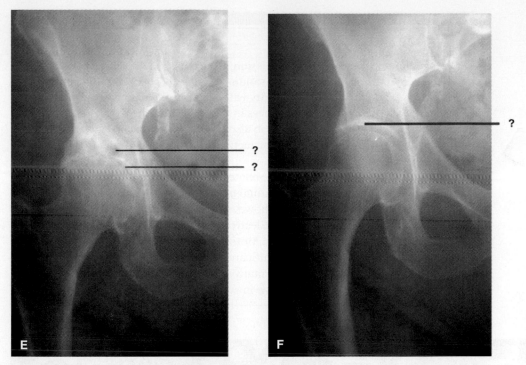

FIGURE 4-6 (Continued)

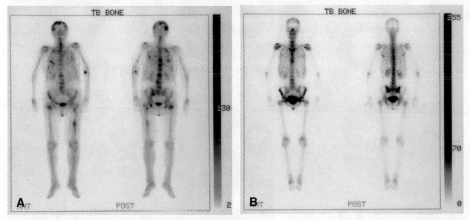

FIGURE 4-7 (**A**) Total body bone scan, obtained 3 hours after i.v. injection of ^{99m}technetium-tagged methylene diphosphonate (MDP), of a female patient with multiple skeletal metastases from carcinoma of the breast. Why does metastatic cancer show up as hot spots on bone scans? (**B**) Comparable bone scan of a male patient with no history of cancer. Background diagnostically uninformative foci of tracer accumulation include the urinary bladder, myeloid tissue, and the shoulder joints. The injection site (median cubital vein) is also evident in **A**. (The answer is discussed in part D4-7 of the Discussion section of this chapter.)

CASE 4-3

Starting about 6 months before admission, Bob Till, aged 69 years, feels "pins and needles" in his legs and cold sensations in his feet. Three months before admission, he experiences some difficulty with walking and also with swallowing, and complains of cramps and weakness in his legs. Later, he notices quick stabs of pain and weakness in his arms. Bob also has a history of cardiac arrhythmia, with sustained episodes of ventricular tachycardia, and for 2 years he has been taking medication for this condition.

During the physical examination, bilateral wasting and muscular weakness are noted in Bob's legs and arms. Cranial nerve function is normal. Tendon reflexes cannot be elicited in the legs; however, pain, temperature, and discriminative touch sensation are all normal. Electromyography indicates some denervation in the distal lower limb muscles. Motor conduction, as measured in the patient's right peroneal nerve, is significantly slower. A sural nerve biopsy obtained using local anesthesia is informative about the underlying cause of the problem. The biopsied nerve is shown in section in parts A and B of Fig. 4-8.

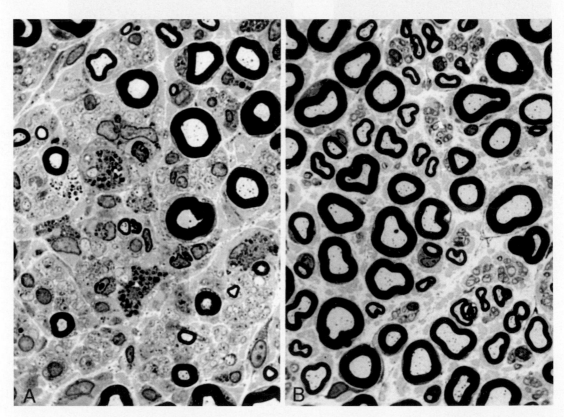

FIGURE 4-8 (**A**) Peripheral nerve biopsy from Case 4-3. (**B**) Normal peripheral nerve biopsy, for comparison with **A**. (**C**) Detail of peripheral nerve biopsy from Case 4-3 (electron micrograph, ×33,800). (**A** and **B** are semithin plastic sections stained with osmium and toluidine blue).

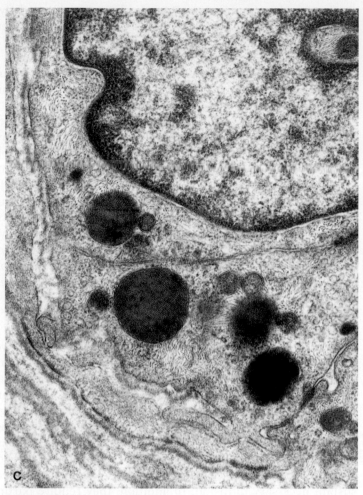

FIGURE 4-8 (Continued)

ANALYSIS
Case 4-3

A How does the nerve in Fig. 4-8A differ from normal?

B Where does the intensely dark-staining material in Fig. 4-8A and 4-8B come from? Why is it there?

C Are the round, dark-staining cytoplasmic structures in Fig 4-8C, a familiar kind of cytoplasmic organelle?

D From your answers to the first three questions, what can you deduce about the way Bob's medication, *amiodarone chlorhydrate*, affected his peripheral nerve function?

(The answers are considered in part D4-8 of the Discussion section of this chapter.)

ESSENTIAL FEATURES OF CONSTITUENT CONNECTIVE TISSUES OF JOINTS AND MUSCLES

The various forms of connective tissue are each described as being (1) ordinary or (2) special. The *ordinary connective tissues* are either *loosely arranged,* ie, areolar, or else *densely arranged,* ie, fibrous. In tendons and ligaments, connective tissue of the dense type is *regularly arranged,* whereas in the other fibrous tissues of joints, the dermis, and capsules of glands and organs, it is *irregularly arranged.* This further classification is based on the orientation of the collagen fibers of the tissue. Bone and cartilage, two of the special connective tissues, are of interest because of their essential support function and roles in locomotion.

Matrix of Loose Connective and Fibrous Tissues

The intercellular molecules of each type of connective tissue are organized into a special *interstitial matrix*. The interstitial matrix of loose connective tissue contains relatively wide *collagen fibers* and somewhat narrower *elastic fibers*. The fibers reinforce a structurally organized soft amorphous gel, comprised of pro-

ANALYSIS
Case 4-4

An elderly patient with fever, dyspnea, and a severe cough feels sharp chest pains on taking deep breaths and when coughing. Three days later, his neck and left shoulder also begin to hurt. The patient thinks the supraclavicular pain is a result of muscle strain from his frequent coughing. What is the alternative explanation?

(The answer is considered in part D4-9 of the Discussion section of this chapter.)

teoglycans, glycosaminoglycans (eg, hyaluronic acid), and glycoproteins, generally referred to as the *ground substance*. At interfaces between loose connective tissue and other tissues, the interstitial matrix is distinctively organized into flat sheets termed *basement membranes*. An essential component in the ground substance of loose connective tissue is *tissue fluid*, which occupies the interconnecting aqueous channels in its gel structure and serves as an ideal medium for the passive diffusion of oxygen, nutrients, and waste products.

Tissue fluid in the ground substance is held (1) in interstices of the extensive hyaluronic acid domains, which constitute a voluminous hydrated gel, and (2) in the aqueous channels that lie between the extended hydrophilic glycosaminoglycan chains of proteoglycan molecules. However, there is an upper limit to the total volume of tissue fluid that can be accommodated within this complex macromolecular meshwork. When excess tissue fluid is produced, eg, under circumstances such as trauma or acute inflammation, pools of free fluid may form in the midst of the gel, and this may become microscopically evident. Accumulation of excess tissue fluid leads to swelling of connective tissue, which is termed *edema* (Gk. *oidema*, a swelling). In *pitting edema*, applied pressure from the fingertips squeezes the excess tissue fluid away from the region and leaves shallow depressions (pits) in the tissue. Such edema can be a clinical sign of impaired venous return, lymphatic obstruction, or decreased colloid osmotic (ie, oncotic) pressure of the plasma.

Tendons and most *ligaments* (ie, dense ordinary connective tissue that is regularly arranged) consist chiefly of parallel bundles of collagen fibers that possess great tensile strength and are highly resistant to stretch. Elastic ligaments, on the other hand, are capable of limited stretch because they are made up of parallel elastic fibers woven together by collagen fibers. Cartilage matrix and bone matrix (described below) have a highly distinctive composition (see Table 4-2), which in the case of elastic cartilage, includes some elastin as well.

Like epithelia, which are avascular and must be nourished by adjacent loose connective tissue, muscles depend on loose connective tissue (*endomysium*) to sustain necessary diffusion. In addition, they require partitions and an outer sheath of strong fibrous tissue (irregularly arranged dense ordinary connective tissue). Known respectively as *perimysium* and *epimysium*, these fibrous components harness the pull of contractions and typically transmit it to a tendon where the extending bundles of collagen become regularly arranged. Morphologically comparable fibrous sheaths exist in peripheral nerves since they possess an *endoneurium* and *perineurium*, together with an *epineurium* in moderate-sized and large nerves. In contrast, the central nervous system (CNS) contains only minimal amounts of connective tissue associated with its tiny blood vessels. In the CNS, the various supporting functions of connective tissue are assumed by a heterogeneous population of neuroglial cells. Bones and cartilages are invested by dense fibrous sheaths, termed *periosteum* and *perichondrium*, and joints are enclosed by *fibrous capsules*. Joint cavities are lined by a *synovial membrane*, which is a connective tissue membrane made up partly of loose and partly of dense ordinary connective tissue.

Connective Tissue Cells

The cells of connective tissue are derived from embryonic mesenchymal cells. They include *fibroblasts, endothelial cells, adipocytes (fat cells)*, and *pericytes*, which are incompletely differentiated cells that persist in adult life as perivascular cells and are capable of producing both fibroblasts and smooth muscle cells. Also present in loose connective tissue are *macrophages, mast cells*, and *plasma cells*, which arise from mesenchyme-derived pluripotential hematopoietic stem cells.

Collagen

The predominant intercellular constituent of connective tissue is *collagen*, which exists in at least 15 different combinations of the 3 α (ie, polypeptide) chains that lie helically intertwined in the collagen molecule. The various types of collagen have characteristic polymer configurations and the distinctive tissue distributions shown in Table 4-1. Basically, the collagens are either fibrillar (eg, types I through III) or non-fibrillar (eg, type IV).

Many of the abundant proline and lysine residues in collagen are hydroxylated; some of the hydroxylysyl residues are also glycosylated. Hydroxylysine and lysine residues participate in the covalent lysyl oxidase-mediated cross-linking process that contributes great strength to the collagen fibril. Because *vitamin C (ascorbic acid)* is one of the cofactors that maintain prolyl hydroxylase and lysyl hydroxylase (the required hydroxylating enzymes) in their active states, a deficiency of this vitamin results in the formation of substandard, weakly cross-linked collagen that is subject to rapid degeneration. This is the underlying problem in *scurvy*.

Collagen is polymerized within the interstitial space from its precursor, *procollagen,* the helically wound α chains of which have non-helical propeptide ex-

TABLE 4-1

SUMMARY OF COLLAGEN TYPES: DISTRIBUTION AND SOURCES

Collagen Type*	Polymer Localization	Cellular Source	Tissue Distribution
I	67 nm-banded wide fibril	Fibroblasts, smooth muscle cells, reticular cells, osteoblasts, and odontoblasts	Abundant as collagen fibers in loose and dense ordinary connective tissue, fibrocartilage, bone, dentin, and cornea
II	67 nm-banded narrow fibril	Chondrocytes and retinal cells	Hyaline and elastic cartilage, nucleus pulposus of intervertebral disk, and vitreous body of eye
III	67 nm-banded narrow fibril	Fibroblasts, reticular cells, smooth muscle cells, endothelial cells, and hepatocytes	Reticular fibers in loose connective tissue, eg, papillary layer of dermis; myeloid and lymphoid tissues; parenchymal organs, eg, liver; blood vessels
IV	Multilayered polygonal lattice	Epithelial cells, endothelial cells, and lens fibers	Basement membranes, eg, glomerular basement membrane, lens capsule of eye; anchoring plaques for anchoring fibrils
V	67 nm-banded narrow fibril	Fibroblasts and smooth muscle cells	Bone, hyaline cartilage, smooth muscle, basement membranes, placental and fetal membranes; co-distributed at low concentration with type I collagen
VI	110 nm-banded narrow fibril	Fibroblasts	Hyaline cartilage, cornea, etc.; widely distributed.
VII	Short fibril composed of a non-staggered array	Uncertain	Anchoring fibrils for epidermal basement membrane
VIII	Uncertain	Vascular and corneal endothelial cells	Endothelial basement membranes, Descemet's membrane of eye
IX	On surface of principal 67 nm-banded fibrils, which are chiefly type II	Chondrocytes	Hyaline cartilage, intervertebral disk
X	Associated with principal 67 nm-banded fibrils	Chondrocytes	Maturing (hypertrophying) cartilage in epiphyseal plates
XI	Incorporated as minor component of 67 nm-banded narrow fibril	Chondrocytes	Hyaline cartilage; co-distributed at low concentration with type II collagen

* Types XII to XV also exist

tensions at their carboxy-terminal and amino-terminal ends. This precursor is synthesized by the rER, where it becomes hydroxylated and glycosylated. The pro-α chains become associated as triple helices, thereby forming procollagen molecules that pass to the Golgi apparatus for packaging into secretory vesicles. The vesicles deliver procollagen to the cell surface where, in the production of most types of collagen, extracellular amino-terminal and carboxy-terminal peptidases called procollagen aminoproteinase and procollagen carboxyproteinase trim the two propeptide extension (registration) sequences from each pro-α chain in the secreted procollagen. In most instances, such extracellular processing of the secreted product enables the collagen molecules thereby produced to undergo self-assembly into fibrils. However, type IV collagen is an exception. Furthermore, in almost all cases, the collagen molecules assemble as a quarter-staggered array in which they overlap by approximately one-quarter of their length. This results in a periodicity of 67 nm in the fibrils (see Table 4-1). An axial periodicity of 67 nm is the hallmark by which collagen fibrils are recognized in the EM (Fig. 4-9). Whereas fibrils of type I collagen aggregate into substantial *collagen fibers,* those of type II collagen remain widely dispersed. Type IV collagen molecules, the triple helix of which contains globular segments, become arranged as a multilayered extended polygonal lattice that gives the appearance of a lamina densa in basement membranes seen at the EM level (Fig. 4-10). Associated with the type IV collagen in basement membranes are the adhesive glycoproteins *laminin, fibronectin,* and *entactin,* along with *heparan sulfate proteoglycans.*

Extracellular peptidase processing is deficient in *Ehlers-Danlos syndrome type VII,* a rare autosomal-dominant inherited disorder of connective tissue that is characterized by hyperextensibility of the joints and skin and an increased risk of congenital dislocation of the hip. Alteration of the cleavage site for procollagen aminoproteinase results in impaired assembly of type I collagen fibers. Other genetic defects affecting collagen assembly or collagen cross-linking produce similar syndromes.

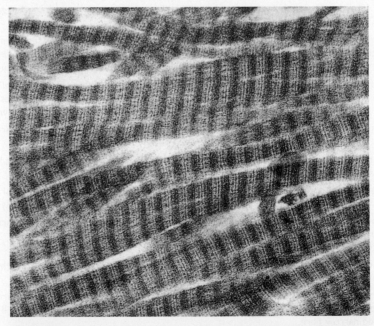

FIGURE 4-9   The distinctive 67-nm axial periodicity of collagen fibrils is due to overlapping quarter-staggered array of their collagen molecules (electron micrograph, ×37,000).

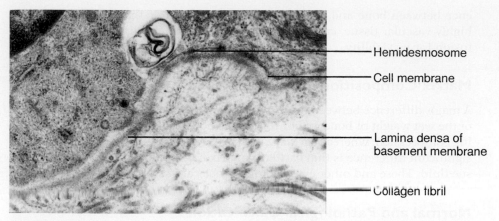

Hemidesmosome

Cell membrane

Lamina densa of
basement membrane

Collagen fibril

FIGURE 4-10 Lamina densa of the basement membrane under the epidermis (electron micrograph).

Elastin

Another matrix protein of clinical interest is *elastin*. This major component of arteries and lungs depends on elastic recoil for its effectiveness. Although lack of recoil due to aging or partial destruction have relatively minor effects on joint and muscle function, they may have a major impact on diastolic blood pressure or the amount of energy required for respiratory movements.

In contrast to collagen fibers, elastic fibers are not constructed of fibrils, nor do they show axial periodicity. They are nevertheless produced from a soluble precursor protein, *tropoelastin*, which in this case polymerizes within a scaffolding of *microfibrils* that become a part of the fibers. Some hydroxyproline but no hydroxylysine is formed, and the molecule does not become glycosylated. Extracellular lysyl oxidase produces tetrafunctional desmosine and isodesmosine cross-links, distinctive amino acid derivatives that are present only in elastin. Labile interactions between the randomly coiled, cross-linked flexible chains of this polymer permit structural deformation and then redistribute the available mechanical energy. *Fibrillin*, one of the glycoproteins in microfibrils, is defective in Marfan's syndrome, an autosomal-dominant connective tissue disorder characterized by dislocation of the lens of the eye, hyperextensibility of joints, and aortic dilatation.

In blood vessels, elastin is present in the form of elastic laminae as well as elastic fibers. *Elastic laminae* are fenestrated sheets of elastin, associated with microfibrils, that are produced by *smooth muscle cells*. Elastic fibers, on the other hand, are produced both by fibroblasts and by smooth muscle cells.

ESSENTIAL FEATURES OF BONE, CARTILAGE AND JOINTS

The two weight-bearing tissues, *bone* and *cartilage*, require unique arrangements (1) to deal with physical stresses and (2) to ensure adequate upkeep. Heavily calcified bone is characterized by having special mechanisms for its efficient maintenance and repair. Some cartilages possess only limited resources for repair, but they remain uncalcified and able to replace deteriorating matrix constituents with minimal expenditure of metabolic energy. The two main subtypes of bone are cancellous (trabecular) and compact (dense). Cartilage exists in three main forms: hyaline, elastic, and fibrocartilage. A fundamental differ-

> **KEY CONCEPT**
>
> Bone is a self-repairing tissue.

ence between bone and the three forms of cartilage is that whereas bone is a highly vascular tissue, cartilage is avascular; hence, it relies on long-range diffusion for its viability.

Matrix Composition in Bone and Cartilage

A major difference between these two types of matrix is that approximately 70% of the wet weight of bone matrix represents bone mineral capable of withstanding compression, whereas cartilage matrix usually remains uncalcified. Another significant difference is that cartilage matrix has a much greater content of tissue fluid. These and other essential differences are summarized in Table 4-2.

Normal and Pathological Calcification

An important metabolic property of bone tissue is that it acts as a storehouse for approximately 99% of the body's total content of calcium, along with approximately 85% of its total phosphorus.

Bone tissue that has not yet become calcified is called *osteoid tissue* or *prebone*. Under normal conditions, the process of *ossification* or *osteogenesis* (meaning bone formation) involves production of organic bone matrix and its ensuing calcification. However, if the local combined ion product of calcium and total free inorganic orthophosphate ions (ie, the $Ca^{2+}.P_i$ product) is insufficient, osteoid tissue does not become adequately calcified. In *rickets* and *osteomalacia*, osteoid tissue accumulates instead of mineralized bone, and weight-bearing long bones are accordingly weak.

BONE MINERALIZATION

Calcification occurs at the interface between osteoid tissue and adjacent calcified bone matrix after a delay of approximately 10 days. It involves (1) binding of extracellular Ca^{2+} to certain matrix constituents, eg, the protein *osteocalcin*, and (2) production by osteoblasts of *alkaline phosphatase*, an enzyme that elevates the local $Ca^{2+}.Pi$ product and hydrolyzes inorganic pyrophosphate, a naturally occurring calcification inhibitor.

In the course of endochondral ossification, which is the kind of prenatal ossification that occurs in pre-formed cartilage models, the protein *chondrocalcin*

TABLE 4-2

INTERSTITIAL MATRIX OF BONE AND HYALINE CARTILAGE: COMPARATIVE COMPOSITION

Content	Bone	Hyaline Cartilage
Mineral (hydroxyapatite, % of wet weight)	70	None except when calcified
Water (% of wet weight)	25	65–80
Collagen (% of organic content)	90 Chiefly type I	40–70 Chiefly type II
Proteoglycan (% of organic content)	Low	8–10 Chiefly in the form of aggregates
Glycosaminoglycans and other proteins (% of organic content)	10	20 (approximately)

and the sulfated glycosaminoglycans in cartilage matrix bind extracellular Ca^{2+}. Also, chondrocytes that hypertrophy produce *matrix vesicles,* small bulbous surface extensions with associated alkaline phosphatase activity. These vesicles accumulate calcium and phosphate ions and have the potential to produce amorphous calcium phosphate. From this initial amorphous form of calcium phosphate, needle-shaped crystals of hydroxyapatite grow out and pierce the limiting membrane of the vesicle, so that they come to lie free in the cartilage matrix.

Matrix vesicles with surface-bound alkaline phosphatase activity also form from the osteoblasts of rapidly growing bone; hence, they are presumed to play an equivalent role as calcification initiators and anti-inhibitors in the mineralization of bone matrix. Alternative mechanisms of calcification may operate interchangeably or synergistically to initiate hard tissue mineralization.

REVIEW ITEM 4-1
Explain why two vitamins are needed for satisfactory bone formation.

PATHOLOGICAL CALCIFICATION

Certain soft tissues are susceptible to *ectopic* (misplaced) *calcification.* Familiar examples include stiffening of heart valves in mitral stenosis and hardening of atherosclerotic plaques (see Chap. 5). Also, necrotic cells accumulate extracellular calcium ions. Ectopic calcification with an added component of tissue fluid or plasma calcium deposition in the interstitial space is termed *dystrophic calcification.* This is the type of calcification that occurs in calcified atherosclerotic plaques, stenosed heart valves, and hardened nodules in breast tissue. Ectopic calcification that results from hypercalcemia, eg, in association with hyperparathyroidism, is described as *metastatic calcification.* A third type of pathological calcification can lead to the formation and growth of crystalline renal calculi (kidney stones) or gallstones in patients who are not hypercalcemic.

Naturally occurring inhibitors of calcification, eg, inorganic pyrophosphate, nucleotides, citrate, and Mg^{2+}, normally afford soft tissues a measure of protection from ectopic calcification.

Types of Bone

Long bones consist of an outer cortex and a central medullary region that contains bone marrow. *Compact* (*dense*) *bone* forms the cortex, whereas the medulla contains *cancellous* (*trabecular* or *spongy*) *bone.* Compact bone develops from pre-existing cancellous bone, which is a lattice-like arrangement (L. *cancellus,* lattice) of bony anastomosing plates and rod-like columns called *trabeculae* (L. for small beams). This type of bone, shown in Fig. 4-11, may be recognized by

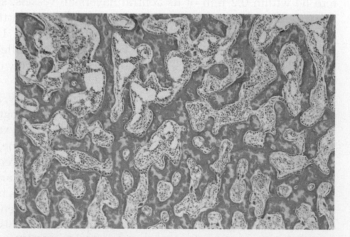

FIGURE 4-11 Cancellous bone, alternatively known as trabecular or spongy bone (low power).

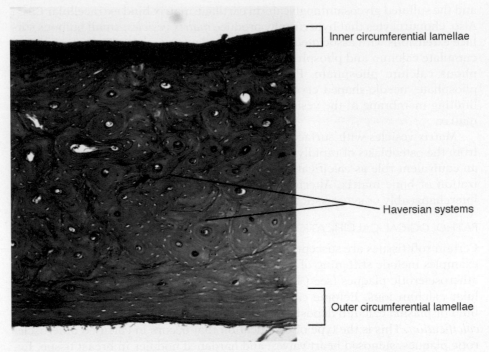

Inner circumferential lamellae

Haversian systems

Outer circumferential lamellae

FIGURE 4-12 Compact bone, alternatively known as dense bone (very low power).

the fact that it has a smaller proportion of matrix than of soft tissue spaces (approximately 1:3). Compact bone, on the other hand, has a greater proportion of matrix than of soft tissue spaces (approximately 9:1). It is built up one layer at a time through the deposition of additional layers of matrix on surfaces of trabeculae. The progressive deposition of new layers of matrix is described as *appositional growth*. It is the only growth mechanism found in bone tissue. Such growth leads to the production of cylindrical arrangements of concentric bony layers (*lamellae*), arrangements that are termed *haversian systems* or *osteons* (Fig. 4-12). The haversian system represents both the structural and the functional unit of compact bone. Because each soft tissue space in cancellous bone is supplied by blood vessels, haversian systems come to contain at least one blood vessel in their central haversian canal (Fig. 4-13). Hence, both types of bone remain richly vascularized. Indeed, bone tissue cannot develop at any site until this has become richly vascularized. All the osteocytes in a haversian system lie within 0.2 mm of its central haversian vessels, so they are adequately nourished by the tissue fluid produced. Nevertheless, for tissue fluid to reach the osteocytes, the spaces in which they lie (their *lacunae*, L. for small pits) must stay interconnected by numerous narrow canals, called *canaliculi*, through which this fluid circulates. Bone viability is accordingly dependent on local integrity of the blood supply.

The bony surfaces bordering on the medullary cavity, and extending from it, are covered by a cell layer termed the *endosteum*, a single layer containing osteogenic (osteoprogenitor) cells and osteoblasts. The external surface of each bone is covered by a tough connective tissue membrane, known as the *periosteum*, consisting of an outer region of dense ordinary irregular connective tissue and an inner cellular layer made up of osteogenic cells and osteoblasts.

Normal stress-bearing compact bone and cancellous bone are often referred to as either *mature bone* or *lamellar bone* (a term that denotes their orderly, layered organization). In contrast, developing bone, and also the rapidly growing cancellous bone that characterizes healing fractures and most bony tumors, does not show this orderly arrangement. Because its collagen fibers are arranged far less regularly, it is sometimes referred to as *woven-fibered* or *woven bone*. Alternatively known as *immature bone*, this type of bone occasionally persists in the alveolar processes, bony labyrinth of inner ear, cranial sutures, and sites of attachment of tendons and ligaments to bones. If formed at other sites, immature bone is regarded as a pathological reactive tissue that will eventually become resorbed and replaced by mature bone. Immature (woven) bone may be recognized by the uneven or closely spaced distribution of its lacunae and by the irregular or streaked staining of its matrix.

In general, the parallel collagen fibers within each lamella of compact (mature) bone lie at an angle to those in adjacent layers. Since collagen can resist tension, this results in a strong construction similar to that of plywood. When seen in H&E sections, the matrix of mature bone stains more evenly and less intensely than that of immature bone. It has a relatively smaller proportion of osteocytes, and these occupy flatter lacunae and are more regularly spaced.

Types of Cartilage

The common type of cartilage is termed *hyaline cartilage*. In H&E sections, this is characterized by having a pale blue or slightly pink, evenly staining matrix and, for the most part, randomly distributed lacunae, each enclosing a chondrocyte. However, since chondrocytes are able to divide, some of the lacunae may be associated in pairs or multiples of two. Known as *cell nests*, such arrangements are a distinctive feature of cartilage that aid in its recognition. The composition of cartilage matrix is given in Table 4-2. Most cartilages are enclosed by a fibrous *perichondrium*. In growing cartilages, this tough connective

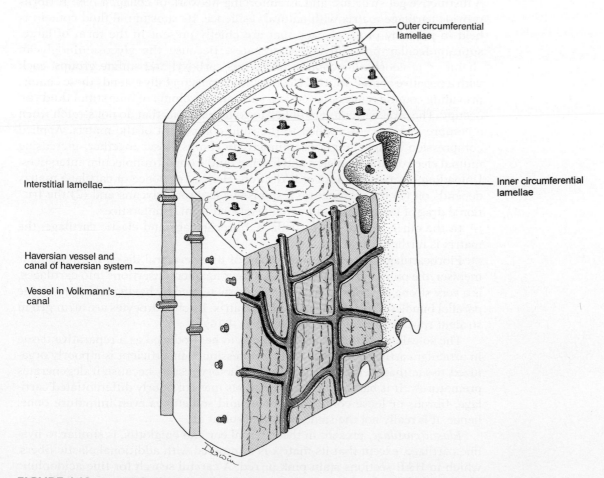

FIGURE 4-13 Basic organization of compact bone.

tissue membrane also possesses an inner chondrogenic layer containing osteogenic cells (discussed below). Articular cartilages are an exception, since they have no perichondrium. Also, because their collagen fibrils have a preferential orientation, the distribution of chondrocytes in articular cartilages is not random. Another site where chondrocytes are arranged in a recognizable pattern (basically, vertical rows) is the epiphyseal plate, ie, the cartilaginous growth plate at each end of a growing long bone (see Fig. 4-18). Articular cartilages and epiphyseal plates are accordingly regarded as specialized forms of hyaline cartilage.

Since chondrocytes are secretory and able to divide, matrix constituents continue to be secreted by daughter cells arising within the cartilage, causing it to expand from within like rising dough. This is termed *interstitial growth*. At the same time, cartilage can grow through the addition of matrix to its outer surface, ie, by apposition. The cells that produce the surface matrix arise as chondroblasts from the chondrogenic layer of the perichondrium. Hence, cartilages are able to grow both interstitially and by apposition.

All forms of cartilage are avascular. Since chondrocytes depend on long-range diffusion for their nutrition, 65–80% of the wet weight of cartilage needs to be water. Much of this water becomes displaced by crystalline calcium phosphate when cartilage matrix calcifies, which is a common occurrence once hypertrophying chondrocytes have produced matrix vesicles. Hyaline cartilages that calcify have a tendency to undergo subsequent replacement by bone, but the calcified deep layer of articular cartilages persists.

PHYSICAL PROPERTIES

A distinctive gel structure and a reinforcing network of collagen type II fibrils provide cartilage matrix with natural resilience. Its substantial fluid content is held in place by proteoglycans that are chiefly present in the form of large, supramolecular proteoglycan aggregates. Because the glycosaminoglycan chains of proteoglycans contain numerous carboxyl and sulfate groups, each with a negative charge, mutual electrostatic repulsion fully extends these chains, providing countless interstices that a substantial volume of interstitial fluid can occupy. The proteoglycans are linked to collagen fibrils that do not stretch when a compressive force is applied to the fluid component of the matrix. Applied compression brings the glycosaminoglycan chains closer together, increasing mutual electrostatic repulsion and forcing fluid from intramolecular interstices. Unloading reverses this loss of hydration. Hence, resilience of cartilage matrix depends on (1) the viscoelastic response of its proteoglycans and (2) the frictional drag of interstitial fluid being displaced from its interstices.

In the other two types of cartilage, fibrocartilage and elastic cartilage, the matrix is further reinforced.

Fibrocartilage, a normal component of intervertebral disks, intra-articular menisci, the pubic symphysis, and tendon or ligament insertions into cartilages, is a very strong type of cartilage that is characterized by having additional large parallel bundles of type I collagen in its matrix. Its chondrocytes are arranged in straight rows between these bundles (Fig. 4-14).

The so-called fibrocartilage that tends to be produced as a reparative tissue in articular cartilage defects when compression is insufficient is a poorly organized tissue that yields clinically unsatisfactory results because it degenerates prematurely. It is basically a heterogeneous mass of poorly differentiated cartilage, fibrous or loose connective tissue, and sometimes even immature bone; hence, it is really not the same type of tissue at all.

Elastic cartilage, present in the external ear and epiglottis, is similar to hyaline cartilage, except that its matrix is reinforced with additional elastic fibers, which in H&E sections stain pink or red. A careful search for fine acidophilic fibers will allow this type of cartilage to be distinguished from calcified carti-

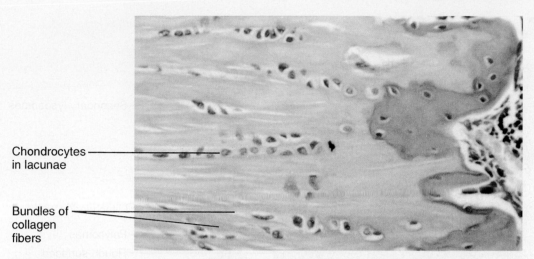

Chondrocytes
in lacunae

Bundles of
collagen
fibers

FIGURE 4-14 Fibrocartilage of a tendon attachment (medium power). A typically straight row of chondrocytes may be recognized at middle left.

lage, irregularly shaped areas of which may appear acidophilic, generally with diffuse edges.

Bone Cells

Bone cells belong to two distinct families. The cells that produce and maintain bone matrix (ie, osteoblasts and osteocytes) arise from osteogenic (osteoprogenitor) cells, which are mesenchyme-derived. The cells that resorb bone (ie, osteoclasts) arise from monocytes produced in myeloid tissue.

OSTEOGENIC CELLS

The endosteum and the deep layer of periosteum contain spindle-shaped stem cells known as *osteogenic* or *osteoprogenitor cells*. Neither of these names has proved satisfactory because they do not convey the two essential facts that these cells are both bipotential and self-renewing. In a vascular environment, some of their progeny differentiate into osteoblasts. In an unvascularized environment, however, their differentiating progeny become chondroblasts instead. These stem cells generally remain quiescent unless there is a requirement for more osteoblasts or chondroblasts, eg, for fracture repair.

OSTEOBLASTS

The metabolically active cells that produce the organic constituents of bone matrix are called *osteoblasts*. These large, rounded, basophilic cells commonly constitute a single layer on surfaces where bone is growing. Non-dividing, mature secretory osteoblasts possess an extensive rER (Fig. 4-15). In H&E sections, their sizable Golgi region often shows up as a negative Golgi image that contrasts with the surrounding basophilia. As noted above, osteoblasts are able to promote calcification of osteoid matrix through the production of matrix vesicles. Osteoblasts are further characterized by having substantial surface-bound *alkaline phosphatase* (ALP) activity. Approximately 50% of the serum ALP is derived from bone tissue; the remainder comes mainly from the liver, kidney, and placenta. An elevated blood level of ALP, in conjunction with relevant clinical findings, can be an indication of excessive osteoblastic activity, profuse bone mineralization, or the occurrence of a bone tumor.

Osteoblasts possess a surface receptor for parathyroid hormone (PTH). Stimulation by this hormone leads to their release of factors that have the ca-

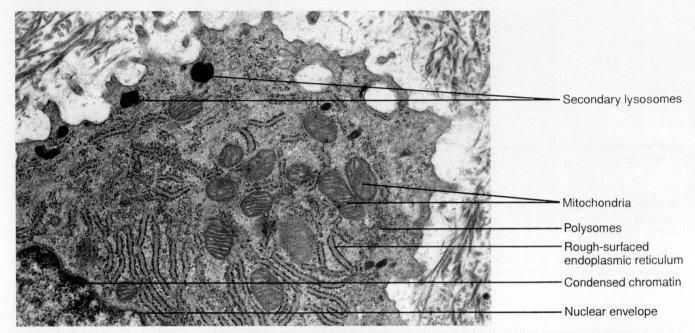

Secondary lysosomes

Mitochondria

Polysomes

Rough-surfaced
endoplasmic reticulum

Condensed chromatin

Nuclear envelope

FIGURE 4-15 Characteristic features of an osteoblast and adjacent osteoid tissue (electron micrograph).

pacity to elicit resorptive activity in osteoclasts. The fact that osteoblasts also secrete collagenase is considered suggestive of some preparative function in readiness for osteoclast-mediated demineralization.

OSTEOCYTES

Osteoblasts that have become buried in the matrix they produced are termed *osteocytes*. A distinctive feature of osteocytes is that they are connected to one another, and also to superficial osteoblasts, by cytoplasmic processes that lie within the narrow canaliculi that link lacunae. Because gap junctions are present between the processes of neighbouring cells, these cells are able to communicate with each other and exchange small molecules. Osteocytes are nondividing cells that are still capable of secreting organic matrix constituents. They are believed to be the cells that maintain bone matrix.

OSTEOCLASTS

For bone to act as an effective storehouse for calcium, an efficient, regulated mechanism is required for the liberation of Ca^{2+} from the matrix. (Figure 4-16 summarizes the manner in which osteoclasts achieve this.) *Osteoclasts* (Gk. *klan*, to break) are large, non-dividing, multinucleated cells that arise through the fusion of monocytes. They are motile cells that, on reaching potential resorption sites, become stationary and develop *ruffled borders* on the surface that is apposed to the bone matrix (Fig. 4-17). Adjacent to each of these borders, a *resorption lacuna* develops. Each lacuna is a small extracellular compartment that is sealed off from the interstitial space through the attachment of a ring-like *clear zone* that encircles the border. The osteoclast produces H^+ and HCO_3^- ions from H_2O and CO_2 through the action of carbonic anhydrase isozyme II (CA in Fig. 4-16). The HCO_3^- ions diffuse into the interstitial space, but a proton ATPase in the membrane of the ruffled border pumps the H^+ ions into the sealed resorption lacuna, acidifying its contents. At the same time, lysosomal hydrolases are discharged through the same border. In the restricted acid environment below the ruffled border, the acid hydrolases begin to degrade organic

KEY CONCEPT

Osteoclasts resorb bone through
focal acidification.

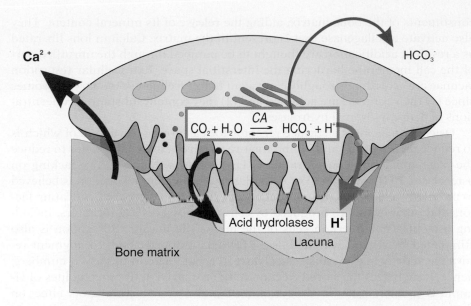

FIGURE 4-16 Mechanism by which osteoclasts liberate calcium from bone matrix (see text for details).

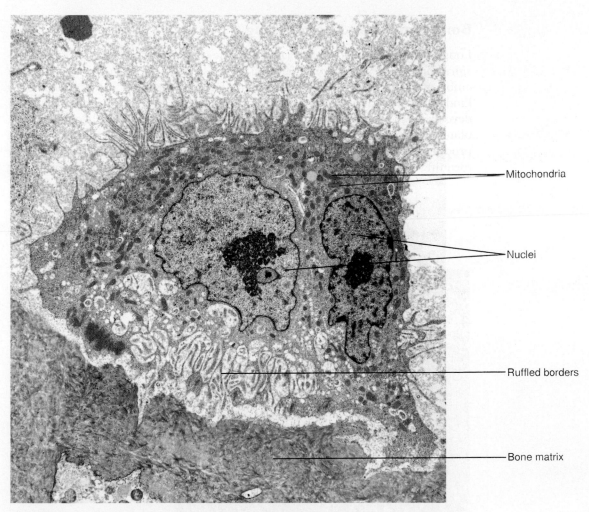

FIGURE 4-17 Distinctive features of an osteoclast (electron micrograph).

constituents of the bone matrix, aiding the release of its mineral content. They also activate a collagenase that is present in the matrix. Calcium ions liberated as a result of acidification are thought to be pumped through the unruffled part of the cell membrane bordering the interstitial space. Extracellular resorption lacunae are accordingly roughly equivalent to intracellular secondary lysosomes since (1) their contents are acidified and (2) they contain substantial concentrations of active lysosomal hydrolases.

Osteoclasts possess a surface receptor for calcitonin, the action of which is to reduce their motility and inhibit their resorptive activity. This helps to reduce the plasma calcium concentration. PTH receptors, however, are lacking on osteoclasts. PTH stimulation of osteoclastic motility and resorption is believed to be chiefly a paracrine response to chemotactic and osteoclast-activating factors and other cytokines produced by cells that possess PTH receptors, including osteoblasts and certain cells of the monocytic lineage. Resorption is also stimulated by several lymphokines. PTH acts indirectly both to augment resorptive activity and to cause osteoclasts to accumulate in increased numbers; hence, it mobilizes the stored calcium in bone matrix. Active metabolites of vitamin D (notably 1,25-dihydroxyvitamin D_3) also exert a stimulatory effect on the formation of osteoclasts from monocytes and promote resorption.

Bone Growth and Remodeling

Long bones develop from embryonic hyaline cartilage models (*endochondral ossification*), whereas flat bones develop from osteogenic cells that arise within an embryonic connective tissue membrane (*intramembranous ossification*). Both kinds of ossification produce cancellous bone, and much of this subsequently develops into compact bone. The flat bones of the cranium first become simple plates of compact bone and then acquire a central region of cancellous bone, producing a sandwich-like arrangement known as the diploë of the skull (Gk. meaning double). Continuing growth of these bones, and any subsequent repair

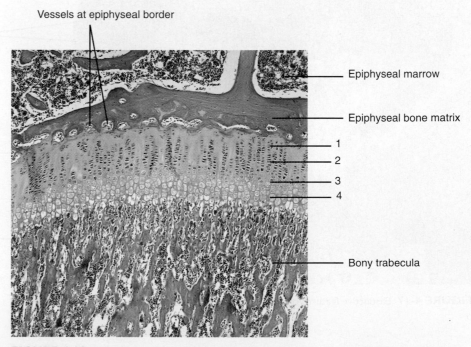

FIGURE 4-18 Constituent zones and the nutritive vessels of an epiphyseal plate (low power). Numbers indicate (1) resting, (2) proliferating, (3) maturing, and (4) calcifying zones.

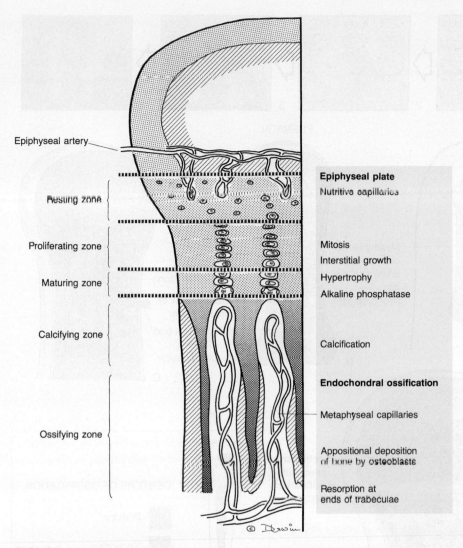

Epiphyseal artery

Resting zone

Proliferating zone

Maturing zone

Calcifying zone

Ossifying zone

Epiphyseal plate
Nutritive capillaries

Mitosis
Interstitial growth
Hypertrophy
Alkaline phosphatase

Calcification

Endochondral ossification

Metaphyseal capillaries

Appositional deposition
of bone by osteoblasts

Resorption at
ends of trabeculae

FIGURE 4-19 Important processes occurring in the region of the epiphyseal plate.

of fractures in them, is exclusively subperiosteal or subendostcal, ie, intramembranous.

Calcification of the midregion of the cartilaginous model of each long bone leads to its central replacement by cancellous bone. The same process occurs, generally postnatally, in the articulating ends (epiphyses) of the bone; hence, the bone acquires a bony shaft (*diaphysis*) with bony *epiphyses* that (1) are separated from the diaphysis by residual cartilages, the *epiphyseal plates,* and (2) are covered by *articular cartilages*. The histological structure of an epiphyseal plate (Fig. 4-18) reflects all the processes involved in endochondral ossification (Fig. 4-19). The same pattern is seen when cartilaginous fracture callus undergoes ossification (discussed below). The process of endochondral ossification is summarized in Fig. 4-20. Whereas progressive deposition of bony lamellae (indicated in red) on trabecular cores of calcified cartilage (indicated in purple) is obviously endochondral ossification, it should be noted that deposition of subperiosteal lamellae under the diaphyseal periosteum is considered intramembranous.

GROWTH

Long bones grow in both length and width. Elongation is a consequence of proliferation of chondrocytes in the proliferating zone of the epiphyseal plates. These chondrocytes are nourished by diffusion from epiphyseal capillaries that

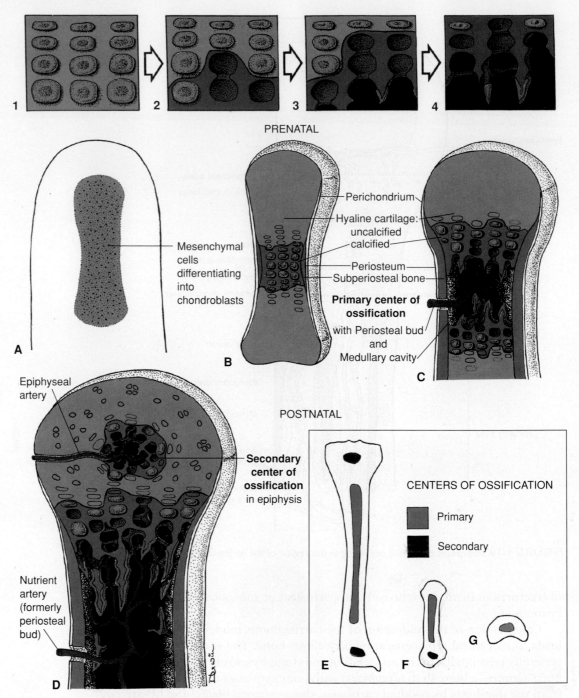

PRENATAL

Mesenchymal
cells
differentiating
into
chondroblasts

A

Perichondrium
Hyaline cartilage:
uncalcified
calcified
Periosteum
Subperiosteal bone
**Primary center of
ossification**
with Periosteal bud
and
Medullary cavity

B

C

POSTNATAL

Epiphyseal
artery

**Secondary
center of
ossification**
in epiphysis

Nutrient
artery
(formerly
periosteal
bud)

D

CENTERS OF OSSIFICATION

Primary

Secondary

E   **F**   **G**

FIGURE 4-20 Endochondral ossification. **A** to **C** represent prenatal stages; **D** to **G** occur postnatally. (**A**) Mesenchymal condensation. (**B**) Calcification in midregion. (**C**) Formation of primary (diaphyseal) center of ossification from periosteal bud. (**D**) Formation of secondary (epiphyseal) centers of ossification from epiphyseal vessels. (**E**) Most long bones have two secondary centers. (**F**) Atypical long bones (eg, phalanges) possess only a proximal secondary center. (**G**) Short bones (eg, lunate) lack secondary centers. (1–4) On the diaphyseal side of the epiphyseal plate, of calcified cartilage matrix begins to break down. Bone becomes deposited on the calcified cartilage remnants, with resulting formation of metaphyseal bony trabeculae.

lie just above the zone of resting cartilage (see Figs. 4-18, 4-19). Soon after new chondrocytes are produced, they hypertrophy and elicit calcification. The calcified cartilage subsequently erodes, and capillary loops grow up into the tunnels that are left behind when the columns of chondrocytes disappear from their lacunae (bottom of Fig. 4-19). In this newly vascularized environment, osteogenic cells from the medullary cavity produce osteoblasts that lay down lamellae of bone matrix on trabecular cores of calcified cartilage. Under the central region of the plate, the bony trabeculae formed on the diaphyseal side of the plate are rapidly resorbed by osteoclasts, but at the periphery they thicken by apposition and produce the compact bone that characterizes the cortex of the metaphyses (the flared regions between the diaphysis and the epiphyses). During further lengthening of the bone, these regions become incorporated into the diaphyseal cortex.

Growth in width is achieved through the addition of subperiosteal lamellae. During active skeletal growth, irregular groove-like protrusions of these lamellae become walls of tunnels that fill in with consecutive layers of matrix, forming additional peripheral haversian systems. Later, the outer surface becomes smoother as a result of deposition of circumferential lamellae (see Figs. 4-12, 4-13). Circumferential lamellae are also deposited over much of the endosteal surface of the diaphysis after the medullary cavity has been widened by osteoclastic resorption (*inner circumferential lamellae* in Figs. 4-12 and 4-13). Some cancellous bone, nevertheless, continues to exist within the medullary cavity. Preferential distribution of its trabeculae along lines of stress provides additional support by transmitting applied loads.

REMODELING

A unique feature of bones is that they undergo *modeling* (*drift*) and lifelong *remodeling*, meaning that their matrix is gradually resorbed and replaced. New bone may be deposited on surfaces that are more appropriate (modeling), or it may have physical properties that are more appropriate (remodeling). Thus, remodeled cranial bones have a central layer of cancellous bone that contains intercommunicating marrow cavities, and when immature bone is remodeled, it becomes replaced by mature (lamellar) bone. All bones tend to weaken and must undergo continual internal remodeling to maintain sufficient strength. The functional unit of the remodeling process in compact bone is termed the

> **REVIEW ITEM 4-2**
>
> What event in bone growth may be recognized in Fig. 4-21? (Consult part D4-10 of the Discussion section of this chapter to confirm your answer.)

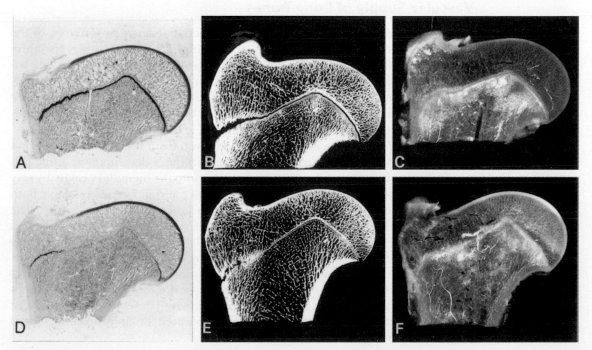

FIGURE 4-21 Proximal epiphysis of humerus (canine, longitudinal section). (**A–C**) Eight months after birth; (**D–F**) 10 months after birth. (**A,D**) Stained with safranin O and fast green. (**B,E**) Microradiographs. (**C,F**) Microangiographs of barium sulfate-perfused preparations.

bone remodeling unit. It consists of (1) a resorption tunnel created by osteoclasts, and (2) an advancing front of osteoblasts that proceed to fill the tunnel with concentric lamellae of osteoid. Such new haversian systems take approximately 3 to 4 months to reach completion. The turnover rate of compact bone that results from internal remodeling is approximately 3% per year. Pieces of lamellar bone from a pre-existing haversian system that persist after the remodeling process are called *interstitial lamellae* (see Fig. 4-13). Cancellous bone shows an even higher rate of turnover (approximately 26% per year), since numerous resorption cavities develop on the extensive surfaces of its trabeculae and subsequently fill in with new lamellae of osteoid.

Normally, the amount of new bone produced during a cycle of bone remodeling compensates fairly precisely for the amount of matrix that was resorbed by osteoclasts. Certain constituents of bone matrix, notably *coupling,* chemotactic, and *bone morphogenetic (osteoinductive) proteins,* ensure this quantitative correlation. When liberated locally from resorbed bone matrix or, in certain cases, generated by bone cells during a resorptive phase, these paracrine and autocrine chemotactic, differentiation, and additional growth factors promote (1) recruitment of osteoblast progenitors, (2) osteoblast differentiation, and (3) secretory activity of osteoblasts. Since bone formation is thereby *coupled* to prior bone resorption, bone turnover should proceed without bone loss.

Osteoporosis

A significant imbalance between bone resorption and bone formation leads to a decline in total bone mass that is known as *osteoporosis.* This can be a result of (1) uncoupling of bone formation and bone resorption, or (2) accelerated resorption that remains uncompensated by sufficient production of new bone. Bone loss is chiefly from endosteal surfaces, and clinical manifestations of lost cancellous bone tend to precede those of lost cortical bone. (For the microscopic appearance of osteoporotic bone, see Fig. 4-5A.)

Vascular Supply of Long Bones

In order to understand orthopedic or reconstructive surgical procedures, or the proper management of bone fractures or joint injuries, it is necessary to appreciate how the various parts of bones are nourished. Even the osteocytes that belong to interstitial lamellae are no more than 0.3 mm from a tissue fluid-producing blood vessel. The vessels in haversian canals (*haversian vessels*) are predominantly wide anastomosing capillaries, but a few are associated arterioles and venules. Blood reaches the diaphyseal arterioles from several sources. The *diaphyseal nutrient artery* (or *arteries*), derived from the periosteal bud that invades the middle of the cartilage model and initiates development of the primary (diaphyseal) center of ossification, passes into the medullary cavity by way of the nutrient canal. As indicated in Fig. 4-22, its multiple branches supply both the bone marrow and at least the inner two-thirds of the diaphyseal cortex. The remainder of the cortex, under most conditions representing substantially less than the outer third, derives nourishment chiefly from blood that is supplied by periosteal arteries. Each epiphysis is supplied by *epiphyseal nutrient arteries* derived from the vessels that initiate development of the secondary (epiphyseal) centers of ossification. Supplementary *metaphyseal nutrient arteries* (branches of adjacent systemic veins) supply the metaphyses. These vessels are derived from periosteal arteries that become incorporated during circumferential growth of the metaphyses.

In general, blood that enters cortical haversian vessels from branches of the diaphyseal nutrient artery flows centrifugally, and then passes from the peripheral cortex into periosteal veins. The metaphyses have their own emissary veins.

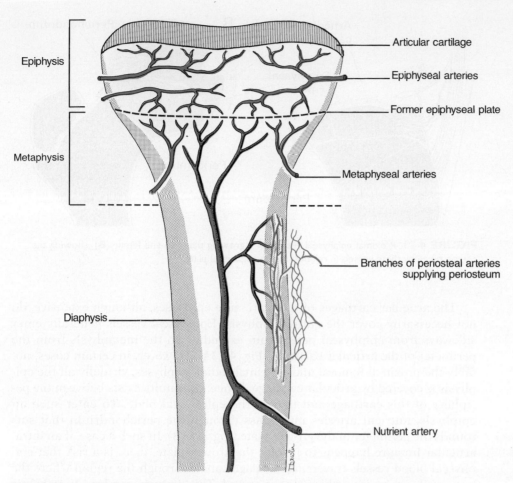

Articular cartilage

Epiphyseal arteries

Former epiphyseal plate

Metaphyseal arteries

Branches of periosteal arteries
supplying periosteum

Nutrient artery

Epiphysis

Metaphysis

Diaphysis

FIGURE 4-22 Basic blood supply of a long bone.

Osteocytes in the outermost diaphyseal lamellae, nevertheless, remain nourished almost entirely from periosteal capillaries that are supplied by periosteal arteries.

By the time of puberty, multiple terminal anastomoses have become established between the various arteries that supply the bone. The cartilaginous epiphyseal plates, which are nourished from capillary loops supplied by the epiphyseal arteries (see Fig. 4-19), become thin and eventually disappear when the rate of chondrocyte proliferation in the epiphyseal plates becomes less than the rate of endochondral ossification. At this stage, full stature is attained. Bony replacement of the growth cartilages permits numerous anastomoses to develop between the nutrient, metaphyseal, and epiphyseal arteries (see Fig. 4-22). Hence, if the principal blood supply coming from the diaphyseal nutrient artery is compromised, eg, as a complication of a fracture, there are enough other arteries providing blood to maintain viability of many of the osteocytes.

CONSEQUENCES OF EPIPHYSEAL SEPARATION

The maturing and calcifying zones of the epiphyseal plates of weight-bearing growing bones remain a site that is not particularly strong. Epiphyseal plate (physial) fractures in children can lead to serious complications, such as premature cessation of growth or angulatory deformity of joints. Avulsion of traction epiphyses tends to be less damaging than the avulsion of weight-bearing epiphyses of the pressure type (eg, the upper or lower femoral epiphysis), many of which (eg, the lower femoral epiphysis) contribute significantly to bone lengthening.

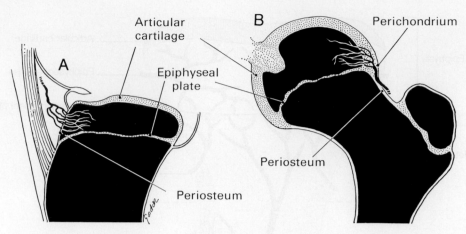

FIGURE 4-23 Proximal epiphyseal vessels of a growing tibia (**A**) and femur (**B**), showing the course taken by these vessels in relation to the epiphyseal plate.

The articular cartilages of most pressure epiphyses, although extensive, do not necessarily cover the entire epiphysis. Epiphyseal vessels generally enter sideways from epiphyseal periosteum extending to the metaphysis from the perimeter of the articular cartilage (Fig. 4-23A). However, in certain cases, notably the proximal femoral and proximal radial epiphyses, virtually all the epiphysis is covered by articular cartilage; hence, continuity exists between the periphery of this cartilage and that of the epiphyseal plate. To enter such an epiphysis, nutrient arteries must pass through the perichondrium that surrounds the perimeter of the growth plate (Fig. 4-23B). In such a case, if an intra-articular fracture happens to involve the growth plate, there is a risk that epiphyseal blood vessels traversing cartilage canals through the region where the two cartilages merge will become ruptured. This, in turn, can lead to ischemic longitudinal growth disturbance or even avascular necrosis of the epiphysis and epiphyseal plate. In contrast, separation of the type of epiphysis shown in Fig. 4-23A, does not isolate the chondrocytes in the epiphyseal plate from their source of nutrition. Moreover, articular cartilage remains viable even in a completely separated epiphysis because its chondrocytes obtain their nourishment by diffusion from synovial fluid. Accordingly, only 15% of injuries involving epiphyseal plates are associated with increased incidence of growth disturbances or angulatory deformities.

Fracture Repair

The repair process in fractures or microfractures of cancellous bone is relatively straightforward. *Bony callus,* the repair tissue, is formed from viable endosteum and unites the fragments. No cartilage is involved. Dead bone, recognizable from its empty lacunae, is resorbed; remodeling restores the appropriate alignment of trabeculae.

The callus produced in healing fractures of long bones can be either bony or cartilaginous, depending on the amount of mobility that occurs at the fracture site. If such mobility is restricted through *functional fracture-bracing* (*cast-bracing*), the callus is primarily bony, particularly the part of it derived from endosteum. Instability of the fracture site results in production of a higher proportion of hyaline cartilage in the callus. This then undergoes endochondral ossification (Fig. 4-24). Initial cartilage formation is chiefly a result of extensive proliferation of periosteal osteogenic cells and differentiation of their progeny in an environment that has not yet become fully revascularized. Subsequent vascularization of this environment converts it into one that supports osteogenesis.

KEY CONCEPT

Postnatal bone repair mimics prenatal bone development.

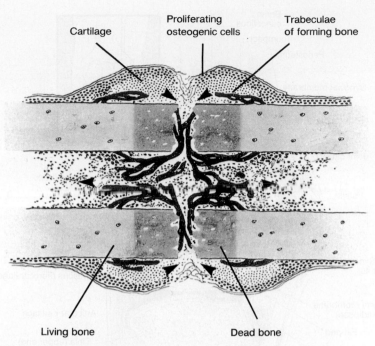

Cartilage   Proliferating osteogenic cells   Trabeculae of forming bone

Living bone   Dead bone

FIGURE 4-24 Healing process in a rib fracture. (Arrowheads denote sites of elongation of trabeculae of the bony callus.)

In bones that have a thick cortex, the numerous osteogenic cells in the lining of haversian canals contribute to production of the callus that unites the cortical regions of the fragments.

After 1 to 2 months, immature cancellous bone unites the fragments. Subsequent replacement by mature bone reconstitutes a cortex, and resorption of bone from the medulla restores the medullary cavity.

Stable internal fixation, eg, by compression plating, promotes direct cortical union through the development of bridging haversian systems. This process is sometimes described as *contact healing.* The results are clinically satisfactory, provided that sufficient time elapses for the initially deposited immature bone to become replaced by mature bone before excessive inappropriate stresses are placed on the fracture site. Because this type of healing takes much longer to reach completion, up to 2 years may be required before clinically satisfactory results are obtained.

Essentially, closely approximated, well-fitted fragments that have been accurately aligned and stably fixed in tight apposition undergo internal remodeling that is largely independent of the occurrence of a fracture. Osteoclasts from nearby viable regions of compact bone randomly create resorption tunnels that sooner or later extend in either direction from one fragment to another. Direct coupling of bone formation to prior resorption ensures that these tunnels subsequently fill in with new bone, and new haversian systems are ultimately formed that effectively peg the fragments together like dowel pins in furniture. Continuing remodeling results in eventual replacement of all the dead bone by mature living bone.

Joints and Joint Problems

The basic structure of a *synovial joint,* ie, the lubricated, freely moving type of joint, is summarized in Fig. 4-25. Its joint cavity is filled with *synovial fluid,* a yellowish viscous fluid that contains hyaluronic acid, an associated lubricating glycoprotein, and a low concentration of suspended leukocytes (<100 cells/mm^3).

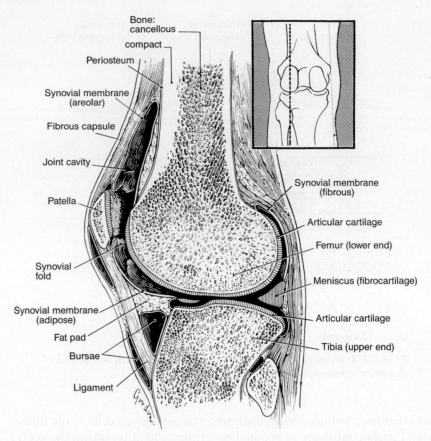

Bone:
cancellous
compact
Periosteum
Synovial membrane
(areolar)
Fibrous capsule
Joint cavity
Patella
Synovial
fold
Synovial membrane
(adipose)
Fat pad
Bursae
Ligament

Synovial membrane
(fibrous)
Articular cartilage
Femur (lower end)
Meniscus (fibrocartilage)
Articular cartilage
Tibia (upper end)

FIGURE 4-25 Tissue components of a synovial joint (knee joint, sagittal section).

These cells are mostly monocytes but also include some lymphocytes, macrophages, and occasional neutrophils. The *synovial membrane (synovium)* lines the joint cavity everywhere, except for the articular cartilages. Its *synovial cells (synoviocytes)* add the lubricating constituents to tissue fluid produced by a capillary plexus in this membrane, which being made of connective tissue, has only a noncontiguous layer of synovial cells at its free surface. When damaged or surgically resected, the synovial membrane regenerates readily.

ARTICULAR CARTILAGE

Postnatal growth of this specialized form of hyaline cartilage (see Fig. 4-6B) is exclusively interstitial since it has no perichondrium. The cartilage consists of three zones. In the *superficial zone*, the chondrocytes are small and their lacunae may be flattened parallel to the articular surface. The *middle* or *transitional zone* represents the region of interstitial growth. In growing cartilages, its proliferating chondrocytes tend to assume a vertical columnar arrangement deep to the articular surface. However, division of chondrocytes becomes a rare occurrence once the articular cartilages have grown, and their vertical columnar arrangement becomes almost random as a consequence of interstitial matrix deposition. The *deep zone* is made up of (1) a *radial layer* of maturing chondrocytes that is rich in proteoglyans, and (2) an underlying layer of *calcified cartilage* that anchors the articular cartilage to subchondral bone.

Articular cartilages are characterized by a distinctive arrangement of type II collagen fibrils that is well suited for distributing the stresses associated with joint function. The fibrils of the superficial zone lie essentially parallel to the articular surface. Those in the deep radial layer extend longitudinally toward the surface, and those of the middle zone arch over and join the horizontal fibrils in the superficial zone. Because articular cartilage is avascular, it relies on simple diffusion from the synovial fluid for most of its nutrients and oxygen.

DEGENERATION AND INJURY

Superficial tears or cracks begin to appear at articular surfaces after the age of 30 and later may become deep fissures. Furthermore, the total number of chondrocytes in the articular cartilages undergoes an age-related decline, suggesting an ultimate loss of proliferative potential.

Osteoarthritis (known also as *degenerative joint disease*) is a common degenerative disorder affecting synovial joints. If the affected joints are weight-bearing, resulting painful disability can make it very difficult for elderly patients to manage. When the condition occurs prematurely or becomes unduly severe, is it regarded as pathological. The essential problem is that articular cartilage matrix begins to yield to compressive loads when its proteoglycan content becomes diminished. An established reason for articular deterioration is progressive, ultimately irreversible loss of proteoglyan from the matrix. Furthermore, articular damage can result in death of chondrocytes. Despite a minimal proliferative response by local viable chondrocytes, with associated production of small quantities of matrix constituents, tissue repair remains mostly ineffective and leaves substantial defects unfilled.

In certain synovial joint injuries, damaged articular cartilages undergo more satisfactory healing if the injured joint is kept in motion, eg, by a mechanical device that ensures slow, continuous passive movement over an appropriate range. Whereas imposed immobilization and continuous elevated hydrostatic pressure both inhibit proteoglycan and protein synthesis, continuous passive joint motion has a stimulatory effect on cartilage matrix production. The intermittent compressive action of such motion produces cyclic variation of the intra-articular synovial fluid pressure and results in pumping effects and increased local blood flow.

From such findings, it may be inferred that any general reluctance to use limbs or synovial joints because of pain, muscular weakness, or habitual inactivity may accelerate or exacerbate degeneration of the articular cartilages.

DISK HERNIATION

Another type of joint with a tendency to degenerate that can also lead to clinical problems (notably, low back pain) is the *anterior intervertebral joint*. The general structure of this joint (the disk that can "slip") is summarized in Fig. 4-26. The *anulus fibrosus,* which surrounds the central *nucleus pulposus,* is essentially a collar made of fibrocartilage. The nucleus pulposus contains a soft, gelatinous matrix with a composition that is basically similar to that of hyaline cartilage. The collagen present in the middle of the nucleus pulposus and the innermost part of the anulus fibrosus is chiefly type II. However, the collagen present at the periphery of the nucleus pulposus and in the outer part of the anulus fibrosus is type I, which is exceptionally strong. When the spine is loaded in compression, the incompressible gelatinous nucleus pulposus becomes pressed against the inextensible anulus fibrosus, acting as a cushion between adjacent vertebral bodies.

After the age of 40, age-related degenerative changes begin to occur in the intervertebral disks, particularly those of the lumbar spine. Loss of water content in the nucleus pulposus, and to a lesser extent in the anulus fibrosus, parallels age-related losses of proteoglycan-associated glycosaminoglycans and proteoglycan aggregates. In pathological degeneration of the disks, these losses become exaggerated, even though they are partly offset by further proteoglycan synthesis. A further age-related change is that tiny fissures start to form between collagen fiber bundles in the anulus fibrosus. Under conditions such as forced spinal flexion, portions of the central soft nucleus pulposus are then inclined to

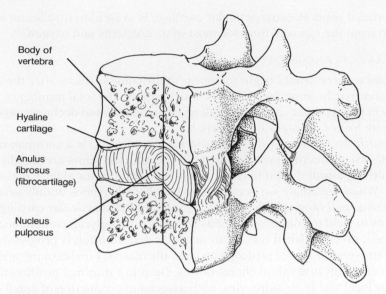

Body of
vertebra

Hyaline
cartilage

Anulus
fibrosus
(fibrocartilage)

Nucleus
pulposus

FIGURE 4-26 Tissue components of an intervertebral disk.

herniate (rupture) through the weakened surrounding anulus, leading to a condition called a *ruptured (prolapsed) disk,* which is more widely known as a "slipped disk." It is fairly common for such herniation to occur along the posterolateral or posterior borders of the lumbar spine, because in this region the anulus fibrosus is comparatively narrow. A commonly associated complication is local compression or stretching of the spinal nerve roots by swollen exuded matrix. As soon as cartilage matrix escapes from the nucleus pulposus, it avidly imbibes tissue fluid, mainly as a consequence of its remaining proteoglycan content. Accompanying inflammation and edema commonly worsen the situation, resulting in severe pain. A possibly dubious consolation is the fact that elderly people have a reduced risk of disk herniation because of the age-related decline in proteoglycan content of their intervertebral disks.

ESSENTIAL FEATURES OF SKELETAL MUSCLE

The voluntary type of muscle associated chiefly with the skeleton is called *skeletal muscle.* Because it exhibits transverse microscopic striations, it is a form of *striated* muscle. Cardiac muscle is the other form. Smooth muscle lacks striations. Cardiac and smooth muscle are described in Chapter 5 in connection with the cardiovascular system. Comparative features of the three different types of muscle are summarized in Table 5-1.

Each *skeletal muscle fiber* is a long, multinucleated cell that arises through fusion from embryonic precursor cells called myoblasts. The functional unit of a skeletal muscle is known as a *motor unit.* It consists of (1) the widely distributed muscle fibers innervated by a lower motor neuron of the spinal cord and (2) the motor neuron itself. All the muscle fibers in the unit contract fully in response to efferent impulses from the neuron. The strength of each muscular contraction is determined by the number of motor units that contribute to it.

Skeletal muscles are histologically a composite of (1) skeletal muscle fibers and (2) their supporting connective tissue. The connective tissue component is organized into epimysial, perimysial, and endomysial sheaths that transmit the pull of contractions, convey nerve fibers, blood vessels, and lymphatics, and nourish the muscle fibers through diffusion.

Internal Organization of Skeletal Muscle Fibers

Figure 4-27, which shows the main structural organization of a skeletal muscle fiber seen at the EM level, may be referred to as often as is necessary for understanding this section. The longitudinal contractile filaments (*myofilaments*) are of two distinct types. The *thin filaments*, 1 μm long and 6–7 nm wide, contain *actin*, together with the *troponin* complex and *tropomyosin*, which are both regulatory proteins that mediate the regulation of contraction by Ca^{2+} ions. The *thick filaments*, 1.5 μm long and 12–15 nm wide, contain *myosin*, an actin-activated, Mg^{2+}-dependent ATPase. When enabled by Ca^{2+} ions to bind to actin, ATP-energized myosin molecules execute an oscillatory swiveling motion, char-

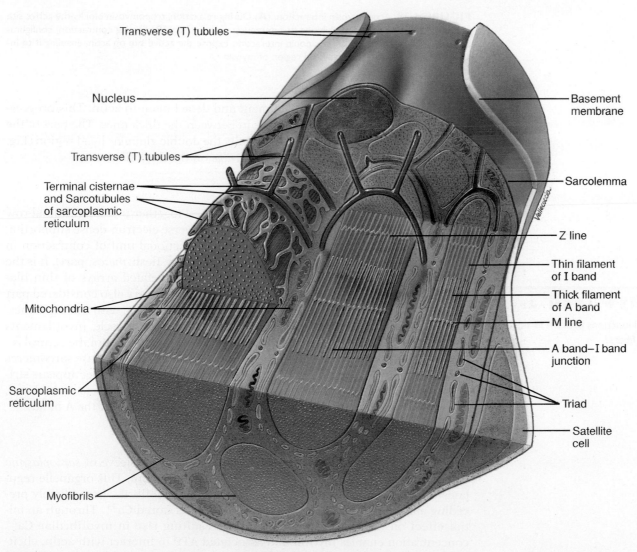

Transverse (T) tubules

Nucleus

Transverse (T) tubules

Terminal cisternae and Sarcotubules of sarcoplasmic reticulum

Mitochondria

Sarcoplasmic reticulum

Myofibrils

Basement membrane

Sarcolemma

Z line

Thin filament of I band

Thick filament of A band

M line

A band–I band junction

Triad

Satellite cell

FIGURE 4-27 Structural details of a skeletal muscle fiber, established through electron microscopy.

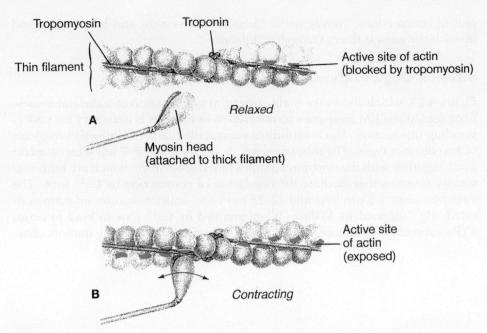

FIGURE 4-28 Actin–myosin interaction. (**A**) During relaxation, tropomyosin blocks the active site (indicated in blue) on actin, inhibiting its interaction with myosin. (**B**) During contraction, configurational changes elicited by Ca^{2+}-troponin interaction expose the active site on actin, enabling it to interact with the double globular head region of myosin.

acterized by rapid cycles of attachment and detachment to actin. This progressively pulls the thin filaments farther in between the thick ones. The part of the myosin molecule that swivels is essentially the double globular head region (Fig. 4-28) that is seen in the EM as a *cross bridge* on the thick filament.

SARCOMERES

The repetitive arrays of thin filaments are joined together in a longitudinal row by lattice-like *Z lines* (Fig. 4-29), which are transverse electron-dense supporting lattices containing the protein α *actinin*. The functional unit of contraction in striated muscles is known as a *sarcomere* (Gk. *sarkos,* flesh; *meros,* part). It is the array of thick filaments, together with the two associated arrays of thin filaments, that lies between two consecutive Z lines (which are also considered part of the sarcomere). A *myofibril* is a long series of sarcomeres, with shared Z lines, that extends the full length of a muscle fiber. In skeletal muscle, myofilaments are restricted to discrete cylindrical myofibrils occupying most of the central region of the fiber. The nuclei lie in the peripheral cytoplasm. Because sarcomeres are transversely aligned in all the myofibrils, the entire muscle fiber appears striated with dark *A bands* and lighter-staining *I bands*. A *Z line* bisects each I band, and an M line interconnects the thick filaments at the center of the A band.

SARCOPLASMIC RETICULUM

Each myofibril is intimately invested with an elaborate sleeve of *sarcoplasmic reticulum* (SR), a derivative of the endoplasmic reticulum. This organelle regulates the all-important Ca^{2+} concentration in the myofibrils. Immediately preceding a muscular contraction, the SR releases its stored Ca^{2+}. Through an initial effect on the troponin complex, the resulting rise in myofibrillar Ca^{2+} concentration enables myosin and associated ATP to interact with actin, eliciting a contraction. Key roles of the SR are, therefore, (1) rapid release of stored Ca^{2+}, initiating contraction and (2) subsequent withdrawal and storage of my-

REVIEW ITEM 4-3

Are cell junctions present in skeletal muscle fibers?

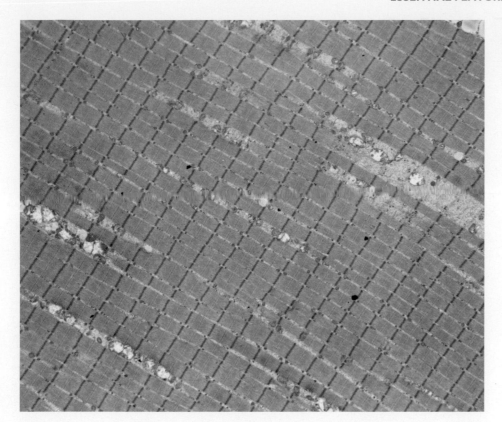

FIGURE 4-29 Myofibrils of a skeletal muscle fiber (electron micrograph, ×3,400).

ofibrillar Ca^{2+}, inducing relaxation. To some degree, the two tasks are spatially separated. Ca^{2+} release occurs chiefly from large *terminal cisternae* of the SR representing the chief site of Ca^{2+} storage. These cisternae border on *transverse (T) tubules,* which are tubular invaginations of the electrically excitable surface membrane (*sarcolemma*). The remainder of the SR, composed of anastomosing *sarcotubules,* is responsible for Ca^{2+} withdrawal through the action of Ca^{2+} ATPase during relaxation. Each T tubule has a terminal cisterna of the SR on either side of it (see Fig. 4-27). The combination of these three components is described as a *triad.* The triads of skeletal muscle fibers lie at the A band-I band junctions, providing maximal Ca^{2+} release into the overlap zone between thick and thin filaments (see Fig. 5-6). Ca^{2+} is released from the SR through a fast *calcium release channel* (known also as the *ryanodine receptor*) that appears as electron-dense particulate structures, formerly known as *junctional feet.* Since the Ca^{2+} release channel lies in intimate association with the *slow Ca^{2+} channel* (known also as the *dihydropyridine receptor*) of T tubules, these electron-dense particles appear to span the gap between each terminal cisterna and its associated T tubule (see Fig. 5-6).

The voltage-gated slow Ca^{2+} channel in the tubular invaginations of the sarcolemma (T tubules) acts as if it instantaneously transmits sarcolemmal depolarization signals to the Ca^{2+} release channel, because the immediate effect of sarcolemmal depolarization is Ca^{2+} release from the terminal cisternae into the cytosol.

Patients with genetic mutations that result in excessively prolonged opening of the Ca^{2+} release channel of the SR when they have been anesthetized with halothane, or have been given the muscle relaxant succinylcholine, have an increased risk of developing muscle rigidity and hyperthermia. This potentially lethal condition, known as *malignant hyperthermia,* is a manifestation of augmented glycolytic and aerobic muscle metabolism in conjunction with prolonged muscular contraction, each elicited by the rising cytosolic Ca^{2+} level.

REVIEW ITEM 4-4

What covers the motor axon terminals of a motor end plate?

Motor End Plate

Voluntary contraction of each skeletal muscle fiber is initiated by efferent nerve impulses that reach its *motor end plate,* ie, the excitatory synapse between axon terminals of a lower motor neuron and the muscle fiber. Firing of impulses by the neuron elicits the release of *acetylcholine,* which binds to a nicotinic acetylcholine receptor that is situated chiefly along the openings of the *junctional folds* in the end plate region of the sarcolemma. Binding of two molecules of acetylcholine to this receptor opens its central transmitter-gated channel, admitting Na^+ and allowing K^+ to leave the muscle fiber. Resulting sarcolemmal depolarization under the end plate generates an end plate potential that spreads as an action potential over the entire sarcolemma, including its T tubular invaginations.

Autoimmune circulating antibodies to the acetylcholine receptor cross-link it, and by inducing its endocytosis downregulate it in the end plate region. Local complement-mediated changes in the postsynaptic membrane (sarcolemma) may also be involved. The reduced receptor concentration leads to progressive and ultimately profound weakness in certain skeletal muscles, a common early sign of which is *ptosis* (drooping of the upper eyelid). Such a cause of muscular weakness is known as *myasthenia gravis* (Gk. *mys,* muscle; *astheneia,* weakness). Since *acetylcholinesterase* is present in the region of basement membrane lying in the synaptic cleft (presumably to counteract any residual acetylcholine), acetylcholinesterase inhibitors are employed in diagnosing and treating this condition.

Muscular Growth, Dystrophy and Repair

A totally different cause of progressive muscular weakness, and one that ultimately becomes fatal because it affects not only skeletal muscles but also the myocardium, is *muscular dystrophy.* Duchenne muscular dystrophy, an X-linked recessive disease affecting boys, is associated with a virtual or total absence of *dystrophin,* a dimeric protein of the membrane cytoskeleton that is believed to be necessary for stabilizing or reinforcing the cell membrane of all three types of muscle fibers and neurons. Current evidence suggests that an important function of dystrophin is to anchor actin-containing filaments of the cytoskeleton to a transmembrane protein complex, ie, an integral cell membrane glycoprotein complex, one glycoprotein of which binds to laminin in the apposed basement membrane.

Among the necrotic and degenerating muscle fibers in dystrophic muscles lie smaller regenerating fibers, characterized by comparatively basophilic cytoplasm and slightly larger nuclei with conspicuous nucleoli. The presence of such regenerating muscle fibers in muscle biopsies is a reliable indication of preceding fiber necrosis. Regenerating muscle fibers, nevertheless, become ultimately outnumbered by necrotic fibers. The source of the new fibers is *satellite* (*myosatellite*) *cells* (see Fig. 4-27) that lie beside skeletal muscle fibers, enclosed by the same basement membrane. Prenatal development of skeletal muscle fibers is normally completed in the first postnatal year. All subsequent normal growth is the result of hypertrophy of these fibers, initially through fusion with additional myoblast-like cells derived from the satellite cells. Later growth and muscular enlargement achieved through exercise involve the addition of new sarcomeres to the ends of myofibrils and the addition of new filaments to the periphery of sarcomeres. When growing myofibrils have reached a diameter of approximately 1 μm, they split longitudinally and form daughter myofibrils, increasing the total number of myofibrils per fiber. Compensation for lost skeletal muscle function as a result of injury is due chiefly to hypertrophy of undamaged muscle fibers. Under most conditions of healing, large defects become filled with a rather disorganized mixture of regenerating muscle fibers (derived from satellite cells) and fibrous scar tissue (produced by fibroblasts). Skeletal muscle is, therefore, regarded as having only a limited regenerative capacity.

ESSENTIAL FEATURES OF NERVOUS TISSUE

Allowing for the fact that substantial coverage of basic and applied aspects of nervous tissue is considered the province of self-contained neuroscience courses, present discussion will be limited to topics that are either fundamentally integrative or generally applicable in understanding medical disorders.

General Organization

Nervous tissue is organized into the various functionally interrelated parts of the nervous system that collectively are responsible for nervous function. The basic functional unit of nervous tissue consists of the cell body of a *neuron*, its various cytoplasmic extensions (*nerve fibers*), and its associated sites of communication with other neurons (*synapses*). *Nerve impulses* represent the means of communication. The part of the nervous system that develops from the neural tube becomes the *central nervous system* (CNS), consisting of the *brain* and *spinal cord*. The remainder of the system, arising mainly from neural crest, constitutes the *peripheral nervous system* (PNS). Functionally, the part of the nervous system concerned with generation and conduction of the afferent impulses (L. *ad*, to; *ferre*, to carry, ie, conducted *toward* the CNS) and elicited efferent impulses (L. *ex*, out of, ie, conducted *away* from the CNS) for *voluntary* motor responses is called the *somatic* (Gk. *soma*, body) *nervous system*. The part of the nervous system involved in an equivalent manner with *involuntary* responses, eg, exocrine secretion and smooth muscle contraction, is called the *autonomic* (Gk. *autos*, self; *nomos*, law) *nervous system* (ANS).

Neurons

Nerve cells (*neurons*) are basically bipolar, pseudounipolar, or multipolar in shape. Except for the ganglion cells in cranial, spinal, and autonomic ganglia and the retina, their cell body (*soma*) is situated in the gray matter of the CNS. In the brain, the layered *gray matter* lies external to the *white matter*, so-called because it consists chiefly of myelinated nerve fibers. In the spinal cord, however, the central H-shaped arrangement of gray matter lies internal to the white matter. Each myelinated nerve fiber in the CNS is a cylindrical, fast-conducting afferent or efferent *axon* (Gk. for axis) that propagates impulses from the cell body of a neuron to the distal end of the axon. The other nerve fibers in the *neuropil* (Gk. *pilos*, felt; meaning the felt-like mass of predominantly unmyelinated nerve fibers that encloses neuronal cell bodies in the gray matter) are *dendrites* (Gk. *dendron*, tree), which in most cases are multiple and branch dichotomously from the cell body in an extensive tree-like arrangement with finely tapered endings. Dendrites conduct the impulses that they receive from other neurons toward the cell body. In the majority of synapses, the *presynaptic terminal* is an axon terminal. The *postsynaptic terminal* may be a dendrite, dendritic spine, neuronal cell body, or axon. Synapses can also be dendrodendritic, dendrosomatic, or soma-somatic.

To maintain the synapses at an axon terminal, which may lie at a distance of 1–2 m from the cell body, *axonal* (*axoplasmic*) transport is essential. *Kinesin*, a microtubule-activated ATPase, translocates membranous vesicles that transport neurotransmitter, enzymes, proteins, and phospholipids required for local synaptic vesicle production in the terminal. Kinesin can propel such vesicles along microtubules at a rate of 5–40 cm per day. This transport occurs in an anterograde direction, ie, away from the cell body. A slower anterograde stream (*axoplasmic flow*) conveys the cytosolic enzymes and cytoskeletal proteins that are needed to maintain the axon terminals. *Cytoplasmic dynein,* another microtubule-activated ATPase, translocates membranous vesicles and organelles along microtubules in a retrograde direction, bringing back to the cell body any unused or recycled materials, eg, excess norepinephrine and synaptic membrane constituents. This retrograde flow has proved useful for the experimental tracing of neural pathways, since EM tracers (eg, horseradish peroxidase) are taken up by endocytosis during the local recycling process that occurs in axon terminals. Phagosomes labeled with the tracer become retrogradely translocated to the neuronal cell body, where their contents are submitted to lysosomal degradation. Findings obtained after injection of such a tracer reveal not only the pathway that these axons follow but also the group of cell bodies (situated, for example, in the brain) to which axons that terminate at the injection site belong. A clinically important effect of retrograde flow is that it can carry toxins and viruses into the CNS. It provides a vulnerable access route for *rabies* virus and viruses that cause *encephalitis* (inflammation of the brain).

Neuroglia

The internal supporting cells of the CNS are collectively known as *neuroglia* or *glial cells* (Gk. *glia,* glue). Like neurons, they arise from neuroectoderm. Often also classified as glial cells are *Schwann cells* and *capsular cells* of ganglia; these are equivalent neural crest derivatives that belong to the PNS. The four types of

REVIEW ITEM 4-5

What is the structure marked (1) in Fig. 4-30? (To confirm your answer, see part D4-11 of the Discussion section of this chapter.)

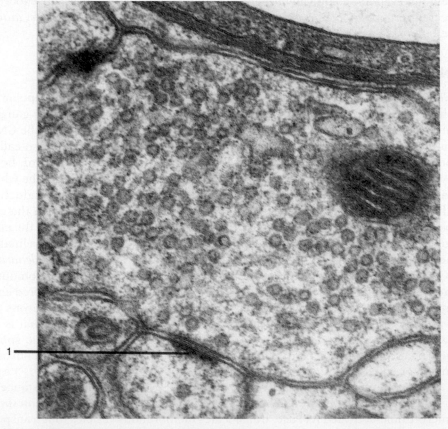

FIGURE 4-30   (Review Item) Identify the structure marked (1).

neuroglia in the CNS are *oligodendrocytes, astrocytes, microglia,* and *ependymal cells.* Collectively, they outnumber the enormous number of neurons by a factor of 10. Besides being supportive in a physical sense, they cooperate in neuronal metabolism and produce myelin that speeds up impulse conduction. *Astrocytomas, glioblastomas,* and other malignant *gliomas* that arise from neuroglia represent approximately one-half of all primary brain tumors.

OLIGODENDROCYTES

These relatively small cells (Gk. *oligos,* small) have cytoplasmic processes that wrap segments of several associated axons with spiral sheets of myelin. Oligodendrocytes are the only cells that produce and maintain myelin in the CNS. A number of oligodendrocytes are required to myelinate each axon. In gray matter, oligodendrocyte nuclei are commonly seen near neuronal cell bodies. In white matter, they lie in rows between bundles of nerve fibers.

ASTROCYTES

These are heterogeneous star-shaped cells (Gk. *astron,* star) with radiating cytoplasmic processes that are reinforced by bundles of intermediate filaments composed chiefly of *glial fibrillary acidic protein* (GFAP), which is an astrocyte marker. The numerous short branching processes of *protoplasmic astrocytes* brace nerve fibers to capillaries in the neuropil of gray matter. *Fibrous astrocytes,* characterized by GFAP-rich processes that are present in smaller numbers, perform a similar function chiefly in white matter. Developmentally, *type I astrocytes,* which resemble protoplasmic astrocytes, may be implicated in creating the special neural microenvironment that induces the formation of continuous tight junctions between the endothelial cells of brain capillaries (discussed below). In postnatal life, however, astrocytes are not required for the maintenance of blood–brain barrier characteristics. The radiating processes of type 1 astrocytes terminate in *astrocyte feet,* which cover most of the capillary surface. In contrast, the majority of astrocyte feet in *type 2 astrocytes,* which apparently correspond to fibrous astrocytes, are associated with nodes of myelinated fibers. Hypertrophied, hyperplastic *reactive astrocytes* produce the cellular scar tissue that characterizes *reactive gliosis (astroglial encapsulation),* the repair process initiated by CNS trauma. Reactive astrocytes are large, phagocytic cells that are believed to arise from residual neuroglial progenitors.

Astrocytes and oligodendrocytes take up the K^+ ions that momentarily pass into the interstitial space during impulse conduction along nerve fibers. Astrocytes are interconnected by gap junctions. They provide nutritional and metabolic support for the neuronal population of the CNS and maintain the ionic microenvironment that these cells require. In white matter, gap junctions also interconnect oligodendrocytes with node-associated astrocytes. Finally, astrocytes constitute an important source of neuronal growth factors, and they also contain substantial amounts of glycogen.

MICROGLIA

These very small glial cells enlarge and become motile and phagocytic in response to injury of the CNS. Postnatally, they can be formed from blood monocytes, so they are widely regarded as diminutive, non-motile resident brain macrophages. Whether their origin is neuroectoderm, pluripotential hematopoietic stem cells, or both, remains a contentious issue.

EPENDYMAL CELLS

These are the low columnar cells, still ciliated during childhood, that constitute the simple epithelial lining (*ependyma*) of the brain ventricles and central canal of the spinal cord. Also, they constitute the covering layer (*choroid plexus epithelium*) of the choroid plexuses, which are situated in the brain ventricles.

REVIEW ITEM 4-6

Where does CSF go after it is produced?

Choroid plexuses are tufted vascularized extensions with the important role of producing cerebrospinal fluid (CSF).

Blood–Brain Barrier

Throughout most of the brain, highly charged molecules, macromolecules, and certain drugs (eg, some of the penicillins) do not reach the interstitial space from the bloodstream. The passage of lipid-soluble molecules, on the other hand, is unimpeded. The morphological basis of this so-called *blood–brain barrier* is the presence of extensive and continuous *tight junctions,* of the *zonula occludens* type, between the perimeters of contiguous endothelial cells of brain capillaries. There is evidence that the special neural microenvironment of the CNS induces these junctions. The degree of sealing by these highly developed junctions is not as great during infancy or under conditions of acute inflammation. No blood–brain barrier exists in the pineal, pituitary, choroid plexuses, or area postrema (vomiting center in the brain stem). However, a comparable barrier does exist in both the retina and the iris, and also in the endoneurium of large peripheral nerves.

Peripheral Nervous System

REVIEW ITEM 4-7

What criteria can be used for distinguishing between sections of autonomic ganglia and sensory ganglia?

Ganglia, peripheral nerves, and *nerve endings* constitute the *PNS. Afferent* components are concerned with sensation, whereas *efferent* components are concerned with responses. Some ganglia are sensory [the *cranial ganglia* and also the *spinal ganglia,* known alternatively as *dorsal (posterior) root ganglia*]. The efferent ganglia of the PNS are also a part of the ANS and, hence, are more commonly known as *autonomic ganglia.*

Peripheral Nerves

The basic histological organization found in peripheral nerves is outlined in Fig. 4-31. Afferent as well as efferent fibers are commonly present in the same fascicle. When cut in longitudinal section, small peripheral nerves may be recognized by the general waviness of their nerve fibers, accentuated by the waviness of elongated associated Schwann cell nuclei (Fig. 4-32). Small peripheral nerves do not possess an epineurium.

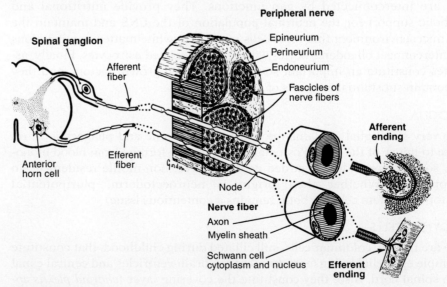

FIGURE 4-31 Essential parts of the peripheral nervous system.

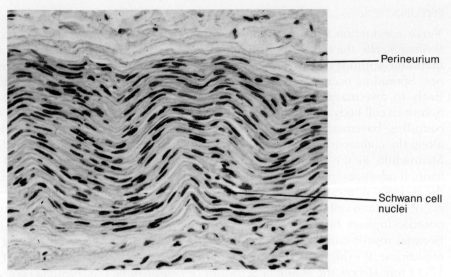

FIGURE 4-32 Peripheral nerve fascicle (longitudinal section).

RESPONSE TO INJURY

Unlike the CNS, the PNS has considerable potential for regeneration. However, post-traumatic recovery is mostly a consequence of renewed axoplasmic flow and axonal transport because it is the axon, not the entire neuron, that regenerates. Under most circumstances, there seems to be virtually no postnatal replacement of neurons, even through mitosis of progenitors or stem cells. Olfactory neurons are a noteworthy exception to the rule, since they can be replaced.

A deleterious effect of prolonged or excessive pressure and crush injuries is that they impair or curtail the essential processes of axonal transport and axoplasmic flow occurring in peripheral axons. Resulting axonal damage is manifested by degeneration of the part of the axon that lies distal to the injury. In some situations where the damaged neurons still remain viable, PNS function may gradually return at a recovery rate of up to 1 mm per day under favorable conditions. Axons that are regenerating under ideal conditions can actually lengthen at a rate of up to 4 mm per day, which corresponds to the rate of axoplasmic flow. Functional recovery, nevertheless, depends on there being a sufficient number of remaining endoneurial sheaths to guide new compensatory axon sprouts to appropriate destinations. When severing of nerves results in axotomy, suturing is necessary for the reconstruction of endoneurial sheaths. Proliferating Schwann cells promote renewed growth of the axon and also play an essential role in the guiding process.

Minimal regeneration of CNS axons, with resulting failure or ineffectiveness of functional recovery following CNS injuries, is believed to be partly due to the absence of Schwann cells and their surrounding basement membranes from the CNS. Furthermore, two of their glial counterparts (namely, oligodendrocytes and mature astrocytes) and certain protein constituents of CNS myelin have been shown to exert an inhibitory influence on axonal growth.

FIRST-DEGREE INJURIES

In contrast to second-degree injuries such as those described in the previous section, first-degree injuries cause only temporary, short-term impairment of nerve function. A common cause is mild or transient pressure applied to a peripheral nerve, which produces a local hypoxia if it compresses the local blood supply. Afferent nerve fibers, in particular, are affected, with resulting paresthesia or numbness.

MYELINATION

Nerve conduction velocity is higher in axons that have become myelinated. *Schwann cells,* the cells responsible for axon myelination in the PNS, show a remarkable aptitude for spreading over the axolemma in a frankly assertive manner. Spreading occurs in a circumferential direction as well as longitudinally. Early in myelination, circumferential spreading has a tendency to haul the Schwann cell body around as well. However, subsequent development of a surrounding basement membrane and associated macular adhering junctions along the endoneurial border of the cell soon anchors the cell body in position. Meanwhile, as the leading edge of the cell continues to progress around the axon, it advances under the myelin that has begun to form along this border. In the process of spirally wrapping an axon, successive circumferential double layers of Schwann cell membrane build up on the axonal surface. Previously interposed cytoplasm becomes squeezed back into the nucleated region of the cell. Because myelin consists of successive double layers of compacted Schwann cell membrane, it exhibits a distinctive and readily recognized linear periodicity of 12–18 nm. Hence, the *sheath of Schwann* or *neurolemma (neurilemma)* consists of (1) an inner myelin region that is part of the *myelin sheath* and (2) an outer region, the *Schwann cell cytoplasm,* which also contains the cell nucleus. Since each Schwann cell wraps an internode, the nodes, which lie 0.3–1.5 mm apart, are positioned *between* consecutive Schwann cells.

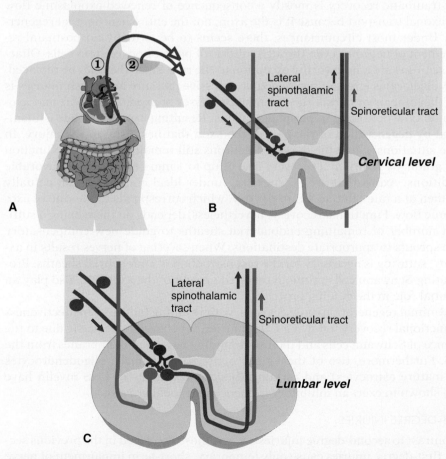

FIGURE 4-33 Pain may be referred to a different site as a consequence of convergence within the spinal cord. (**A**) The patient's supraclavicular pain in Case 4-4 actually represents referred pleuritic pain (see part D4-10 of the Discussion section of this chapter). (**B**) Pathway of converging somatic and visceral afferent impulses that enter the spinal cord at the cervical level. (**C**) Pathways of converging somatic and visceral afferent impulses that enter at the lumbar level.

Myelin, which is a highly efficient electrical insulator, is a lipid–protein complex consisting of approximately 75% lipids (cholesterol, phospholipids, and glycolipids) and 25% proteins (notably myelin-associated glycoprotein and myelin basic proteins). Because lipid constituents are all extracted by the fat solvents used in routine section preparation and staining, myelin appears only as empty spaces in H&E sections. *Unmyelinated fibers* are associated as small groups with Schwann cells. Each unmyelinated fiber occupies a superficial trough in the Schwann cell cytoplasm and, hence, is freely exposed to tissue fluid. The Schwann cells that are associated with unmyelinated axons do not produce a surface *myelin-associated glycoprotein,* which is required for axons to undergo the process of myelination. This glycoprotein is, however, present as an integral membrane protein on the surface of the Schwann cells that myelinate and also on oligodendrocytes.

In *multiple sclerosis* and *Guillain-Barré syndrome (peripheral polyneuropathy)*—which represent major demyelinating diseases of the CNS and PNS, respectively—impulse conduction becomes either profoundly impaired or blocked.

Referred Pain

Visceral and deep pain impulses are generally only poorly localized and, in some cases, their sites of origin are inaccurately perceived by the brain. A pain that has been erroneously attributed to a wrong site is called a *referred pain*. Visceral pain that seems reasonably localized is sometimes referred to other sites as well, in which case it is often called a *radiating pain*. For a straightforward example of pain referral, see Analysis (Case 4-4) and part D4-9 of the Discussion section below. Figure 4-33 shows the neural pathways involved in the case.

CASE DISCUSSIONS

D4-I (CASE 4-I)

At first glance, the sections shown in parts A and B of Fig. 4-1 might seem fairly normal. The tissues seen here lie beyond the borders of an abscess cavity that became lined with new vascular connective tissue (granulation tissue). The close association between cancellous bone and substantial areas of hyaline cartilage is one clue that this bone tissue lies just under the epiphyseal growth plate. The site from which it was obtained is further indicated by the fact that the bony trabeculae have pale-blue cores of calcified cartilage, which may be considered evidence of endochondral ossification.

The marrow spaces lying between the trabeculae are filled with a fibrous tissue that contains inflammatory cells, mostly small lymphocytes and plasma cells. This finding is compatible with a diagnosis of *chronic recurrent multifocal osteomyelitis* although only one major focus was found. *Osteomyelitis,* which is bone inflammation due to a pyogenic (pus forming) organism, may also involve the bone marrow. The synovial biopsy was sampled from the synovium, ie, the *synovial membrane* made of connective tissue that lines the joint capsule. It revealed a nonspecific mild *acute synovitis,* which probably explains the large volume of joint effusion present (70 mL of fluid instead of the normal amount of <5 mL). Evidence of bone resorption is found in the fibrous tissue that occupies the marrow spaces in this biopsy (see Fig. 4-1C). Small granulomas are also present, and some of the multinucleated giant cells have walled off fragments of dead bone from the surrounding tissue (see Fig. 4-1D).

Chronic recurrent multifocal osteomyelitis is a protracted but largely indolent condition that is characterized by occasional exacerbations with long intervening remissions. Attempts to isolate the responsible organism are invariably unsuccessful, and antibiotic therapy may fail to bring about clinical improvement. The bloodstream is one route by which infecting bacteria may enter the bone. Irregularly dilated sprouts of tiny medullary blood vessels extend into the lowermost region of the growth plate (ie, the zone of calcifying cartilage). These vessels are fragile and hemorrhage easily, so tiny pools of infected extravasated blood can collect under the growth plate. Because such infected foci are confined they may become regions of bone necrosis. In the initial phase, acute inflammation generally leads to abscess formation, with focal bone resorption and compensatory formation of new bone at the abscess margins. Bacteria may spread through the bone by way of its canals and canaliculi and gain access to the nearest joint cavity. The chronic inflammatory phase that follows the acute phase is characterized by lymphocytic infiltration and the development of granulomatous foci. Although the clinical course of this condition may be very prolonged, the long-term prognosis is good. In this case, however, the chronic inflammation just under the epiphyseal growth plate caused premature closure of the right growth plate, with resulting shortening of the right leg.

D4-2 (CASE 4-2)

Sites of major bone destruction with *neovascularization* (new blood vessel formation) and newly formed calcified matrix (tumor bone) can indicate bone cancer. Certainly, the numerous mitotic figures (see Fig. 4-2C) present in such a small area of the biopsy does not suggest normal bone tissue, nor is anything suggesting bone recognizable in this field other than the stromal appearance of the cells. Parts B and D of Fig. 4-2 show that some bone matrix is, in fact, present even though the biopsy consists largely of the cells seen in part C. Taken together, these various components indicate that this lesion is a differentiated *osteosarcoma* (*osteogenic cell sarcoma*).

Further histological evidence that this is a malignant tumor is seen in Fig. 4-2D. In addition to bony trabeculae covered with osteoid (*upper left*) and an artery cut in longitudinal section (*bottom left*), a vein is present (*bottom right*). This vein has osteoid-covered bone tissue within its lumen. Tumor cells probably gained access to small blood vessels in the malignant stroma and grew by extension into this larger vessel, where they produced a mass of tumor matrix.

The irregular bony trabeculae seen in Fig. 4-2B are made up of pink superficial layers of osteoid tissue deposited on cores of immature tumor bone, which may be recognized from its purple staining and relative abundance of randomly distributed lacunae.

Patients with osteosarcoma have a relatively high incidence of lung and bone metastases. In view of the generally poor prognosis associated with this type of cancer, Jeff's negative chest x-ray and CT scan appear to be encouraging. The chances of succeeding with a limb-salvaging procedure and a long-lasting prosthetic implant, however, are not good.

D4-3 (FIG. 4-3)

Although the bone tissue shown in Fig. 4-3 arose in a skeletal muscle, scarcely anything seen here suggests such an unusual location. Osteogenic differentiation has occurred within a scar site remaining from the earlier muscle injury, and this has resulted in *heterotopic ossification* within the muscle. Bone production in injured muscles is fairly common and is known as *myositis ossificans*.

A difference between the bony trabeculae formed at the periphery of this site and those seen in Fig. 4-1 is that the trabeculae produced in muscle lack blue cores of calcified cartilage. This appearance could indicate that any preexisting cartilage was all replaced, but it is also consistent with the occurrence of intramembranous ossification within the muscle. Why previous muscle damage would result in local osseous metaplasia (changed differentiation) is not clear. However, it may be significant that the ossifying peripheral region of the site is well vascularized, and it is clear that a variety of different factors are capable of inducing the production of heterotopic bone.

It may be noticed that the peripheral bony trabecula seen in Fig. 4-3B is growing by apposition on one surface only. The other surface is being eroded. Thus, the left border is characterized by the presence of a pale-pink layer of osteoid tissue with associated osteoblasts, whereas the right border shows bone matrix being etched by multinucleated osteoclasts.

Since this region of localized heterotopic ossification is an entirely benign type of growth, surgical removal is not essential. Heterotopic bone may vanish in due course without intervention.

D4-4 (FIG. 4-4)

The tumor seen in the neck region of the left humerus is a *chondrosarcoma* (see Fig. 4-4A). Tumor *cartilage* appears as a glistening, homogeneous, and translucent lobulated mass. In contrast, the adjacent normal bone tissue appears either dense, opaque, and whiter (*compact bone*) or else trabecular with marrow spaces (*cancellous bone*). Malignant chondrocytes, together with the cartilage matrix they produced, extend into the neighboring soft tissues. Extensive bone erosion may be recognized at this site. Distal to it, a smaller mass of cartilage lies in the medulla of the humerus. Chondrosarcomas grow relatively slowly but commonly metastasize to the lungs. Blue-stained matrix, large cell nests, and chondrocyte lacunae are all recognizable in Fig. 4-4B.

D4-5 (FIG. 4-5)

The appearance of the iliac crest biopsy shown in Fig. 4-5A,C is consistent with a clinical diagnosis of *osteoporosis*. Careful comparison with an iliac crest biopsy from a normal age-matched person (see Fig. 4-5B,D) reveals a loss of supporting cancellous bone and a reduction in thickness of bone cortex in this patient. However, the differences found in such histological sections (see Fig. 4-5A,B) are generally subtle and rarely very striking.

Osteoporotic vertebral bodies that have similarly lost many of their internal supporting trabeculae are susceptible to crush fractures. Vertebral (spinal) osteoporosis, therefore, commonly results in kyphosis (Gk. kyphōsis, humpback ie, forward curvature of the thoracic spine).

The type of osteoporosis that affects postmenopausal women is chiefly a consequence of accelerated bone resorption. The complex result of declining estrogen levels is imbalance between bone resorption and bone formation. Stress protection due to a lack of physical activity (eg, in sedentary occupations or lifestyles) further predisposes postmenopausal women to osteoporosis and, hence, fractures.

High estrogen levels, bisphosphonates, or calcitonin reduce bone resorption without significantly increasing bone formation. Maintenance on sodium fluoride diminishes bone resorption and modestly stimulates osteogenesis, retarding the loss of cancellous bone in this type of osteoporosis; however, its effect is insufficient to increase the total bone mass. Also, adverse effects of fluoride such as weight-bearing pain may occur. Calcium supplementation and reasonable levels of physical activity help to retard bone loss in osteoporotic patients.

D4-6 (FIG. 4-6)

The articular cartilage of the femoral head (illustrated in Fig. 4-6A) has become abraded and now constitutes only an incomplete layer over the subchondral bone. The articular cartilage in major weight-bearing joints (eg, the hip and knee) is particularly susceptible to degenerative changes. Loss or degradation of proteoglycans from cartilage matrix reduces the tissue's resistance to compression, and resulting frictional wear of the softened, non-resilient matrix at major synovial joints can lead to *osteoarthritis,* the condition illustrated here. Degenerating softened articular cartilages that are repeatedly compressed develop fibrillations (microscopic vertical splits) on their free surface (see Fig. 4-6A). If deeper fissures form, synovial fluid may be squeezed down into fibrosed marrow spaces in the subchondral bone tissue, where it may collect as subchondral bone cysts (see Fig. 4-6C,E). The stress-bearing region of the plate of subchondral bone thickens (see Fig. 4-6E), becoming less resilient; under ordinary circumstances, any repair tissue that forms is reparative poorly differentiated cartilage (sometimes described as "fibrocartilage"), not articular cartilage. The end result is that the weight-bearing joints become progressively denuded of their articular cartilage. The femoral head shown in Fig. 4-6D, for example, has lost almost all its articular cartilage. Its weight-bearing surface is smoothly polished (*eburnated*) bone. Only the part labeled (?) still retains its covering of articular cartilage. A great deal of pain may be experienced when such joints are submitted to the full weight of the body. To relieve pain and keep the patient ambulatory, implantation of a suitable metallic joint prosthesis (*replacement arthroplasty*) often becomes necessary. Loss of articular cartilage can be recognized radiographically as a narrowing of the joint space normally seen in joint x-rays (compare parts E and F of Fig. 4-6). *Osteophytes* (bony spurs covered with cartilage) commonly grow out of the epiphyses at the margins of their articular surfaces, restricting the joint's mobility; this may lead to angular deformities, eg, *genu varum* (bow-leggedness) in patients with degenerating knee joint cartilages.

D4-7 BONE SCANS (FIG. 4-7)

Cells of certain cancers tend to metastasize to bones, eg, as a result of dissemination to red marrow of parts of the axial skeleton. The tumor cells present in these bony metastases commonly produce factors that augment local osteoclastic activity. However, in some cases (eg, prostatic carcinoma), they trigger an osteoblastic response, and the associated osteosclerotic lesion is unrelated to prior resorption.

Sites of significantly increased matrix turnover are readily detectable with radionuclide-labeled diphosphonates, which resemble pyrophosphate in structure and adsorb to bone mineral. However, radiologically detectable osteolytic lesions are not evident in bone scans when the coupled osteoblastic response is impaired. In many cases (eg, breast cancers), the metastatic tumor cells elicit a mixed osteoclastic and osteoblastic response, partly because coupling proteins released from the matrix during the process of resorption counteract the effects of this process by eliciting secretion of further matrix constituents, and partly because tumor cells release osteoblast-stimulating growth factors.

D4-8 (CASE 4-3)

Amiodarone chlorhydrate, a benzofuran derivative, is used in the management of cardiac arrhythmias and angina pectoris. However, some patients who are maintained on a prolonged course of this drug develop a reversible, *iatrogenic* (treatment-induced, from Gk. *iatros,* physician) *peripheral neuropathy.* Careful comparison between parts A and B of Fig. 4-8 leads to the conclusion that in this patient's peripheral nerves, myelin has been lost from some nerve fibers, particularly larger ones. *Myelin*, a lipid–protein complex that increases axonal conduction velocity by insulating much of the axolemma, is stained black by osmic acid. The osmium also renders myelin electron dense in electron micrographs. Because the myelin present in peripheral nerves is formed from successive double layers of Schwann cell membrane, it has a characteristic lamellar appearance at the EM level. In addition, it is sometimes possible to recognize the spiral arrangement that results from growth of the inner border of Schwann cells around the axon during myelination.

It is necessary to examine and interpret Fig. 4-8C for the next clue. It shows endothelial cells of a small blood vessel in the connective tissue component of the nerve. Their cytoplasm contains some large granule-like inclusions. The lamellated or loose-textured content of these structures is unlike that seen in familiar cytoplasmic organelles. The fact that many of them contain lamellae of electron-dense material is perhaps enough to suggest a lipid content that is somehow related to myelin. Yet, the endothelial cells in which these unusual granules are seen neither produce conspicuous storage granules nor form myelin. Cytoplasmic inclusions with contents that seem unfamiliar or unusual for the cell type concerned are commonly some sort of secondary lysosome. Similar granule-like inclusions may be present in the patient's Schwann cells, perineurial fibroblasts, or intraneural macrophages. These inclusions are believed to represent intracellular accumulations of breakdown products that are related to myelin.

The biopsy indicates a decreased number of large myelinated nerve fibers in the patient's peripheral nerves. Thinning of the myelin sheath, segmental demyelination, and subsequent axonal degeneration are only partly compensated for by axonal regeneration and remyelination. Impaired motor conduction suggests that peripheral myelin remains inadequately replaced through remyelination. Skeletal muscle biopsies taken from patients with amiodarone neuropathy show considerable variability in muscle fiber diameter and contain angular atrophic muscle fibers. These changes indicate denervation atrophy of some of the muscle fibers.

The underlying mechanism of amiodarone neuropathy is still unclear. However, it is known that this drug inhibits two lysosomal enzymes, namely, *phospholipases A1* and *A2*. It is, therefore, likely that the distinctive residual bodies (secondary lysosomes) found in various cell types in the peripheral nerves of these patients contain undegraded phospholipids. As far as Schwann cells are concerned, it would seem that their essential role in maintaining myelin sheaths of peripheral axons becomes substantially impaired by inhibition of these two enzymes. The resulting net loss of myelin slows axonal conduction, and this is manifested as a motor or sensorimotor neuropathy. Amiodarone-induced demyelination is also believed to contribute to axonal degeneration and resulting denervation atrophy of muscle fibers.

D4-9

Pain impulses are sent to the brain by afferent neurons, the cell bodies of which lie chiefly in the spinal ganglia. In contrast to cutaneous pain, which is accurately localized by the somatosensory cortex, most deep somatic or visceral pain is perceived as being diffuse and poorly localized. Also, the site at which visceral pain is perceived is not necessarily the site of origin of the pain impulses. Bizarre painful sensations of this type are known as *referred pains*. Some of them are projected to sites that lie at some distance from their source.

As a complication of *pneumonia*, the patient in Case 4-4 developed inflammation (*pleuritis* or *pleurisy*) in the central region of the diaphragmatic parietal pleura. This pleuritis elicited pain impulses in the afferent fibers of the phrenic nerve supplying the region (see Fig. 4-33A). Afferent fibers in the phrenic nerves enter the spinal cord at the same cervical level (primarily C3 to C5) as the supraclavicular nerves carrying afferent fibers from the neck and shoulder. They enter at this level because the diaphragm develops from mesoderm of the head and neck region, and subsequently shifts to a more caudal position between the thoracic and abdominal cavities. Pains of this type are referred from the viscera to body wall tissues or other more superficial tissues that arise from the same body segment, ie, tissues with the same segmental nerve supply as the organ in which the pain impulses originated. Visceral pain that is referred to the corresponding dermatome is perceived as somatic pain.

The pathways taken by convergent somatic and visceral afferent impulses entering the spinal cord at cervical and lumbar levels are shown in Fig. 4-33B,C. In cases where pain is referred, it is likely that the brain misinterprets the source of the afferent impulses converging on the lateral spinothalamic and spinoreticular tracts.

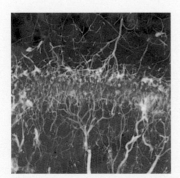

FIGURE 4-34 Proximal epiphyseal growth plate region of a humerus, showing multiple anastomoses between the metaphyseal and epiphyseal vasculatures at the site of the growth plate (microangiograph of canine humerus).

D4-10

In Fig. 4-21, the chief difference between the upper row of preparations (A–C) and the lower row (D–F) is that *epiphyseal closure* is occurring in the (D–F) group. Bony replacement of the growth cartilage (epiphyseal plate) is particularly evident in D; articular cartilage remains intact. Bony bridging between the primary and secondary centers of ossification (epiphyseal union) is particularly evident in E. Closure is confirmed in F, which discloses that vascular anastomosis has occurred between epiphyseal and diaphyseal vessels. Further details of this anastomosis are shown in Fig. 4-34. In the metaphyseal region, increasing consolidation of the cortical bone is also evident (compare E with B).

D4-11 (FIG. 4-30)

This is an example of an *axodendritic chemical synapse*, ie, the common kind of directed synapse. The direction of neurotransmission may be surmised from the presence of synaptic vesicles, along with a mitochondrion, in the large presynaptic terminal in the upper part of the micrograph. In addition, postsynaptic thickening of the postsynaptic membrane is evident.

BIBLIOGRAPHY

Bone and Joints

Aarden EM, Burger EH, Nijweide PJ. Function of osteocytes in bone. J Cell Biochem 55: 287, 1994.

Benjamin M, Evans EJ. Fibrocartilage. J Anat 171:1, 1990.

Bullough PG. Atlas of Orthopedic Pathology with Clinical and Radiologic Correlations, ed 2. New York, Gower Medical Publishing, 1992.

Clark JM. The organization of collagen fibrils in the superficial zones of articular cartilage. J Anat 171:117, 1990.

Gardener DL. Problems and paradigms in joint pathology. J Anat 184:465, 1994.

Hall BK, ed. Bone: A Treatise, vol 5. Fracture Repair and Regeneration. Boca Raton, Fla., CRC Press, 1991.

Hall BK, Newman SA. Molecular Biology of Cartilage. Boca Raton, Fla., CRC Press, 1991.

Holtrop ME. Light and electron microscopic structure of osteoclasts. In: Hall BK, ed. Bone: A Treatise, vol 2. The Osteoclast. Boca Raton, Fla., CRC Press, 1990, p 1.

Hunziker EB. Growth plate structure and function. In: Woessner JF, Howell DS, eds. Joint Cartilage Degeneration: Basic and Clinical Aspects. New York, Marcel Dekker, Inc., 1993.

Hunziker EB. Mechanism of longitudinal bone growth and its regulation by growth plate chondrocytes. Microsc Res Tech 28:505, 1994.

Kuettner KE, Aydelotte MB, Thonar EJ-MA. Articular cartilage matrix and structure: A minireview. J Rheumatol 18(suppl 27):46, 1991.

Mitlak BH, Nussbaum SR. Diagnosis and treatment of osteoporosis. Annu Rev Med 44:265, 1993.

Mundy GR. Bone Remodeling and Its Disorders. London, Martin Dunitz Ltd., 1995.

Poole CA. The structure and function of articular cartilage matrices. In: Woessner JF, Howell DS, eds. Joint Cartilage Degeneration: Basic and Clinical Aspects. New York, Marcel Dekker, Inc., 1993.

Prestwood KM, Pilbeam CC, Raisz LG. Treatment of osteoporosis. Annu Rev Med 46:249, 1995.

Rosenberg ZS, Shankman S, Steiner GC, Kastenbaum DK, Norman A, Lazansky MG. Rapid destructive osteoarthritis: Clinical, radiographic, and pathologic features. Radiology 182:213, 1992.

Salter RB. Continuous Passive Motion (CPM): A Biological Concept for the Healing and Regeneration of Articular Cartilage, Ligaments, and Tendons. Baltimore, Md., Williams & Wilkins, 1993.

Sevitt S. Bone Repair and Fracture Healing in Man. Edinburgh, Churchill-Livingstone, 1981.

Väänänen HK. Pathogenesis of osteoporosis. Calcif Tissue Int 49(Suppl):S11, 1991.

Woessner JF, Howell DS, eds. Joint Cartilage Degeneration: Basic and Clinical Aspects. New York, Marcel Dekker, Inc., 1993.

Muscle

(For further references on cardiac and smooth muscle, see Chap. 5.)

Ashcroft FM. Ca^{2+} and excitation-contraction coupling. Curr Opin Cell Biol 3:671, 1991.

Byers TJ, Kunkel LM, Watkins SC. The subcellular distribution of dystrophin in mouse skeletal, cardiac, and smooth muscle. J Cell Biol 115:411, 1991.

Campion DR. The muscle satellite cell: A review. Int Rev Cytol 87:225, 1984.

Drachman DB. Myasthenia gravis. N Engl J Med 298:136,186, 1978.

Ervasti JM, Campbell KP. Membrane organization of the dystrophin-glycoprotein complex. Cell 66:1121, 1991.

Hilton-Jones D, Squier MV. Dystrophin-associated protein complex: Clinical implications. Lancet 341:528, 1993.

Huxley HE. Sliding filaments and molecular motile systems. J Biol Chem 265:8347, 1990.

Huxley HE. A personal view of muscle and motility mechanisms. Annu Rev Physiol 58:1, 1996.

Jorgensen AO, Shen AC-Y, Arnold W, McPherson PS, Campbell KP. The Ca^{2+}-release channel/ryanodine receptor is localized in junctional and corbular sarcoplasmic reticulum in cardiac muscle. J Cell Biol 120:969, 1993.

Pasternak C, Wong S, Elson EL. Mechanical function of dystrophin in muscle cells. J Cell Biol 128:355, 1995.

Petrof BJ, Shrager JB, Stedman HH, Kelly AM, Sweeney HL. Dystrophin protects the sarcolemma from stresses developed during muscle contraction. Proc Natl Acad Sci U S A 90:3710, 1993.

Nervous Tissue

Bolser DC, Hobbs SF, Chandler MJ, Ammons WS, Brennan TJ, Foreman RD. Convergence of phrenic and cardiopulmonary spinal afferent information on cervical and thoracic spinothalamic tract neurons in the monkey: Implications for referred pain from the diaphragm and heart. J Neurophysiol 65:1042, 1991.

Bunge RP, Bunge MB, Bates M. Movements of the Schwann cell nucleus implicate progression of the inner (axon-related) Schwann cell process during myelination. J Cell Biol 109:273, 1989.

Thomas WE. Brain macrophages: Evaluation of microglia and their functions. Brain Res Rev 17:61, 1992.

Vale RD. Intracellular transport using microtubule-based motors. Annu Rev Cell Biol 3:347, 1987.

Vallee RB, Bloom GS. Mechanisms of fast and slow axonal transport. Annu Rev Neurosci 14:59, 1991.

Wilkin GP, Marriott DR, Cholewinski AJ. Astrocyte heterogeneity. Trends Neurosci 13:43, 1990.

Review Items: Cross References

Information relevant to the Review Items listed in this chapter may be found in the following pages of Cormack, DH. Essential Histology. Philadelphia, J.B. Lippincott, 1993:

REVIEW ITEM	PAGES AND FIGURES
4-1	180–181
4-3	230
4-4	219 and Fig. 10-6
4-6	204–205
4-7	205, 211

CHAPTER 5

Cardiovascular and Lymphatic Systems

CASE 5-1

For the last 2 years, Millie Garcia, aged 42 years, has been distressed by shortness of breath that she experiences when she exerts herself. Strenuous activity makes her cough. Sometimes her sputum looks pink and frothy, and on several occasions in recent months it has been flecked or streaked with red blood. Millie often gets palpitation, attacks of which are becoming increasingly frequent. One day, she coughs up a small quantity of red blood in her sputum. She decides that it is time to seek medical advice.

Millie's medical history indicates that at the age of 9 she had rheumatic fever. A chest x-ray shows that her heart is enlarged. Auscultation of the heart and echocardiography indicate that she has valvular disease. Figure 5-1 shows her mitral valve after its surgical excision.

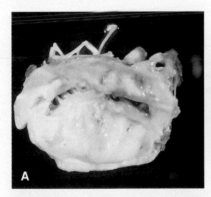
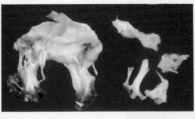
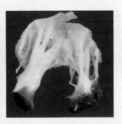

A   B   C

FIGURE 5-1 (**A**) Photograph of the mitral valve in Case 5-1 (atrial aspect of the closed valve). This patient's mitral valve is characterized by having limited mobility and a narrow, crescent-shaped orifice. Small, flat calcified nodules known as vegetations may be discerned along the line of cusp apposition. (**B**) Photograph of the component cusps of this mitral valve, showing the atrial aspect of its large, semicircular anterior cusp on the left and the three component scallops (lateral, central, and medial) of its shallower posterior cusp on the right, together with their attached chordae tendineae. The thickened free edge of the anterior cusp shows several calcified fibrous nodules. Its thickened chordae tendineae may be seen to advantage in **C**, which illustrates the ventricular aspect of the anterior cusp. Some retraction, shortening, and irregular thickening has also occurred in the posterior cusp.

ANALYSIS
Case 5-1

A What tissues are normally found in a cusp (leaflet) of the mitral valve?

B What is the chief cardiac problem in patients who have recurring bouts of rheumatic fever?

C Which other cardiac valves are also commonly affected in rheumatic fever?

D What is known about the cause of valve deformity in this condition?

E What caused this patient's dyspnea and cough?

F What caused this patient's episode of overt hemoptysis?

G Which parts of this patient's heart do you think are enlarged?

(The answers to these questions are considered in part D5-1 of the Discussion section of this chapter.)

CASE 5-2

Mervyn Brown, aged 61 years, is a corpulent, highly strung business executive. His blood pressure is 170/95. In recent years, he has been preoccupied with not feeling well and the fact that his younger brother, who also had hypertension, died unexpectedly at the age of 52. Just before an important appointment, he becomes short of breath even though he is not hurrying. Ten days later, he experiences a transitory loss of vision in his left eye and develops a headache on the same side. He resolves both to cut back his cigarettes to one pack per day and to avoid overexertion.

Mervyn suffers an 8-minute episode of severe chest discomfort, of apparent cardiac origin, and is admitted to hospital. In response to questioning, he recalls a previous episode of epigastric pain, associated with profuse sweating and profound fatigue, that occurred a few weeks ago. While he is in the coronary care unit, he develops other complications, including severe dyspnea. His condition fails to improve with therapy and he does not survive. Some representative regions of his myocardium, together with the appearance of its posterior interventricular artery, are shown in Figs. 5-2 and 5-3A,B.

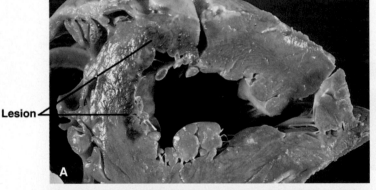

Lesion

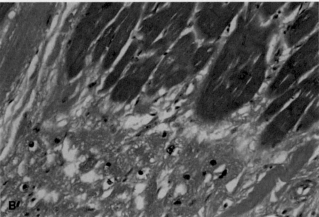

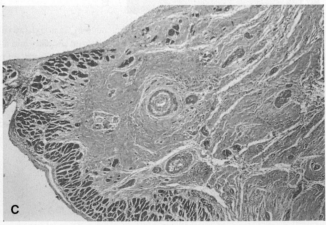

FIGURE 5-2 (**A**) Appearance of cut surface of the heart in Case 5-2. (**B**) Histological appearance of the red area seen in the left ventricular wall in **A**. (**C**) Section of a different part of the left ventricle in same patient's heart.

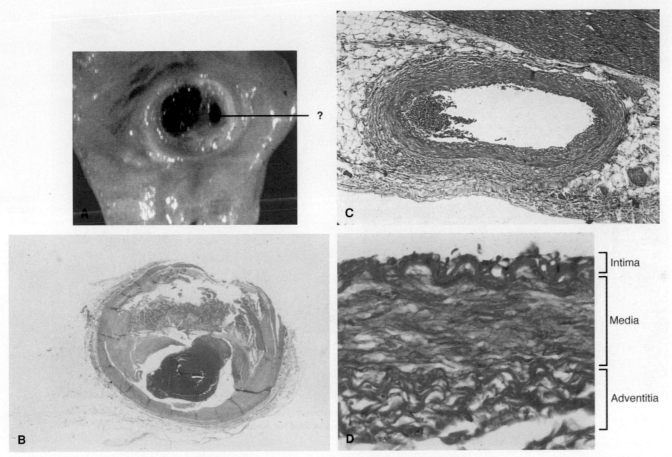

FIGURE 5-3 (**A**) Posterior descending branch of the right coronary artery (posterior interventricular artery) from Case 5-2. [The feature labeled (?) is potentially informative.] (**B**) Section of the posterior interventricular artery from Case 5-2 (low power). (**C**) Section of a normal coronary artery (posterior interventricular artery, low power). (**D**) Details of the wall in a normal coronary artery (posterior interventricular artery, medium power).

ANALYSIS
Case 5-2

A Are any normal cardiac muscle fibers distinguishable in parts B and C of Fig. 5-2?

B What does part B of Fig. 5-2 reveal about part A of this illustration? What does part C show? Can you account for any significant differences between parts B and C of this illustration?

C How did the changes seen in Fig. 5-3A,B cause the reddish lesion seen in the left ventricular wall in Fig. 5-2A?

D What is the likely cause of this patient's transitory visual disturbance? What other risks did he have?

E Figure 5-4 shows another example of a coronary artery. Which layers of its wall show histological changes?

(The answers are considered in part D5-2 of the Discussion section of this chapter.)

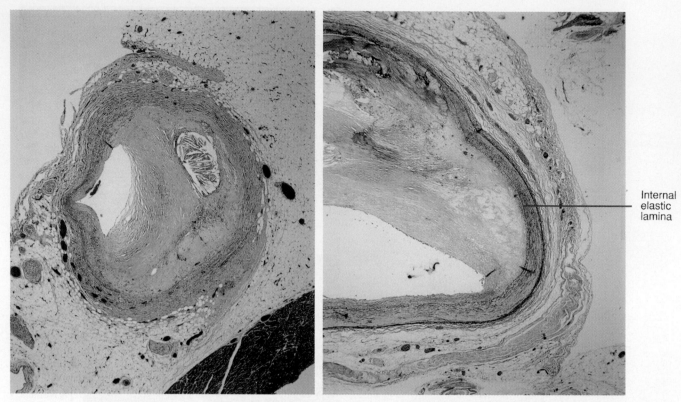

Internal elastic lamina

FIGURE 5-4 What changes have occurred in these coronary arteries? (**A**) Low power, trichrome stain. (**B**) Higher magnification, stained for elastin (*black*).

ESSENTIAL FEATURES OF CARDIAC MUSCLE

Cardiac muscle constitutes the muscular walls of the heart (*myocardium*). This specialized type of muscle is also present in the pulmonary vein and superior vena cava. In contrast to the motor neuron-dependent arrangement by which contraction is elicited in skeletal muscles, each contraction of the myocardium is triggered by the *spontaneous* depolarization of cardiac *pacemaker cells*. Cardiac contractions are, therefore, considered to be *intrinsic* (ie, *myogenic*) as well as *involuntary*.

The functional unit of the myocardium is the *cardiac muscle fiber*. Each cardiac fiber is a series of muscle cells that are joined end to end by unique structures known as *intercalated disks*. At an intercalated disk, more than one cardiac muscle cell may be attached to the adjacent cell (Fig. 5-5). Cardiac muscle fibers, therefore, branch and anastomose with each other. Also, some of these fibers (eg, Purkinje fibers) are wider than usual and possess fewer myofibrils because they are specialized for conduction rather than contraction.

The endomysium that lies between the muscle fibers is highly vascular and each fiber has a surrounding basement membrane. Because cardiac muscle cells do not divide and satellite cells (ie, repair cells) are absent, *cardiac muscle does not regenerate*. Each cardiac muscle cell possesses one or two central nuclei (generally only one). Recognition of (1) central nuclei, (2) striations, and (3) intercalated disks permits a positive identification of this type of muscle. Branching is not very easy to recognize.

Every constituent cell of the myocardium participates in each rhythmic wave of contraction that progresses through the heart. The force of contraction de-

REVIEW ITEM 5-1

What types of cell junctions are found in cardiac muscle fibers? Why are such junctions necessary?

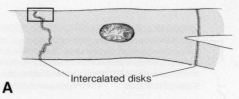

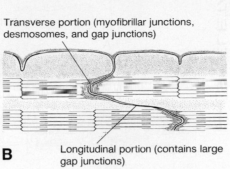

Intercalated disks

A

Transverse portion (myofibrillar junctions, desmosomes, and gap junctions)

B

Longitudinal portion (contains large gap junctions)

FIGURE 5-5 (**A**) Cardiac muscle cell in a cardiac muscle fiber. (**B**) Components of an intercalated disk (area indicated in **A**, enlarged).

pends on both intracellular Ca^{2+} concentration and myocardial ATP production. Also, the heart rate is modulated on a continuous basis.

Calcium Handling

Two clinically important differences between cardiac muscle cells and skeletal muscle cells are (1) the inherent automaticity of pacemaker cells and (2) the absolute dependence of cardiac muscle cells on Ca^{2+} derived from external sources for triggering of their contraction. Without extracellular Ca^{2+}, the heart cannot beat. Figure 5-6 compares some of the details of Ca^{2+} handling in skeletal and cardiac muscle fibers and summarizes some key structural and functional differences between these two types of muscle.

Structural and Functional Organization of Cardiac Muscle Fibers

Figure 5-7 summarizes the chief structural features that may be seen at the EM level in cardiac muscle fibers (Fig. 5-8). It may help to compare Fig. 5-7 with Fig. 4-27, which shows corresponding details in a skeletal muscle fiber.

Essentially, the *intercalated disks* between component muscle cells have transverse portions with adhering (anchoring) junctions and longitudinal portions with gap junctions. The abundant gap junctions in cardiac muscle fibers ensure direct electrical conduction, enabling waves of depolarization to spread from cell to cell over the entire myocardium. Because of these gap junctions, the entire myocardium performs as a functional unit.

In cardiac muscle cells, the myofibrils are arranged peripheral to the nucleus, anastomose with each other, and are of somewhat variable diameter. Their repetitive pattern of sarcomeres and molecular composition are, nevertheless, the same as in skeletal muscle (see Chap. 4). The transverse portions of an intercalated disk lie at the level of Z lines, but the disk may follow a stepwise course as it traverses the muscle fiber (Figs. 5-5 and 5-8, *inset*).

The T tubules of a cardiac muscle cell, together with the remainder of the sarcolemma, admit the triggering amount of Ca^{2+} necessary for each myocardial contraction and are, accordingly, comparatively wide. Unlike their corresponding position in skeletal muscle (ie, the borders between A and I bands), T tubules of cardiac muscle are situated opposite Z lines. The sarcoplasmic reticulum (SR) of cardiac muscle is less extensive than that of skeletal muscle. It con-

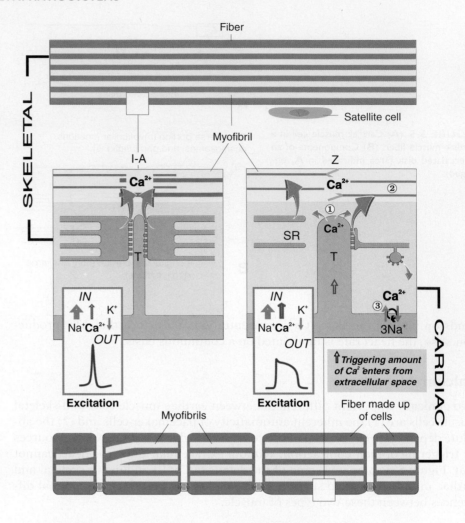

Notes: Gap junctions conduct depolarization along fiber
① Extracellular Ca² triggers internal Ca²⁺ release
② Force of elicited contraction ∝ myofibrillar [Ca²]
③ Ca²/3Na⁺

FIGURE 5-6 Comparative summary of structure and function in skeletal and cardiac muscle. Respective sources of Ca^{2+}, redistribution of intracellular Ca^{2+} (*represented as purple arrows*) in excitation–contraction coupling, and some other major differences are emphasized. All the Ca^{2+} ions required for a full contraction are supplied by the extensive sarcoplasmic reticulum (SR) in skeletal muscle fibers. In contrast, the Ca^{2+} ions held in the SR of cardiac muscle cells are not released until a triggering amount of Ca^{2+} has entered the cell from the extracellular fluid (1). The sarcolemma and T tubules of a cardiac muscle cell have a voltage-dependent "slow" Ca^{2+} channel that opens during the plateau phase of the action potential (*see excitation panel for cardiac muscle*), admitting the Ca^{2+} that triggers Ca^{2+} release from the SR. They also have a voltage-sensitive gated channel that during contraction exchanges extracellular Ca^{2+} for intracellular Na^+ (3). The brief action potential in skeletal muscle ensures a rapid response to efferent impulses and facilitates voluntary control of contraction. The longer action potential in cardiac muscle prolongs opening of the voltage-dependent "slow" Ca^{2+} channel and protects against tetanization.

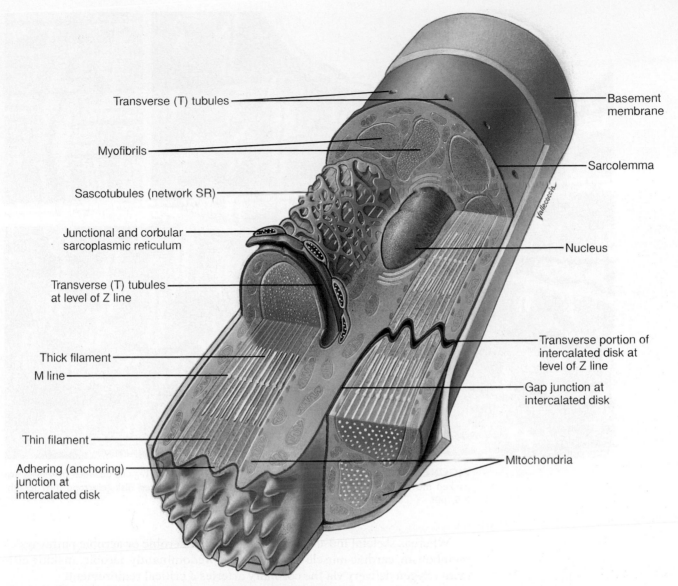

Transverse (T) tubules

Myofibrils

Sascotubules (network SR)

Junctional and corbular
sarcoplasmic reticulum

Transverse (T) tubules
at level of Z line

Thick filament

M line

Thin filament

Adhering (anchoring)
junction at
intercalated disk

Basement
membrane

Sarcolemma

Nucleus

Transverse portion of
intercalated disk at
level of Z line

Gap junction at
intercalated disk

MItochondria

FIGURE 5-7 Structure of a cardiac musce fiber, as established by electron microscopy.

sists chiefly of anastomosing sarcotubules (*network SR*) and lacks the distinctive, large terminal cisternae that constitute a key component of the triads of skeletal muscle. Nevertheless, lying in close apposition with the sarcolemma and T tubules are regions of *junctional SR* that are provided with Ca^{2+} release channels. Bulbous and saccular distentions of the SR (shown at *middle right* in Fig. 5-6, next to junctional SR) are similarly provided with Ca^{2+} release channels. Termed *corbular SR*, these distentions are considered additional storage and release sites for Ca^{2+}.

The total amount of Ca^{2+} that can be sequestered in the three regions of the SR is substantially smaller than in skeletal muscle. Moreover, Ca^{2+} release (and resulting access to the myofibrils) depends on entry into the cytosol of a triggering amount of Ca^{2+} from the extracellular space (see Fig. 5-6). In contrast, skeletal muscle fibers are self-sufficient with respect to Ca^{2+}, since their extensive SR can store enough Ca^{2+} for a full contraction and release it all in response to an action potential.

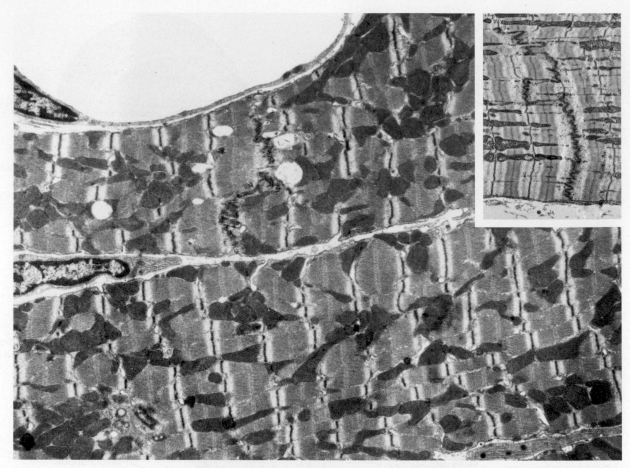

FIGURE 5-8 Cardiac muscle (electron micrograph, ×6,500). The regions between myofibrils are packed mostly with mitochondria. (*Inset*) Portion of an intercalated disk (electron micrograph, ×5,100).

Whereas skeletal muscle can utilize either anaerobic or aerobic pathways of metabolism, cardiac muscle metabolism is predominantly aerobic, making efficient oxygen delivery via the coronary arteries a critical requirement.

A summary of the comparative features of cardiac, skeletal, and smooth muscle is given in Table 5-1.

ESSENTIAL FEATURES OF THE HEART

The walls of the heart are made up of (1) a lining connective tissue layer called the *endocardium*, (2) the cardiac musculature or *myocardium*, and (3) a covering connective tissue layer known as the *epicardium*. Deep to the lining endothelial membrane of the endocardium, the loose connective tissue commonly contains adipocytes. The epicardium consists of adipocyte-containing fibroelastic connective tissue and a covering mesothelium. The *pericardium* is a fibrous sac with a serous lining that encloses a narrow potential space (the *pericardial cavity*). As may be seen in Fig. 5-9, the visceral layer of serous pericardium is the same membrane as the epicardial mesothelium.

A roughly triangular mass of fibrous connective tissue known as a *trigonum fibrosum* is continuous with fibrous supporting rings that resist dilatation at the origins of the aorta and pulmonary artery. The mitral and tricuspid valves are supported by similar fibrous rings. The various fibrous components are con-

TABLE 5-1
TYPES OF MUSCLE: COMPARATIVE FEATURES

Feature	Skeletal Muscle	Cardiac Muscle	Smooth Muscle
Structural characteristics	Fiber = multinucleated cell	Fiber = branching row of cells	Fiber = cell
	Peripheral nucleus	Central nucleus	Central nucleus
	Cells interconnected by fibrous sheaths	Cells interconnected by intercalated disks	Cells interconnected by connective tissue
	Myofibrils composed of sarcomeres	Myofibrils composed of sarcomeres	No myofibrils or sarcomeres
	T tubules situated at A band-I band interface	T tubules (wider) situated at Z lines	Caveolae randomly situated
	Extensive SR (sarcotubules and large terminal cisternae)	Less extensive SR (sarcotubular network, junctional, and corbular)	Small, simple sarcotubular SR
Regulation of contraction	Voluntary regulation of full contraction in each fiber by efferent impulses from a lower motor neuron	Involuntary regulation of pacemaker-generated heart rate by autonomic nerve impulses reaching S-A and A-V nodes	Involuntary regulation of contraction by autonomic nerve impulses reaching innervated cells*
			Other contraction-eliciting stimuli are hormones and stretch
	Force of contraction depends on no. of motor units participating	Force of contraction depends on the internal Ca^{2+} concentration	Force of contraction is Ca^{2+}-modulated; partial contraction can be maintained in each cell
	Actin–myosin interaction is regulated by troponin	Actin–myosin interaction is regulated by troponin	Actin–myosin interaction is regulated by calmodulin and caldesmon
Excitation	Motor nerve impulses elicit depolarization	Spontaneous depolarization of pacemaker cells spreads because of gap junctions	Elicited depolarization of innervated cells spreads because of gap junctions
Source of the Ca^{2+} needed for contraction	Released from SR	Triggering amount of extracellular Ca^{2+}; remainder released from SR	Triggering amount of extracellular Ca^{2+}; remainder released from SR
Growth and regeneration	Growth through hypertrophy	Growth through hypertrophy	Growth through hypertrophy and hyperplasia
	Limited regeneration from myoblasts arising from satellite cells; muscle fibers do not divide	Does not regenerate; lacks satellite cells; muscle cells do not divide	Regenerates readily both through mitosis and also from pericytes

*Whereas in visceral smooth muscles only a small proportion of the muscle cells are directly innervated, in multiunit smooth muscles all of them are directly innervated.

nected with each other and also with the membranous part of the interventricular septum. Myocardial muscle fibers insert into this fibrous mass, so it is sometimes described as the *skeleton* of the heart. The microscopic structure of *heart valves* is considered in part D5-1 of the Discussion section of this chapter.

Cardiac Impulse Conduction

A distinctive feature of the cardiac *pacemaker cells* of the sinoatrial (S-A) node is their intrinsic rhythm of *spontaneous depolarization*. This is largely attributable to a slow inward passage of extracellular Ca^{2+} due to increased Ca^{2+} membrane conductance during diastole. The steady rise in internal net positive charge gradually depolarizes the cell membrane from -90 mV (relative to the cell exterior) to -50 mV, the threshold potential at which an action potential is generated. Subsidiary pacemaker cells that can assume pacemaker function exist in

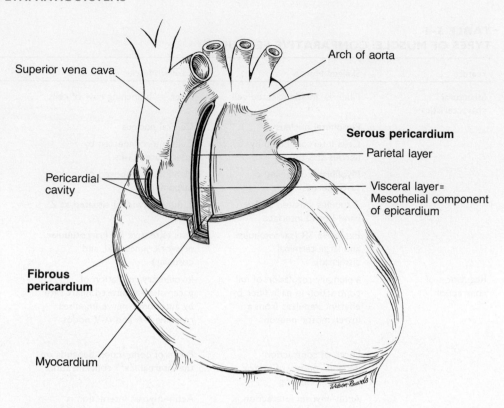

FIGURE 5-9 The membranous layers enclosing the myocardium.

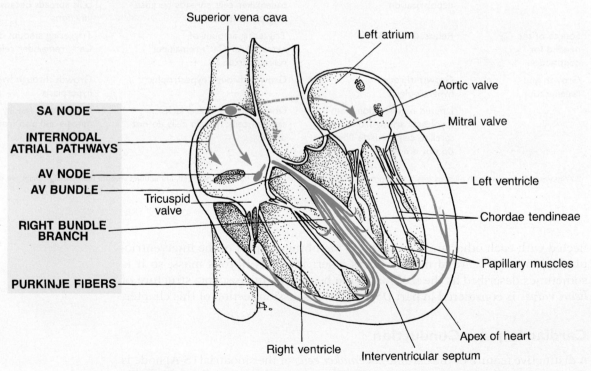

FIGURE 5-10 The cardiac impulse-conducting pathways (seen in a coronal plane).

the atrioventricular (A-V) node, and latent pacemaker cells exist in other parts of the cardiac conducting system, but their spontaneous depolarization rate is slower.

Under ordinary circumstances, depolarization of the myocardium commences at the *S-A node*, which is situated in the right wall of the superior vena cava at its junction with the right atrium (Fig. 5-10). A wave of depolarization is initiated that is conducted by the *internodal atrial pathways* to the *A-V node*, which lies in the lower part of the interatrial septum, near the opening of the coronary sinus. Here, conduction is momentarily delayed, providing time for atrial depolarization to approach completion. Ensuing rapid conduction by *Purkinje fibers* extending from right and left branches of the *A-V bundle* (*bundle of His*) then leads to successive depolarization of the lower region of the inter-ventricular septum, papillary muscles, apical ventricular myocardium and, finally, the upper region of the ventricular myocardium and interventricular septum. The entire impulse-conducting system of the heart is made up of cardiac muscle cells that are specialized for initiating or conducting waves of depolarization and that are coupled electrically by gap junctions.

Autonomic Regulation of Heart Rate

Cardiac sympathetic fibers supply all parts of the heart, chiefly the S-A and A-V nodes and other parts of the conducting system, but also the remainder of the myocardium. *Vagal parasympathetic fibers* supply the two nodes and, primarily, the atrial musculature. Noradrenergic sympathetic stimulation increases the heart rate and increases the force of cardiac contraction. Cholinergic parasympathetic (vagal) stimulation decreases the heart rate and decreases the force of atrial myocardial contraction. Normal vagal tone reduces the heart rate from an intrinsic rate of approximately 100 beats per minute to a resting rate of 68–75 beats per minute.

Myocardial Infarction: Clinical Manifestations

Depending on which sides of the heart become functionally impaired after myocardial infarction, the patient may show signs of left heart failure, right heart failure, or some combination of these. In *left heart failure*, obvious consequences of severe damage to the muscular walls of the left ventricle are (1) dilatation of this ventricle and (2) incomplete emptying of this ventricle during systole. The part of the left ventricular myocardium that survives generally shows evidence of compensatory hypertrophy. Incomplete emptying of the left ventricle also raises the left ventricular diastolic pressure, which elevates the left atrial and pulmonary venous pressures, with resulting pulmonary congestion.

Equivalent changes of the right ventricular wall are seen in *right heart failure*, which may occur when the right ventricular myocardium is severely damaged or when there is pulmonary hypertension, eg, as a consequence of (1) pulmonary congestion in patients with left heart failure or (2) pulmonary disease. Right heart failure leads to systemic congestion, increased venous pressure, and resulting dependent edema, seen chiefly in the ankles (or the presacral region in bedridden patients).

ESSENTIAL FEATURES OF SMOOTH MUSCLE

The functional unit of smooth muscle is the *smooth muscle cell*, known also as a *smooth muscle fiber*. For a comparative summary of the main structural and functional features of smooth muscle cells, see Table 5-1. Their organization as

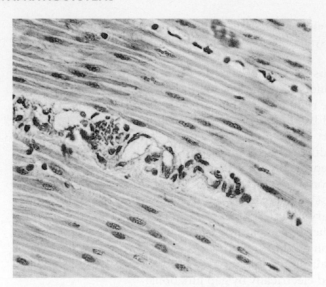

FIGURE 5-11 Smooth muscle fibers in a bundled arrangement with intervening loose connective tissue.

bundles (Fig. 5-11) or helical (circular) and longitudinal *layers* is important for (1) restricting the luminal diameter of tubes and hollow viscera, and (2) propagating peristaltic waves of contraction.

Although contraction is comparatively slow in this type of muscle, it can be partial as well as indefinitely prolonged in each cell, and requires minimal ATP expenditure. Furthermore, in addition to the *contractile* phenotype of smooth muscle cells, there is a *synthetic* phenotype that produces elastin, collagen, and the other interstitial constituents of arterial walls.

Smooth muscle cells contain thin and thick filaments, but the filaments are not arranged in sarcomeres, and Z lines are lacking (Fig. 5-12). Compared with striated muscle fibers, smooth muscle cells contain a higher proportion of actin relative to myosin. Contraction is elicited when a rise in the cytosolic Ca^{2+} concentration causes *calmodulin* to combine with an inactive enzyme precursor to

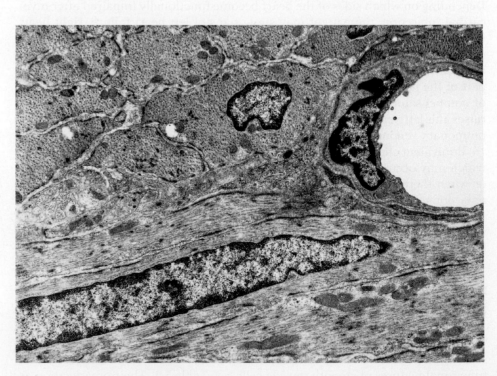

FIGURE 5-12 Smooth muscle cells cut in longitudinal and transverse section (electron micrograph). The vessel at upper right is a capillary.

produce activated *myosin light-chain kinase*. By phosphorylating the myosin, this enzyme promotes myosin assembly into thick filaments, brings about interaction between myosin and actin, and initiates an ATP-dependent contraction. Relaxation is a consequence of ensuing myosin dephosphorylation. Another Ca^{2+}-dependent regulator of smooth muscle contraction, *caldesmon*, is a thin filament constituent.

The SR, only minimally represented in smooth muscle cells, lacks cisternae and consists entirely of sarcotubules. Associated spherical surface invaginations called *caveolae* are considered to be the counterpart of T tubules, which are not present in smooth muscle cells. As in cardiac muscle, depolarization is conducted from cell to cell by gap junctions.

Smooth muscle cells possess the muscarinic type of *cholinergic receptor* and two distinct classes of *adrenergic receptors*, designated α and β, each of which has subtypes.

The structural arrangement through which the contractile forces generated in smooth muscle cells are applied is summarized in Fig. 5-13. Essentially, contractile forces generated when thin filaments slide between thick filaments are transmitted to structures called *dense bodies* that, like Z lines, contain α actinin. Some of the dense bodies lie in the cytoplasm and others are attached to the cell membrane. Intermediate filaments as well as thin filaments are attached to the dense bodies. They transmit the tensile forces produced to the superficial dense bodies, which are then pulled inward (Fig. 5-13B). The regions of cell membrane that lie between superficial dense bodies balloon out, and the long axis of the cell shortens.

ESSENTIAL FEATURES OF BLOOD VESSELS AND LYMPHATICS

The chief histological features of the various blood vessels are summarized in Table 5-2. The wall structures of some major blood vessels are compared in Figs. 5-14 and 5-15.

In arteries, most of the elastin produced by smooth muscle cells is deposited in the form of *fenestrated elastic laminae. Elastic fibers* are, nevertheless, assembled as well. Loss of elastin, particularly from elastic arteries, leads to arterial dilatation. Permanent dilatation (eg, aortic *aneurysm*) is potentially dangerous because it can lead to internal splitting or rupture of the vessel wall and uncontrollable hemorrhage.

The outer region of the wall of large and medium-sized blood vessels (in particular, those vessels that have a substantial adventitia or media or that carry deoxygenated blood) is sustained by small nutrient vessels termed *vasa vasorum*. In the thoracic aorta, vasa vasorum supply the outer two thirds of the media as well as the adventitia. In large muscular arteries, the vasa vasorum extend in only as far as the periphery of the media. In large veins, they supply the muscular adventitia, and in medium-sized veins that possess a fairly substantial wall (eg, femoral and saphenous veins), they supply the adventitia and at least the outer half of the muscular media. Vasa vasorum are more plentiful in veins than in arteries. The walls of veins also contain an abundance of lymphatic capillaries, which provides a potential route for the spread of disseminating cancer cells.

Veins are provided with *valve leaflets* that are similar in construction to those of the heart. However, poorly supported superficial veins of the lower extremity have a tendency to become dilated, eg, as part of the aging process. Venous

Relaxed

Intermediate   Thin
filaments   filaments

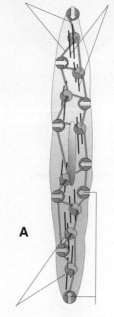

A

Internal   Superficial
dense   dense bodies
bodies

Contracted

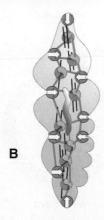

B

FIGURE 5-13 Essential basis of smooth muscle contraction.

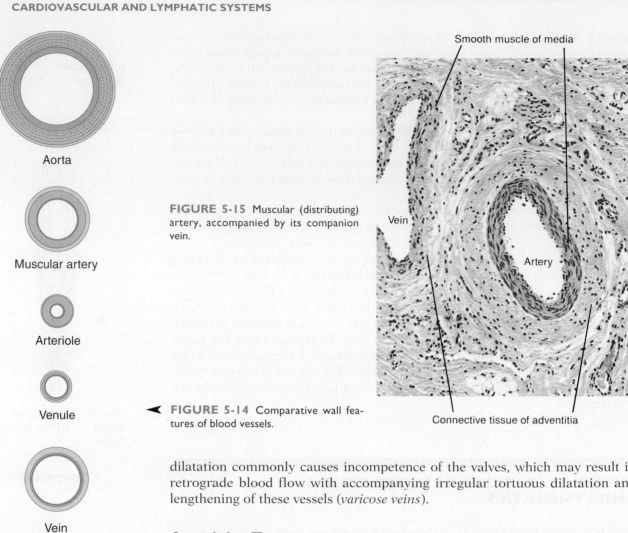

Aorta

Muscular artery

Arteriole

Venule

Vein

Vena cava

FIGURE 5-15 Muscular (distributing) artery, accompanied by its companion vein.

Smooth muscle of media

Vein

Artery

Connective tissue of adventitia

◄ **FIGURE 5-14** Comparative wall features of blood vessels.

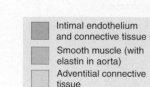
Intimal endothelium and connective tissue

Smooth muscle (with elastin in aorta)

Adventitial connective tissue

dilatation commonly causes incompetence of the valves, which may result in retrograde blood flow with accompanying irregular tortuous dilatation and lengthening of these vessels (*varicose veins*).

Arteriolar Tonus

One of the main determinants involved in the regulation of systemic blood pressure is the total peripheral resistance to blood flow. An important component of the peripheral resistance is the degree of partial contraction (*tonus*) in the smooth muscle cells in the media of arterioles. Increased arteriolar smooth muscle tonus (ie, arteriolar vasoconstriction) significantly contributes to essential hypertension that is vascular resistance-dependent. A further increase in peripheral resistance may occur if the muscular media undergoes hypertrophy that leads to permanent constriction of the arteriolar lumen. (Some key regulators of vascular smooth muscle tone are listed in Table 5-3.)

Atherosclerotic Plaques

In muscular (distributing) arteries, the intima is normally very thin, basically consisting of endothelium, its basement membrane, and the internal elastic lamina. Intimal thickening is considered suggestive of *endothelial injury*, and additional finding of *monocytes, macrophages*, or *smooth muscle cells* is considered indicative of development of *atherosclerotic (atheromatous) plaques*. These plaques can predispose to (1) formation of local or spreading and splitting ("dissecting") aneurysms and (2) platelet aggregation, with ensuing thrombosis and an associated heightened risk of regional infarction. A general outline of the key stages that contribute to the atherosclerotic process is given in Table 5-4. (For additional information, *see* Case 5-2 Analysis and part D5-2 of the Discussion section of this chapter.)

KEY CONCEPT

Roughly half the total vascular peripheral resistance is exerted by arterioles in large muscle masses.

TABLE 5-2
BLOOD VESSELS AND LYMPHATICS: CHIEF FUNCTIONAL ROLES AND WALL STRUCTURE

Vessel	Functional Roles	Intima	Media	Adventitia
Elastic artery	Conveys blood from the heart and maintains diastolic pressure	Endothelium, elastic laminae, smooth muscle cells, and fibroblasts	Elastic laminae with smooth muscle cells; vasa vasorum	Thin layer of connective tissue; vasa vasorum
Muscular (distributing) artery	Supplies body site with required volume of oxygenated blood	Endothelium and internal elastic lamina	Smooth muscle cells with elastin; vasa vasorum	Thick layer of connective tissue; vasa vasorum
Medium vein	Conveys blood toward the heart	Endothelium and minimal amount of connective tissue; valves	Smooth muscle cells and connective tissue; vasa vasorum	Relatively thick layer of connective tissue, with some smooth muscle cells; vasa vasorum
Large vein	Returns blood to the heart	Endothelium and connective tissue	Smooth muscle cells; vasa vasorum	Thick layer of connective tissue, with longitudinal bundles of smooth muscle; vasa vasorum
Arteriole	Regulates local blood flow and reduces blood pressure	Endothelium and internal elastic lamina	Smooth muscle cells (one or two layers)	Thin layer of connective tissue
Venule	Collects blood from capillaries	Endothelium and pericytes	Smooth muscle cells (single layer)	Very thin layer of connective tissue
Metarteriole	Regulates blood flow through capillaries	Endothelium	Smooth muscle cells (one discontinuous layer)	Extremely thin layer of connective tissue
Capillary	Produces tissue fluid; facilitates extracellular exchanges through transcytosis and diffusion	Endothelium (continuous or fenestrated) and pericytes	Not represented	Minimal amount of connective tissue
Lymphatic capillary	Collects excess fluid from the interstitial space	Endothelium (with a discontinuous or absent basement membrane)	Not represented	Extremely thin layer of connective tissue, with anchoring filaments
Large lymphatic	Conveys lymph toward lymphatic ducts	Endothelium and connective tissue; valves	Thin layer of smooth muscle cells and connective tissue	Fairly thin layer of connective tissue, with some smooth muscle cells

Microcirculation

The components of the terminal vascular bed that may be recognized easily in sections are arterioles, venules, and capillaries (Fig. 5-16). Arterial vessels that are <100 μm in overall diameter are called *arterioles*. Their distinguishing features include (1) a muscular media characterized by *one or two circular (helical) layers of smooth muscle cells* (Fig. 5-16B), (2) a wall thickness that approximates the luminal diameter, and (3) a reasonably distinct internal elastic lamina, at least in the larger arterioles (Fig. 5-16A). *Venules* are thin-walled vessels, 8–100 μm in diameter, that possess either a single layer of associated smooth muscle cells (which constitute the media of *muscular venules*) or a single layer of associated pericytes (which lie in the intima of *postcapillary* and *collecting venules*). *Capillaries* are vessels with a luminal diameter of 8–10 μm. External to their endothelium lies a discontinuous layer of intimal pericytes that are enclosed by the endothelial basement membrane (Fig. 5-17). The endothelium of endocrine capillaries and renal glomeruli is typically *fenestrated*. Delivery of arterial blood to capillary beds is regulated by *arterioles* and *metarterioles*. Since distal ends of metarterioles empty into venules (Fig. 5-18), metarterioles are able to function as bypass channels and capillary beds may fill only intermittently.

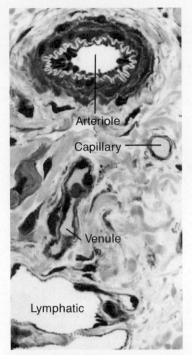

Arteriole

Capillary

Venule

Lymphatic

Endothelial cells

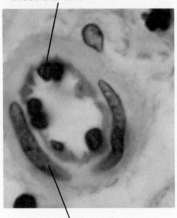

Smooth muscle cells

FIGURE 5-16 (**A**) Arteriole, capillary, venule, and lymphatic. (**B**) Arteriole (higher magnification).

TABLE 5-3
KEY REGULATORS OF PERIPHERAL VASCULAR TONUS

		Vasoconstrictor	Vasodilator
Systemic regulators		Impulses from noradrenergic sympathetic vasoconstrictor nerve fibers (important regulatory mechanism in all body parts)	Impulses from cholinergic sympathetic vasodilator nerve fibers (subsidiary in skeletal muscle)
			Impulses from cholinergic parasympathetic vasodilator nerve fibers (a few body parts, eg, penis)
		Norepinephrine	
		Epinephrine (other body parts)	Epinephrine (heart, skeletal muscles, lungs, and liver)
		Vasopressin ($=$ antidiuretic hormone)	Vasodilator drugs, eg, glyceryl trinitrate (nitroglycerin)
		Angiotensin II (a renin-generated product)	Kinins
Local regulators			Metabolites (eg, CO_2, H^+, K^+, lactate, and adenosine in cardiac muscle)
		Endothelin (from endothelial cells)	Nitric oxide ($=$ endothelium-derived relaxing factor)
		Serotonin (from aggregated platelets)	Histamine (eg, in acute inflammation)
		Thromboxane A_2	Lipoxin A
		Leukotrienes (eg, in allergic inflammation)	
		Prostaglandin $F_{2\alpha}$	Prostaglandins E_1, E_2, D_2, I_2, and I_3

Basement membrane   Pericyte process

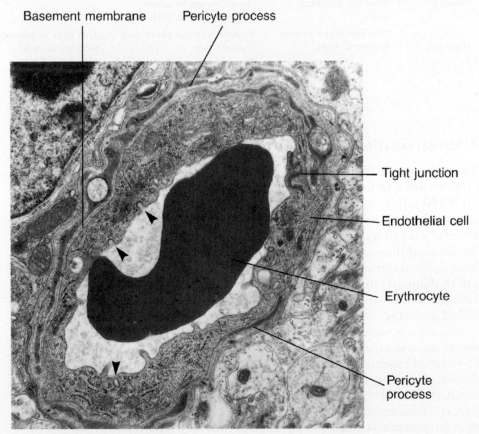

Tight junction

Endothelial cell

Erythrocyte

Pericyte process

FIGURE 5-17 Capillary (electron micrograph). Arrowheads indicate coated pits, where endocytosis is occurring.

TABLE 5-4
ATHEROSCLEROTIC PROGRESSION IN ARTERIAL WALLS

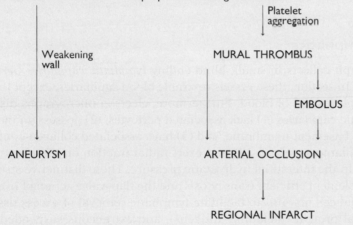

INTACT WALL

↓

Endothelial damage admits monocytes, T lymphocytes, and LDL.

Damage is potentially reversible because endothelial cells can proliferate and migrate.

Damage triggers production of cytokines and growth factors.

↓

FATTY STREAK

Further production of cytokines and growth factors by endothelial cells, smooth muscle cells, and monocytes/macrophages, eg, PDGF, FGF, TGF-β, IL-1*.

Lipid-laden, proliferating motile macrophages accumulate in the intima (monocyte-derived *foam cells*).

Smooth muscle cells migrate from media to intima, where they proliferate and accumulate lipid (additional *foam cells*).

T lymphocytes (some CD8+, others CD4+) produce cytokines and growth factors.

↓

FIBROUS PLAQUE

Continuing production of cytokines and growth factors, notably by endothelial cells, smooth muscle cells, and macrophages.

Continuing proliferation of smooth muscle cells and macrophages.

Accumulation of ECM* constituents, eg, collagen, proteoglycans, elastin, and glycoproteins, produced by smooth muscle cells and endothelial cells.

Accumulation of extracellular lipid.

Surface ulceration with central necrosis of the plaque and ensuing calcification.

```
                                              | Platelet
                                              | aggregation
                                              ↓
            | Weakening                   MURAL THROMBUS
            | wall                             |
                                              ↓
                                           EMBOLUS
                                              |
                                              ↓
    ANEURYSM                            ARTERIAL OCCLUSION
                                              |
                                              ↓
                                        REGIONAL INFARCT
```

*ECM = extracellular matrix; FGF = fibroblast growth factor; IL-1 = interleukin 1; LDL = low density lipoprotein; PDGF = platelet-derived growth factor (also produced by endothelial and smooth muscle cells); TGF-β = transforming growth factor-beta.

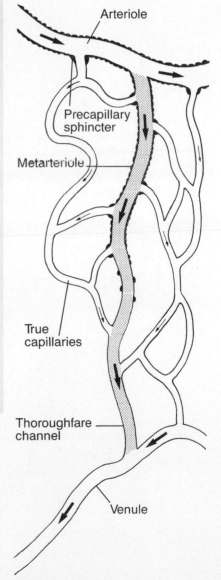

FIGURE 5-18 Constituent vessels of the microcirculation.

- Arteriole
- Precapillary sphincter
- Metarteriole
- True capillaries
- Thoroughfare channel
- Venule

**REVIEW ITEM
(FIG. 5-19)**

Identify, as precisely as possible, the type of blood vessel seen in Fig. 5-19. (To confirm your answer, see Part D5-3 of the Discussion section of this chapter).

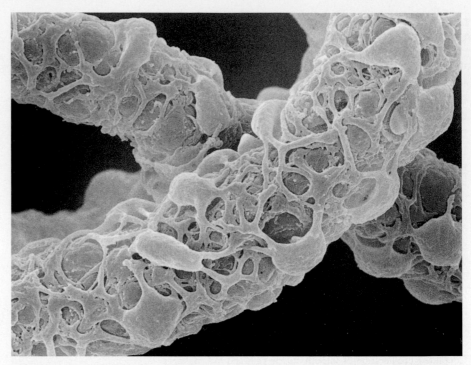

FIGURE 5-19 Unidentified vessel (scanning electron micrograph, ×2,300). See Review Item.

Lymphatics

Lymph collects in small, blind-ending *lymphatic capillaries* (*terminal lymphatics*). In section, these vessels resemble blood capillaries, except that they contain lymph instead of blood. Furthermore, electron micrographs disclose that lymphatic capillaries (1) lack associated pericytes, (2) possess an incomplete or absent basement membrane, and (3) have associated collagen-containing anchoring filaments (Fig. 5-20) that exert radial traction on these vessels if there is a rise in the interstitial hydrostatic pressure. These distinctive structural features supplement efficient transcytosis and the flap–valve action of overlapping endothelial cell margins to facilitate lymphatic removal of excess tissue fluid, interstitial protein (including antigens), and extraneous suspended particles. The negative intraluminal hydrostatic pressure that draws excess tissue fluid into lymphatic capillaries is apparently generated by contractile activity of the lymphatic endothelium. Under conditions of local edema, the radial traction transmitted by anchoring filaments is increased, and this holds these small thin-walled vessels open and promotes lymphatic drainage.

The thin-walled, medium-sized *lymphatics* (see Fig. 5-16A) that receive lymph from the lymphatic capillaries have some smooth muscle cells in their media and adventitia. Like veins, larger lymphatics are provided with flap-like valve leaflets. Peristaltic contractions supplement the effects of external compression and propel lymph toward the thoracic duct and right lymphatic duct. Originating in the abdomen as the *cisterna chyli*, the *thoracic duct* enters the thorax and opens into the junction between the left internal jugular and subclavian veins. The right lymphatic duct opens into the corresponding junction on the right side.

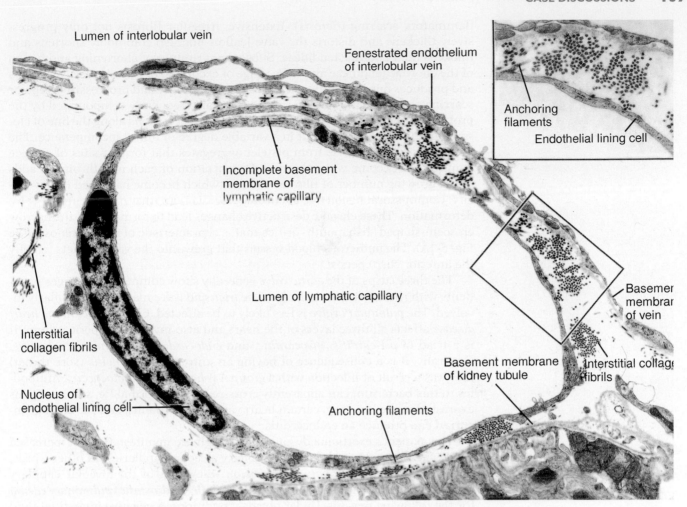

Lumen of interlobular vein

Fenestrated endothelium
of interlobular vein

Anchoring
filaments

Endothelial lining cell

Incomplete basement
membrane of
lymphatic capillary

Interstitial
collagen fibrils

Lumen of lymphatic capillary

Basemen
membran
of vein

Nucleus of
endothelial lining cell

Basement membrane
of kidney tubule

Interstitial collage
fibrils

Anchoring filaments

FIGURE 5-20 Lymphatic capillary (electron micrograph, ×10,000). *(Inset)* Area indicated by box,
seen at twice the magnification.

CASE DISCUSSIONS

D5-1 (CASE 5-1)

The cusps of the mitral valve are strong, thin, membranous leaflets with a core
of dense irregular connective tissue. Their central fibrous plate contains numerous elastic fibers that are relatively abundant in the subendothelial tissue on
the atrial side of the leaflet. On each side, this fibrous tissue is covered by a thin
layer of loose connective tissue with overlying endothelium. The central fibrous
tissue is continuous with the fibrous core of the attached chordae tendineae and
also with the fibrous ring that surrounds the valve orifice. Normally, only the
base of the valve leaflet is vascularized, and smooth muscle cells are restricted
to the base of the leaflet.

A major clinical problem in patients with recurring bouts of rheumatic fever
is gradual but progressive restriction of the orifice of the mitral valve, ie, *mitral
stenosis.* The leaflets (anterior and posterior cusps) of this valve typically undergo a series of changes. An initial phase of *inflammation* and accompanying
vascularization in the leaflets is followed by a more protracted phase of postin-

flammatory scarring (*fibrosis*). Extensive, irregular fibrosis not only progressively thickens and distorts the valve leaflets but also commonly shortens and thickens their chordae tendineae. Subsequent rupture or shortening and fusion of the chordae tendineae alters the range of excursion of the mitral valve leaflets and produces mitral insufficiency. Decreased mobility and progressive irregular scarring or calcification of the valve leaflets are frequently compounded by the protrusion of small abnormal nodules known as *vegetations* along the line of closure, and these changes result in a variable degree of mitral incompetence. The protruding nodules arise from platelet aggregates that form at sites of surface damage and become white thrombi. Organization of each new thrombus adds to the growing number of fibrous nodules, which become hardened if they calcify. Commissural fusion due to chronic fibrosis is another major cause of valve deformation. These chronic destructive changes lead to formation of the narrow crescent-shaped "fish mouth" orifice that is characteristic of mitral stenosis (see Fig. 5-1A). The numerous blood vessels that grew into the valve leaflets (chiefly the anterior cusp) persist.

The three cusps of the *aortic valve* generally show comparable changes in patients with rheumatic heart disease. The *tricuspid valve* may also be similarly involved. The *pulmonary valve* is less likely to be affected. Chronic *rheumatic heart disease* affects all three layers of the heart and also involves the pericardium. It is a triad of *pericarditis, myocarditis,* and *endocarditis* with *chronic valvulitis.* Generally, it is a consequence of having an untreated *pharyngitis* (sore throat) that was a result of infection with a *group A β-hemolytic streptococcus*. Antibodies to this bacterium can apparently cross-react with normal (ie, self-) antigens expressed in the heart, eg, certain heart valve glycoproteins, and the damage incurred can produce an endocarditis.

This patient's exertional dyspnea and cough are manifestations of increased hydrostatic pressure within her pulmonary alveolar capillaries. In other words, they are signs of *pulmonary hypertension*. Elevation of the alveolar capillary pressure >30 mm Hg can result in *hemodynamic (hydrostatic) pulmonary edema* for the following reasons. Under normal conditions, a negative interstitial fluid pressure exists in the lungs, chiefly as a consequence of osmotic withdrawal of much of the interstitial water by pulmonary intravascular plasma proteins. However, substantial elevation of the hydrostatic pressure in the alveolar capillaries increases the rate of transudation of pulmonary interstitial fluid. As soon as the total volume of interstitial fluid produced exceeds the maximal volume of lymph that can leave the lungs, *pulmonary interstitial edema* develops. Moreover, if the alveolar capillary hydrostatic pressure becomes sufficiently elevated to disrupt tight junctions between the alveolar capillary endothelial cells, an additional plasma protein-containing transudate is formed. In patients with severe pulmonary hypertension, this transudate may also contain some erythrocytes. Disruption of alveolar epithelial tight junctions, or other loss of integrity of the alveolar epithelium, substantially raises the total extravascular fluid volume of the lungs. Histologically, the resulting *alveolar edema* may be recognized by the fact that some of the pulmonary alveoli and small airways contain edema fluid. Because this fluid contains some plasma protein, it stains light pink in H&E sections. If, in addition, the accumulating edema fluid also contains erythrocytes, the expectorated sputum may look blood-streaked as well as frothy. Alveolar edema is generally detectable as "wet" rales and rhonchi or as a diffuse haziness in chest x-rays (radiographs).

Patients with pulmonary hypertension commonly develop anastomoses between their pulmonary veins and bronchial veins, and this can lead to development of *bronchial vein varicosities*. Because such varicosities carry blood that is under substantial hydrostatic pressure, they are inclined to rupture and hemorrhage, resulting in *hemoptysis*.

Restriction of the orifice of the mitral valve, *mitral stenosis*, impedes left ventricular inflow during diastole and reduces left ventricular output. Resulting elevated left atrial pressure causes enlargement of the left atrium. Because the pulmonary veins open into the left atrium, pulmonary venous pressure is also elevated. Increased hydrostatic pressure is transmitted through the pulmonary microcirculation to the pulmonary arteries and the patient has *pulmonary hypertension*. Elevated pulmonary arterial pressure predisposes the major pulmonary arteries to development of atherosclerotic plaques. It also increases right ventricular systolic pressure, and this leads to enlargement of the right ventricle. Hence, in mitral stenosis, both the left atrium and the right ventricle are dilated. Because left atrial dilatation increases the chances of forming reentrant loops, it predisposes such patients to palpitation (ie, *atrial fibrillation*).

D5-2 (CASE 5-2)

Cardiac muscle fibers may be recognized by their central nuclei and more or less circular appearance in transverse section. A number of brightly stained, intact cardiac muscle fibers can be seen in the top half of Fig. 5-2B. Cardiac muscle fibers are also discernible (under lower magnification) near the endocardial surface seen on the left side of Fig. 5-2C. Viable muscle fibers generally stain dark red.

In this patient, myocardial ischemia led to destruction of part of the posterior region of the interventricular septum. The adjoining portion of the posterior wall of the left ventricle was also severely damaged. In addition, some involvement of the posterior wall of the right ventricle was noted in the autopsy report. Hence, the reddish lesion seen in Fig. 5-2A represents a *subendocardial posteroseptal myocardial infarct*.

The clinical presentation in this case is somewhat atypical since chest discomfort was reported instead of crushing chest pain. Furthermore, it appears not to have been the patient's first heart attack. The medical history and Fig. 5-2C, suggest that a previous myocardial infarction occurred several weeks before admission when the patient experienced acute epigastric pain and profound fatigue. The occurrence of chest pains after the development of a myocardial infarct is suggestive of ischemia at an additional site in the viable myocardium.

Careful comparison of parts B and C in Fig. 5-2 indicates that B is a more recent infarct than C. The tissue adjacent to the surviving muscle fibers in B is *granulation tissue*, a relatively cellular and vascular form of loose connective tissue that constitutes the initial repair tissue. The majority of its cells are fibroblasts, along with occasional residual dead neutrophils. Neither striations nor nuclei are distinguishable in the damaged muscle fibers after a few days. In contrast to the granulation tissue in part B, the repair tissue seen in part C of Fig. 5-2 is a dense connective tissue consisting chiefly of collagen fibers. This stronger type of scar tissue takes at least 1 month to form.

Figure 5-3A,B shows the underlying reason for the infarction. In contrast to a normal coronary artery (see Fig. 5-3C,D), this patient's posterior interventricular artery has a partly occluded lumen resulting from the development of an atherosclerotic plaque. The internal elastic lamina has been penetrated by smooth muscle cells (see Fig. 5-4B), and the intima has become greatly thickened by progeny of these migrating cells and by interstitial matrix that they have produced.

The fact that this patient had a *transient ischemic attack* (TIA) that interfered with his vision suggests atherosclerotic involvement of his carotid arteries as well. The cerebral emboli that precipitate such attacks mostly arise from mural thrombi that develop in association with atherosclerotic plaques in the carotid or vertebral arteries. However, a cerebral embolus can also arise from a mural thrombus that has formed in the heart, eg, in association with a myocardial infarct.

In general, the danger of a small embolus is that it can cause regional infarction through acute arterial occlusion. A large embolus arising from a massive source, eg, from a mural thrombus in the left atrium or left atrial appendage of a patient with mitral stenosis (see Case 5-1), can cause occlusion at the bifurcation of the aorta if it impacts at this site (*saddle embolism*).

To minimize enlargement of mural thrombi forming over myocardial infarcts, one of which was transmural, this patient was given a course of anticoagulant therapy. Nevertheless, he subsequently developed pulmonary edema with persistent severe dyspnea, a manifestation of ventilation–perfusion imbalance and reduced pulmonary compliance. Pulmonary hypertension can develop if a posteroseptal myocardial infarction results in left ventricular failure.

In Mervyn's case, no information exists about the additional possibility of *venous thrombosis*, eg, in a proximal leg vein. Impairment of venous blood flow by venous thrombi contributes to approximately 70% of cases of symptomatic *pulmonary embolism*, one of the possible precipitating causes of severe dyspnea.

Widespread atherosclerotic involvement of this patient's arteries correlates with his genetic constitution and essentially stressful lifestyle. Atherosclerosis remains the leading cause of death in North America, Japan, and Europe. Its earliest recognizable stage, the *fatty streak*, is very common. This lesion is interpreted as an early response to endothelial damage, such as that resulting from hypertension, hyperlipidemia, or smoking. Progression to an advanced lesion known as the *fibrous plaque* is a consequence of various cellular and tissue interactions, many of which appear to be mediated by growth factors, as shown in Table 5-4. Figure 5-4 shows microscopic evidence of several of these changes.

D5-3 (FIG. 5-19)

The vessels seen in Fig. 5-19 have been prepared by a method that shows their external (stromal) surface in three dimensions. Stellate surface cells revealed through the selective removal of associated connective tissue fibers and basement membranes are obviously not spindle-shaped smooth muscle cells. The long, branched cytoplasmic processes extending from their generally ovoid cell bodies collectively constitute a lacy sheath around the endothelium. Each ovoid cell body measures approximately 4–5 μm in its longest diameter. Hence, the luminal diameter of these vessels may be estimated as approximately 10 μm. The presence of so many spidery *pericytes* along the external border of vessels with a caliber of approximately 10 μm suggests that such vessels are *postcapillary venules* (the important vessels from which leukocytes and plasma emerge in the acute inflammatory reaction).

BIBLIOGRAPHY

Ashcroft FM. Ca^{2+} and excitation-contraction coupling. Curr Opin Cell Biol 3:671, 1991.

Basha BJ, Sowers JR. Atherosclerosis: An update. Am Heart J 131:1192, 1996.

Byers TJ, Kunkel LM, Watkins SC. The subcellular distribution of dystrophin in mouse skeletal, cardiac, and smooth muscle. J Cell Biol 115:411, 1991.

Fitzgerald D, Lazzara R. Functional anatomy of the conduction system. Hosp Pract 23(6):81, 1988.

Hughes AD, Schachter M. Hypertension and blood vessels. Br Med Bull 50:356, 1994.

Jorgensen AO, Shen AC-Y, Arnold W, McPherson PS, Campbell KP. The Ca^{2+}-release channel/ryanodine receptor is localized in junctional and corbular sarcoplasmic reticulum in cardiac muscle. J Cell Biol 120:969, 1993.

Lehman W, Moody C, Craig R. Caldesmon and the structure of vertebrate smooth muscle thin filaments: A minireview. Ann N Y Acad Sci 599:75, 1990.

Lilly LS, ed. Pathophysiology of Heart Disease. Philadelphia, Lea & Febiger, 1993.

Lindsay J, Hurst JW, eds. The Aorta. New York, Grune & Stratton, 1979.

Motta PM, ed. Ultrastructure of Smooth Muscle. Boston, Kluwer Academic Publishers, 1990.

Ogata T, Yamasaki Y. High-resolution scanning electron microscopic studies on the three-dimensional structure of the transverse-axial tubular system, sarcoplasmic reticulum and intercalated disc of the rat myocardium. Anat Rec 228:277, 1990.

Roden DM, George AL, Jr. The cardiac ion channels: relevance to management of arrhythmias. Annu Rev Med 47:135, 1996.

Ross R. The pathogenesis of atherosclerosis: An update. N Engl J Med 314:488, 1986.

Ross R. The vessel wall. In: Fozzard HA, Haber E, Jennings RB, Katz AM, Morgan HE, eds. The Heart and Cardiovascular System: Scientific Foundations, ed 2, vol 1. New York, Raven Press, 1992, p 163.

Ryan TJ. Structure and function of lymphatics. J Invest Dermatol 93(Suppl):18S, 1989.

Wissler RW. Update on the pathogenesis of atherosclerosis. Am J Med 91(suppl 1B):3S, 1991.

Woolf N. Pathology of atherosclerosis. Br Med Bull 46:960, 1990.

Review Items: Cross References

Information relevant to the Review Item listed in this chapter may be found in the following page of Cormack, DH. Essential Histology, JB Lippincott, 1993:

REVIEW ITEM	PAGES
5-1	227

CHAPTER 6

Lungs

CASE 6-1

Mike Higgins has smoked one to two packs of cigarettes per day for almost 30 years. Now at the age of 61, he suffers from a recurrent cough that started 3 years ago. Even though he feels short of breath when he has to hurry or climb stairs, he is not bothered by a lot of sputum and has no inclination to seek medical advice.

On physical examination 3 years later, it is noted that Mike takes an abnormally long time to exhale, even during quiet breathing. A chest x-ray reveals that he has a depressed diaphragm level and marked pulmonary hyperinflation. His serum α_1-antitrypsin (α_1-AT) level is significantly decreased. Potential hepatic involvement is investigated by obtaining a transdermal needle biopsy of his liver. Mike is strongly advised to give up smoking.

After another 2 years, chronic organizing pneumonia is diagnosed in the left lower lobe. Mike subsequently develops acute bronchopneumonia, from which he fails to recover.

The general and histological appearance of Mike's right lung (upper lobe) may be seen in Fig. 6-1A,B. A liver section stained with diastase/PAS is shown in Fig. 6-2.

ANALYSIS
Case 6-1

A What major pulmonary change is evident in Fig. 6-1A,B?

B What prolonged expiration time in this patient?

C Why does this patient's liver have the histological appearance shown in Fig. 6-2 when it has been stained with diastase/PAS?

D Until Mike developed pneumonia, what chiefly impaired his pulmonary function?

(To confirm your answers, see part D6-1 of the Discussion section of this chapter; reference to Fig. 6-16 may also be helpful.)

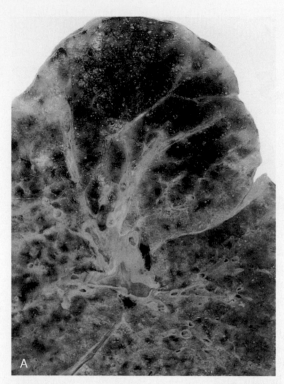

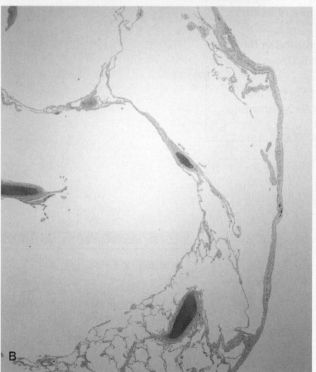

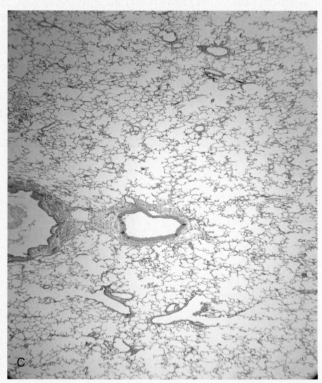

FIGURE 6-1 (**A**) Photograph of lung in Case 6-1. (**B**) Section of lung from Case 6-1 (very low power). (**C**) Section of a normal lung for comparison with **B** (very low power).

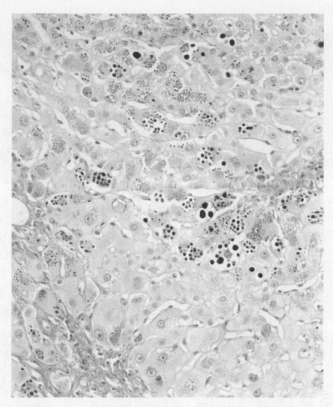

FIGURE 6-2 Liver section from Case 6-1. (Diastase/PAS stain.)

CASE 6-2

Maria Sanchez, aged 44 years, is unconscious and febrile on admission. Her blood pressure is 150/100. Pulse is 110/min and regular. Body temperature is 39.5°C. Respiratory rate is 20/min; bilateral respiratory rales are noted. Chest x-ray shows consolidation in both lungs. She does not smoke.

Maria was hospitalized a few months ago for investigation of left-sided abdominal pain. At that time, fever and green sputum were noted, and the chest x-ray indicated a left lower lobe pneumonia. Her condition stabilized with appropriate antibiotics and she was discharged. Maria also has a long history of polymyositis and has been maintained on low-dose steroid therapy for many years.

Other complications arise after re-admission. Maria survives only for 3 months. Microbiological cultures grown postmortem from her lung tissue yield a heavy mixed growth of Pseudomonas aeruginosa, Fusarium species (a fungus), and additional aerobic organisms. No anaerobes are isolated.

Some of the histological changes found in this patient's lungs are illustrated in Fig. 6-3. The pathologist noted that this patient also had chronic pancreatitis and fat necrosis surrounding the head of the pancreas. The cause of death was established as pneumonia and pancreatitis, with fat necrosis, resulting from cytomegalovirus (CMV) infection.

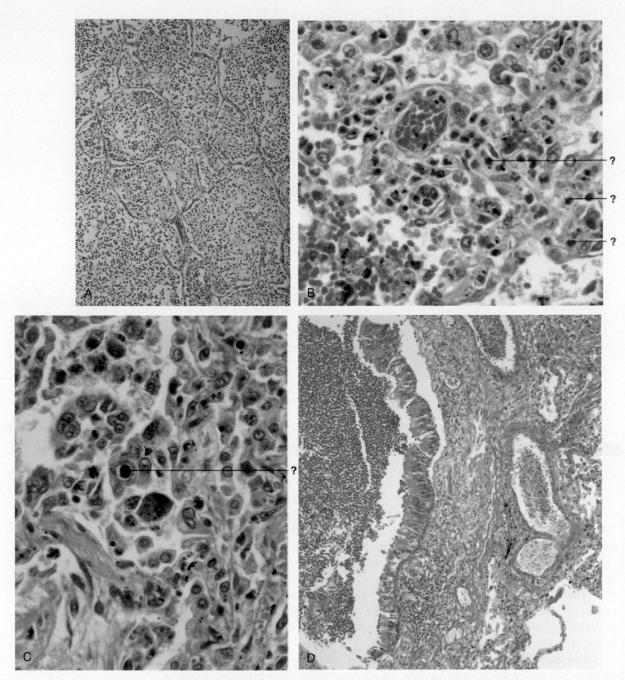

FIGURE 6-3 (**A**) Lung section from Case 6-2 (low power). (**B**) Details of an interalveolar wall in Case 6-2 (medium power). (**C**) Another part of the section seen in **A** (medium power). (The items labeled (?) in **B** and **C** are potentially informative.) (**D**) What structure is recognizable on the left side of this field, and what fills its lumen? (See part D6-2 of the Discussion section of this chapter for a detailed description.)

ANALYSIS
Case 6-2

A How does the microscopic appearance of this patient's lungs (Figs. 6-3) differ from normal?

B Where do the majority of erythrocytes lie in the lung tissue shown in Fig. 6-3B?

C What is the significance of the heavily stained structure in the middle of the nucleus of the epithelial cell shown in Fig. 6-3C?

D Why does this patient have a fever?

E Does anything in this patient's history suggest that she may be at increased risk of picking up infections?

(The answers are considered in part D6-2 of the Discussion section of this chapter.)

CASE 6-3

Gloria Bainton, aged 68 years, has an 11-month history of persistent, nonproductive, wheezy coughing. Over the same time period, her vitality waned and her body weight dropped. She has smoked the equivalent of one pack of cigarettes per day for 40 years.

A chest x-ray reveals a 5-cm mass in the upper lobe of the right lung (Fig. 6-4). Bronchoscopy and mediastinoscopy produce negative results. Since the patient is considered well enough to recover from major surgery, a right pneumonectomy is performed. Enlarged peribronchial lymph nodes are also excised. The histological appearance of a portion of resected lung tissue is shown in Fig. 6-5.

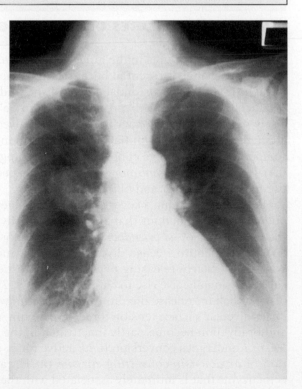

FIGURE 6-4 Chest x-ray from Case 6-3. Postero-anterior projection.

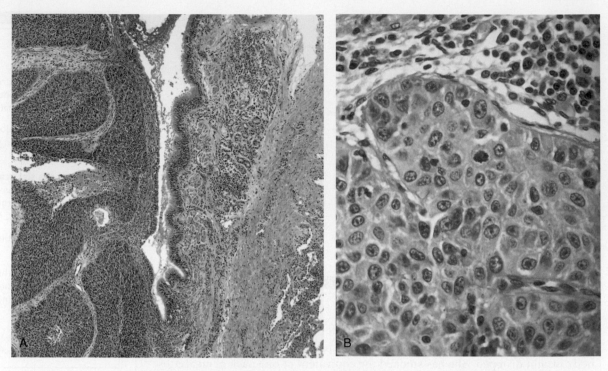

FIGURE 6-5 Resected lung tissue from Case 6-3. (**A**) Low power. (**B**) Cells in the resected mass seen under medium power.

Figure 6-6 is an additional pictorial item for analysis.

ESSENTIAL FEATURES OF THE LUNGS

A variety of key features in the lungs facilitate gas exchange between blood and air. This exchange is essential because atmospheric oxygen is an indispensable element in the body's oxidative metabolism, and carbon dioxide, continuously produced as a metabolic byproduct, needs to be eliminated. Ventilation is precisely matched to pulmonary perfusion and alveolar gas exchange is extremely efficient, enabling substantial metabolic demands to be met. The *conducting components* of the lungs condition the incoming air and enable it to replenish the alveolar air; the *respiratory components* expedite essential gas diffusion between the alveolar air and blood plasma.

Besides performing a key role in the exchange of blood gases, the lungs carry out a variety of functions that are not necessarily (or strictly) respiratory. Thus, the many types of *neuroendocrine (Kulchitsky or K) cells* scattered through the airway epithelium release diverse products, including serotonin, calcitonin, bombesin (gastrin-releasing peptide), somatostatin, and leu-enkephalin. Such cells occasionally give rise to carcinoid tumors. *Type II pneumocytes* in the alveolar epithelium release dipalmitoyl *phosphatidlycholine*, the surfactant that reduces alveolar surface tension forces. Serotonin, norepinephrine, acetylcholine, and bradykinin become partly inactivated in the pulmonary circulation. *Angiotensin I* undergoes conversion to its active form, *angiotensin II*, through the action of *angiotensin-converting enzyme* (ACE), a dipeptidyl carboxypeptidase ectoenzyme that is intimately associated with the luminal surface of pulmonary (and certain other) *endothelial cells. Bronchus-associated lymphoid tissue* (*BALT*) maintains mucosal immunity in the airways.

ANALYSIS
Case 6-3

A Which features of Fig. 6-5A indicate that this section is from a lung?

B Which other cells do the bright pink-stained cells in Fig. 6-5B resemble morphologically? What is the origin of the bright pink-stained cells in this illustration?

C Why is enlargement of peribronchial lymph nodes in this 40-pack/year smoker significant?

(To confirm your answers, see part D6-3 of the Discussion section of this chapter.)

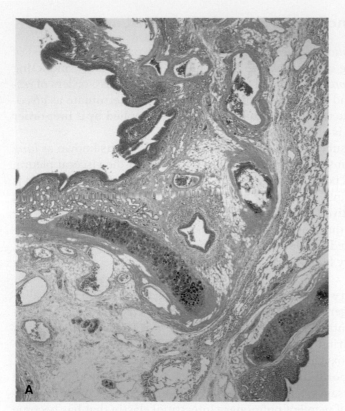

FIGURE 6-6 (A) Bronchus from a patient who has a long history of recurring bouts of sinusitis and bronchitis. She produced purulent sputum and required almost continual therapy with antibiotics. (B) Normal bronchus for comparison with A.

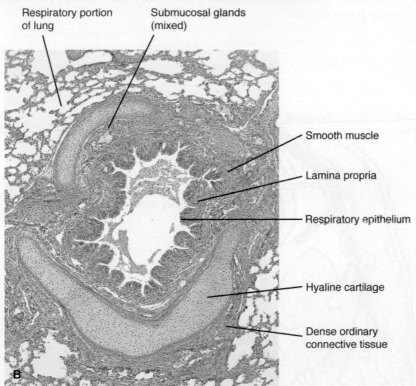

Respiratory portion of lung

Submucosal glands (mixed)

Smooth muscle

Lamina propria

Respiratory epithelium

Hyaline cartilage

Dense ordinary connective tissue

ANALYSIS
Fig. 6-6

What changes do you observe in this patient's bronchi (Fig. 6-6A)? What do such changes indicate?

(The answers are considered in part D6-4 of the Discussion section of this chapter.)

Structural and Functional Organization of the Lungs

The *structural organization* of each lung is based on approximately *23 orders of dichotomous branching* of the airways. These include 16 orders of conducting passages (*bronchi* and *preterminal* and *terminal bronchioles*), three orders of *respiratory bronchioles,* and three orders of *alveolar ducts,* and terminate as *alveolar sacs* and *alveoli.* The unit of gas-exchanging tissue supplied by a first-order respiratory bronchiole is termed the *lung acinus.*

Also, fibrous septa subdivide each lung into anatomical units known as *lung lobules* (Fig. 6-7). When seen with the unaided eye through the visceral pleura, these lobules appear as polygonal areas up to 1.5 cm in diameter. Each lobule is supplied by a preterminal bronchiole and contains approximately 20–30 lung acini. Thinner connective tissue septa incompletely subdivide the lung lobule into *secondary lobules* that have a diameter of approximately 1 mm. Each secondary lobule is supplied by a terminal bronchiole and contains two lung acini. Many of the pulmonary lymphatics and veins follow the course of interlobular septa (see Fig. 6-7).

The main pulmonary blood supply delivers deoxygenated blood to the alveolar capillaries for oxgenation. This *pulmonary arterial circulation* is complemented by a supplementary *bronchial arterial circulation.* The *bronchial arteries* follow the general distribution of the bronchial tree and supply walls of conducting passages with oxygenated blood from the systemic circulation.

A functionally important component of the lungs (notably the visceral pleura, conducting passages, and interalveolar walls) is *elastin.* Expiratory outflow is largely a result of recoil of pulmonary interstitial elastin that has become stretched during inspiration.

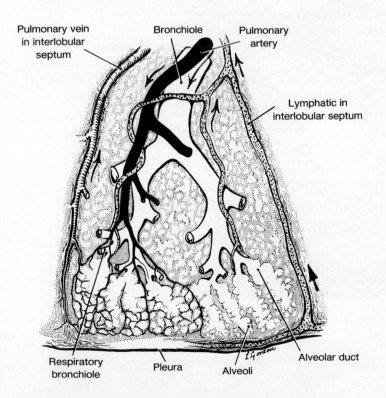

FIGURE 6-7 Basic organization of a peripheral lung lobule.

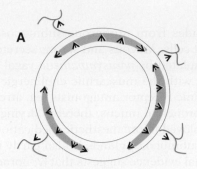

A

Bronchial walls supported chiefly by cartilages that resist bending and compression; supplemental radial traction.

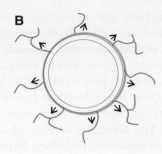

B

Radial traction of bronchiolar walls by elastic fibers in interalveolar walls.

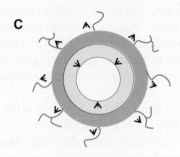

C

Submucosal, peribronchial, or peribronchiolar edema encroaches on lumen and reduces radial traction.

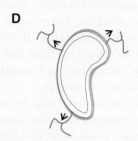

D

Radial traction on bronchiolar walls is decreased if interstitial elastin is depleted (eg, in emphysema).

FIGURE 6-8 (**A,B**) Tissue components that provide support for the walls of bronchi and bronchioles, respectively. (**C**) Airflow is significantly obstructed if these conducting passages become edematous. (**D**) Bronchioles are more inclined to become compressed if their associated elastin is destroyed.

Conducting Components

The respiratory conducting passages include the *trachea, bronchi,* and *bronchioles*. The wall structure of the trachea is essentially similar to that of bronchi, except that the C-shaped trachcal cartilages have a posterior gap traversed by the *trachealis* muscle, which is smooth.

Bronchi

Intrapulmonary conducting passages with a diameter >1 mm are known as *bronchi* (see Fig. 6-6B). A distinctive feature of the bronchi is that their walls are supported with irregular plates of *hyaline cartilage*. The tracheobronchial epithelial lining, *pseudostratified ciliated columnar epithelium,* contains abundant *goblet cells*. Mucus production by these surface cells is supplemented by secretory activity of underlying *submucosal mixed glands*. Bundles of *smooth muscle* also are present in the submucosa.

The histological organization of bronchi clearly safeguards against collapse (Fig. 6-8A). The bronchial lumen can, nevertheless, become obstructed by (1) excessive amounts of mucus from hypertrophied submucosal glands, or (2) encroachment by the wall when there is inflammatory edema (Fig. 6-8C).

MUCUS PRODUCTION

Tracheal and bronchial mucus exudes from numerous submucosal mixed glands as well as from surface goblet cells. Mucous and serous secretory activity of the submucosal glands is stimulated by *parasympathetic* vagal impulses through interaction of acetylcholine with the muscarinic cholinergic receptor on mucous and serous cells. Muscarinic receptor antagonists (eg, atropine and scopolamine) decrease but thicken bronchial mucus, thereby "drying" the airway mucosa and, hence, may be employed in preanesthetic medication.

The secretory activity of airway submucosal glands is also partly regulated by *sympathetic* impulses. Experimental evidence suggests that α_1-noradrenergic impulses inhibit serous secretion and that β_2-noradrenergic impulses may stimulate mucus secretion. In addition to water, ions, and mucus, *bronchial fluid* (ie, the mixed secretion of surface and glandular cells) contains IgA, proteoglycans, and the antimicrobial neutrophil-derived agent, lactoferrin.

Factors that commonly predispose to respiratory disorders and complications include (1) *chronic airway obstruction*, due for example to persistent bronchoconstriction, perpetuating inflammatory edema, chronic secretion of mucus, or accumulation of thickened bronchial mucus, and (2) *ciliary loss* or *decreased ciliary motility*, due for example to toxic damage by cigarette smoke or ciliary immotility in immotile cilia syndromes, with resulting impairment of mucociliary clearance.

The extremely thick bronchial mucus produced by patients with the inherited autosomal recessive disease *cystic fibrosis* (CF) results from an absence, or in certain cases defective functioning, of an outwardly directed chloride channel known as the *cystic fibrosis transmembrane conductance regulator* (CFTR). This channel protein is a normal component of the luminal domain of the cell membrane of both secretory and absorptive epithelial cells. Several mutations of the CFTR gene impair the channel's capacity to transfer Cl^- in response to increasing intracellular concentrations of cyclic AMP. Other mutations preclude incorporation of the channel protein into the cell membrane. It has been proposed that the marked desiccation of airway mucus occurring in CF is a manifestation of impaired water secretion. This seems to be related to an electrolyte imbalance that results from (1) decreased Cl^- transport into the lumen and (2) increased uptake of Na^+ from the lumen, which is probably an indirect effect of (1). The pulmonary conducting passages become progressively obstructed and distended with secretions, predisposing to bacterial infection and chronic inflammation.

Bronchioles

Tubular intrapulmonary conducting passages that are <1 mm in diameter are called *bronchioles* (Fig. 6-9). Their walls are characterized by the absence of both cartilage and submucosal glands. Except in the largest preterminal bronchioles, their epithelial lining is simple columnar. The smallest bronchioles possess a low columnar epithelium that lacks goblet cells and cilia. Helical bundles of *smooth muscle* are peripheral to the lamina propria, which is particularly rich in elastin.

During inspiration, expansion of the thoracic cavity causes distention of the gas-exchanging air spaces in the lungs. This produces elastic tension in the interalveolar walls, including those that are attached to the perimeter of bronchioles (see Fig. 6-8B). As a consequence, bronchioles become progressively distended in inspiration. Expiration is brought about by elastic recoil of the pulmonary elastin; hence, it is generally passive. At the end of expiration, enough pulmonary elastic tension remains to maintain a negative intrapleural

---

REVIEW ITEM 6-1

How are cilia constructed and how do they utilize ATP to generate motility?

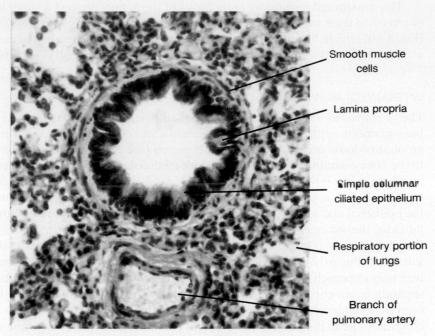

Smooth muscle cells

Lamina propria

Simple columnar ciliated epithelium

Respiratory portion of lungs

Branch of pulmonary artery

FIGURE 6-9 Bronchiole and accompanying branch of the pulmonary artery.

pressure (approximately −5 mm Hg), and this continues to hold bronchioles open. *Forced expiration* brought about by active participation of the abdominal and internal intercostal muscles tends to *compress* bronchioles.

The tendency for bronchioles to undergo (1) compression during forced expiration, or (2) constriction when bronchiolar smooth muscle tonus increases, becomes more evident when there is a decrease in the radial traction exerted by stretched elastic fibers on the perimeter of the bronchiolar wall (see Fig. 6-8C). Pathological conditions that lead to *loss of pulmonary elastin* (see Case 6-1) significantly increase airway resistance to expiratory outflow.

BRONCHIAL AND BRONCHIOLAR TONUS

Tonic *contraction* of bronchial and bronchiolar smooth muscle is increased by *parasympathetic* vagal cholinergic stimulation. Bronchial tonus is also increased by circulating catecholamines through α-noradrenergic stimulation. Furthermore, certain leukotrienes act as potent bronchoconstrictors.

β^2-*Noradrenergic stimulation*, on the other hand, induces *relaxation* of bronchial and bronchiolar smooth muscle cells. A β_2 agonist (eg, salbutamol administered as an aerosol) is, therefore, generally effective as a bronchodilator for alleviating bronchospasm.

In addition, substance P elicits *contraction*, whereas vasoactive intestinal peptide (VIP) brings about *relaxation*.

Components Involved in Gas Exchange

The pulmonary *alveolus* is conventionally viewed as being the basic *structural unit* of respiratory gas exchange. Alveoli (L. *alveolus*, small hollow space) are spherical *air spaces*—approximately 250 μm in diameter—that are separated from each other by delicate *interalveolar walls* (*septa*). However, the *functional unit* of gas exchange is considered to be the *lung acinus* (defined above), because in some respiratory diseases (eg, panacinar emphysema) the acinus becomes affected as a whole.

> **KEY CONCEPT**
>
> Radial traction counteracts compression of bronchioles in expiration.

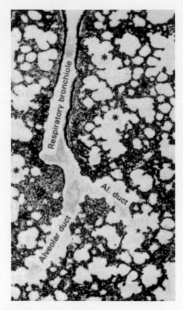

FIGURE 6-10 Respiratory bronchiole leading to two alveolar ducts. Examples of alveolar sacs are marked with asterisks.

The constituent *respiratory bronchioles* of the acinus possess a small number of alveoli in their walls. Respiratory bronchioles lead directly into *alveolar ducts* (Fig. 6-10) which, like alveoli, represent *air spaces*. Composite air spaces termed *alveolar sacs* border on the alveolar ducts and open into alveoli (Fig. 6-10).

INTERALVEOLAR WALLS

The *interalveolar walls* have a distinctive sandwich-like construction, with simple squamous epithelial cells (*type I pneumocytes*) on each side and a minimal amount of loose connective tissue in between (see Fig. 6-15C). The connective tissue layer contains an extensive network of alveolar capillaries, numerous elastic fibers, a few interstitial cells (eg, fibroblasts), some reticular fibers (collagen type III fibrils), and substantial supporting basement membranes produced by the epithelial and endothelial cells (Figs. 6-11, 6-12). Where alveolar capillaries lie close the surface, the epithelial and endothelial basement membranes are fused. As a consequence, the *alveolar–capillary* barrier at these sites is only 0.2 μm thick (Fig. 6-12). The barrier thickness in other regions of the interalveolar wall may approach 2.5 μm due to the presence of interstitial cells and fibers and separate basement membranes (*upper left* in Fig. 6-11; bottom of Fig. 6-12), but even so, the interalveolar interstitial space is minimal. Furthermore, the nearest lymphatics lie in the peribronchiolar and perivascular connective tissue sheaths and interlobular septa (see Fig. 6-15A).

The *alveolar epithelium* is made up of flat *type I pneumocytes* and rounded *type II pneumocytes*, which are the source of *pulmonary surfactant*. Tight junctions are present between the type I pneumocytes and also between type I and type II pneumocytes (Fig. 6-13). Attached to these epithelial cells are *alveolar*

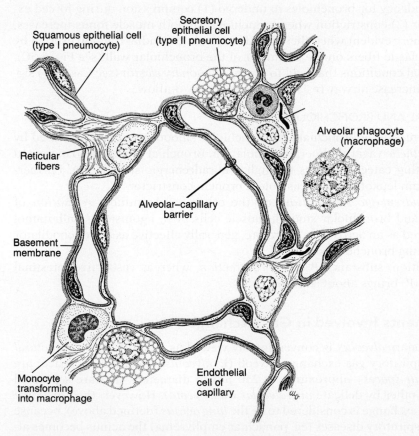

FIGURE 6-11 Basic organization of the interalveolar wall.

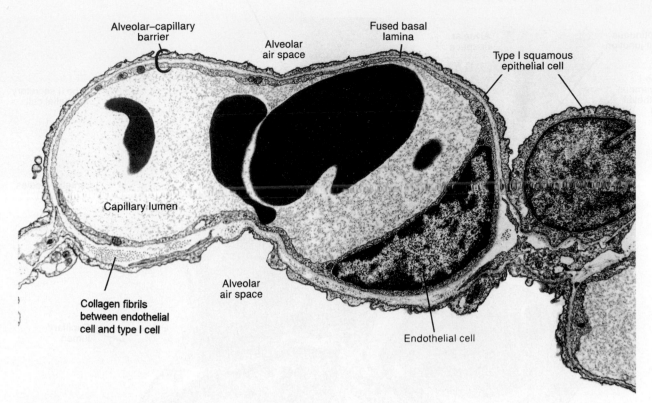

FIGURE 6-12 Alveolar capillary in an interalveolar wall (electron micrograph).

macrophages that move around and phagocytose any particulate material that may be present. Alveolar macrophages that have engulfed erythrocytes released in recurring microhemorrhages (eg, in pulmonary congestion) contain the hemoglobin-derived pigment *hemosiderin*. The sputum of patients with congestive heart failure commonly contains *"heart failure" cells*, which are alveolar macrophages that stain positively for iron.

PULMONARY SURFACTANT

Unlike type I pneumocytes, which are non-dividing, terminally differentiated cells, type II pneumocytes can give rise to type I cells in addition to more type II cells. Type II cells are characterized by the presence of distinctive secretory granules called *lamellar bodies* (Figs. 6-13, 6-14), which in LM sections may appear as tiny intracellular extracted lipid spaces. These secretory granules contain a phospholipid-rich, electron-dense lamellar material, which in human type II cells is concentrically arranged in whorls. As soon as this phospholipid-rich surfactant material becomes extruded by exocytosis, it spreads across the surface of the thin film of tissue fluid that covers the alveolar epithelium (Figs. 6-14, 6-15C). The remainder of the phospholipid-containing lipoprotein passes into the subphase, where it becomes part of a lipoprotein complex, which serves as a storage pool for surfactant. The distinctive tubular organization of this subphase complex somehow suggested the name *tubular myelin* (TM in Fig. 6-14), but it is not related to myelin.

Pulmonary surfactant is a detergent-like complex of phospholipids (chiefly *dipalmitoylphosphatidylcholine,* known also as *lecithin*), proteins, and carbohydrates. The strong attractive force between water molecules in the thin film of tissue fluid that lines alveoli inherently produces a high *surface tension*. However, by diminishing intermolecular attraction at the film surface, pulmonary

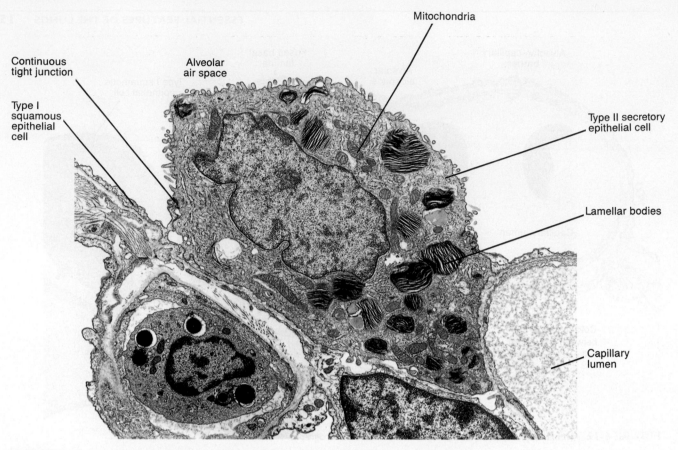

Continuous
tight junction

Type I
squamous
epithelial
cell

Alveolar
air space

Mitochondria

Type II secretory
epithelial cell

Lamellar bodies

Capillary
lumen

FIGURE 6-13 Type II pneumocyte (canine) and neighbouring components in the interalveolar wall.

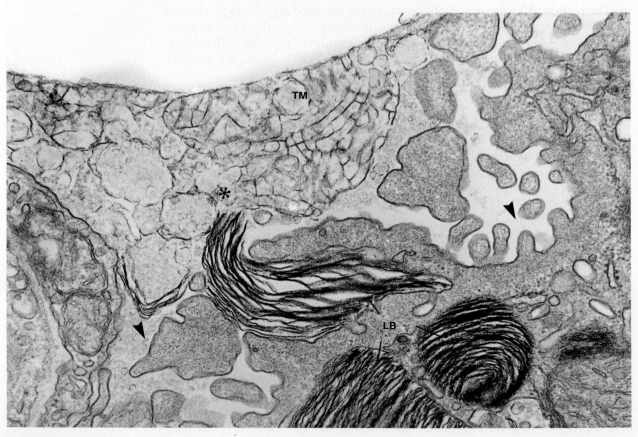

TM

*

LB

FIGURE 6-14

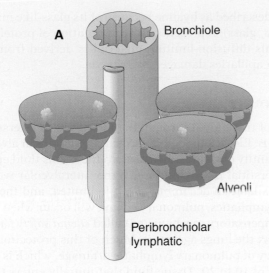

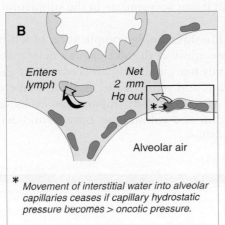

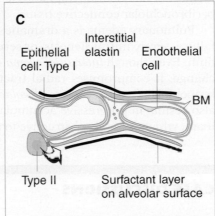

* *Movement of interstitial water into alveolar capillaries ceases if capillary hydrostatic pressure becomes > oncotic pressure.*

FIGURE 6-15 (**A**) Lung components that are involved in pulmonary edema. (**B**) Normal fluid balance in the interalveolar and peribronchiolar interstitium. The small net mean filtration pressure that drives tissue fluid from the alveolar capillaries is estimated to be approximately 2 mm Hg (based on pulmonary arterial pressure = 22/11 mm Hg, mean alveolar capillary hydrostatic pressure = 9 mm Hg, pericapillary interstitial hydrostatic pressure = −4 mm Hg, alveolar capillary oncotic pressure = 25 mm Hg, and pericapillary interstitial oncotic pressure = 14 mm Hg). (**C**) Functionally important structural features of interalveolar walls (*boxed-in* area indicated in **B**). In addition, numerous alveolar macrophages are present on the free surfaces of the walls (as indicated in **A**). A superficial film of tissue fluid, situated between the epithelial cells (ie, type I and II pneumocytes) and the surfactant layer, bathes the epithelial cells and macrophages. (BM = epithelial and endothelial underlying basement membranes; *arrow* denotes production of surfactant by type II pneumocytes.)

surfactant decreases this tension. Under conditions where surface tension remains inadequately reduced, alveoli show a tendency to collapse during expiration; and the surfaces that become apposed, adhere to each other.

NEONATAL IDIOPATHIC RESPIRATORY DISTRESS SYNDROME (RDS)

Immaturity of type II pneumocytes at birth can result in severe dyspnea and neonatal cyanosis. It is a common complication of premature deliveries and cesarean sections. Under normal circumstances, type II cells secrete effective amounts of surfactant by week 31 of gestation. Babies born after week 37 seldom develop the syndrome. Maturation of type II pneumocytes in fetal lungs may be assessed by estimating the lecithin-sphingomyelin ratio in the amniotic fluid. An L:S ratio of 2:1 is indicative of full maturation.

This syndrome generally results in collapse of some of the alveoli (*atelectasis*). RDS is specifically recognized by the presence of an extraneous alveolar surface layer, known as a *hyaline membrane*, that impairs respiratory gas exchange. Indeed, RDS was previously called *hyaline membrane disease*. The sur-

◄ **FIGURE 6-14** Exocytosis of surfactant by a type II pneumocyte (electron micrograph of perfusion-fixed lung, ×58,700). At the *asterisk,* phospholipid is being discharged from a lamellar body (LB). An electron-dense layer of this product is just discernible on the surface of the pool of alveolar tissue fluid at top left. The phospholipid is also becoming incorporated into tubular myelin (TM).

face layer, which is described as hyaline because of its glass-like microscopic appearance (Gk. *hyalos*, glass), represents an accumulation of protein-rich, fibrin-containing fluid. This diffusion-limiting material is derived from plasma that leaks from alveolar capillaries damaged by hypoxia.

Pulmonary Edema

Normal movement of tissue fluid through the interalveolar interstitium is summarized in Fig. 6-15B. Elevation of the hydrostatic pressure in alveolar capillaries increases the quantity of tissue fluid they produce. This fluid enters the minimal amount of interstitial matrix present in the interalveolar walls. Since the interstitial space available to accommodate it is limited, and the interalveolar walls are devoid of lymphatics, pulmonary edema will occur when the combined effect of several compensatory mechanisms called *edema safety factors* becomes insufficient to protect the lungs against it. Much of this protection is due to the remarkable efficiency of pulmonary lymphatic drainage, which is capable of increasing by a factor of 10 to 20. Tissue fluid that initially enters the interalveolar interstitial spaces passes readily into the peribronchiolar, perivascular, interlobular, or subpleural lymphatics; and it can accumulate in the subpleural and peribronchiolar connective tissue.

Pulmonary edema is a dramatic, life-threatening complication of left heart failure, severe mitral stenosis, or severe injury of the alveolar capillary endothelium. Even though *interstitial edema* only marginally impairs respiratory gas exchange, it compromises radial traction and reduces the luminal diameter of bronchioles (see Fig. 6-8C). *Alveolar edema* critically impairs gas exchange. It also results in progressive accumulation of a voluminous edema fluid-derived foam, which is highly obstructive to airflow.

CASE DISCUSSIONS

D6-1 (CASE 6-1)

It is evident from Fig. 6-1A,B that a large number of alveoli are missing from this patient's lungs. Furthermore, many of the remaining alveoli are greatly overexpanded. This condition, *emphysema,* is the consequence of substantial and irreversible damage to the interalveolar walls. Such extensive destruction significantly decreases the surface area available for gas diffusion, and Mike's prolonged expiration and shortness of breath on exertion are commensurate with the pulmonary damage sustained.

Expiration is highly dependent on elastic recoil of the lungs. A significant proportion of their elastin is situated in the interalveolar walls. Depletion of pulmonary elastin can result in overinflation of the lungs, with noticeable expansion of the thoracic cavity. Bronchioles resist the tendency to collapse during expiration, chiefly because of the radial traction exerted on them by tension in the elastic fibers that lie in the attached, partly stretched interalveolar walls (see Fig. 6-9B). However, the total number of intact elastic fibers pulling radially on the bronchioles is significantly reduced in patients with emphysema, and this results in airflow obstruction during expiration (see Fig. 6-9D).

If diastase is employed for a preliminary digestion of stored glycogen in hepatocytes, PAS staining discloses any glycoproteins that may also be present. The cytoplasmic PAS-positive globules seen in hepatocytes in Fig. 6-2 are α_1-AT (α_1-antiproteinase) that has been synthesized. Instead of being secreted, however, most of it stays in the rER. This results in an α_1-AT deficiency. α_1-AT is a plasma α_1-globulin. It is a broadly acting *antiprotease* with *antielastase* activity that acts as a protective agent and keeps most of the elastin intact. In people who receive only the *Z allele* for this enzyme, the gene product tends to polymerize intracellularly instead of following the usual secretory pathway, and much of it remains trapped within cells (see Fig. 6-2). Abnormally low levels of this enzyme can, therefore, indicate inheritance of the Z allele, eg, in the homozygous ZZ condition.

Figure 6-16 is a compilation of the chief reasons for Mike's emphysema, and the following points summarize what is shown.

1. The amount of intact elastin remaining in the lungs reflects the overall balance between (1) elastin-degrading proteases and (2) antiproteases, as indicated in the mauve panel, right of center in Fig. 6-16. In Case 6-1, the balance point is skewed toward degradation because the patient has low α_1-AT levels.
2. In this patient, the α_1-AT activity that normally restricts protease activity is low for at least two reasons, indicated on the *left* in Fig. 6-16. First, Mike's liver section illustrates that an inherited deficiency of this enzyme can be due to its inability to leave hepatocytes as a secretory product (see Fig. 6-16, *bottom left*). Secondly, Mike is a compulsive and excessive smoker, and the reactive free radicals present in cigarette smoke can inactivate this enzyme (see Fig. 6-16, *upper left*).
3. Cigarette smoking, certain inhaled particles, and lung infections represent only a few of the causes of pulmonary inflammatory changes that involve macrophages and leukocytes, chiefly neutrophils (see Fig. 6-16, *upper right*). Neutrophils are attracted chemotactically by a great many agents, one of which is elastin fragments. They release a potent elastase and also free radicals, both of which potentially are highly damaging to lung tissue.

D6-2 (CASE 6-2)

The lung tissue assessed in Case 6-2 shows several changes that are indicative of *acute bronchopneumonia* and also *focal organizing bronchopneumonia*. During the postmortem examination, marked mucosal congestion was noted in the trachea and major bronchi, and both lungs were unusually heavy as well as being firm on palpation. Diffuse alveolar damage is seen in these sections (see Fig. 6-3A,B), and many bronchioles are tightly plugged by neutrophil-containing pus and cell debris (see Fig. 6-3D). Some small bronchioles and their associated alveolar ducts are filled with a newly derived vascular loose connective tissue (granulation tissue). Extensive intra-alveolar hemorrhage is evident (see Fig. 6-3B). Foci of recognizable acute pneumonia with associated neutrophils can also be identified (see Fig. 6-3B).

In seeking the ultimate diagnosis, an important clue lies in the appearance of nuclei such as that indicated in Fig. 6-3C. Too large to be a nucleolus, the central heavily stained structure is a *nuclear inclusion*. The presence of such large inclusions in nuclei of fairly large cells is highly suggestive of a *cytomegalovirus* (CMV) infection. Inclusion bodies indicative of a CMV infection can also be present in the cytoplasm, but they are rarely as conspicuous as those in the nucleus. The viral infection was confirmed in this instance by (1) immunostaining with peroxidase-labeled antibody to CMV and (2) postmortem isolation of CMV from the patient's lungs. Pseudomonas and several other aerobes were also isolated.

The body's usual response to bacterial infections and most other types of infections is to develop a *fever*. Pseudomonas aeruginosa is a gram-negative aerobic bacterium that opportunistically infects immunosuppressed patients, and this patient was chronically immunosuppressed for several years by the low doses of steroid that she received for her polymyositis. Gram-negative bacteria can produce a fever in two ways. First, they may release pyrogenic (fever-causing) *exotoxins*. These bring about a release of cytokines that can produce a fever.

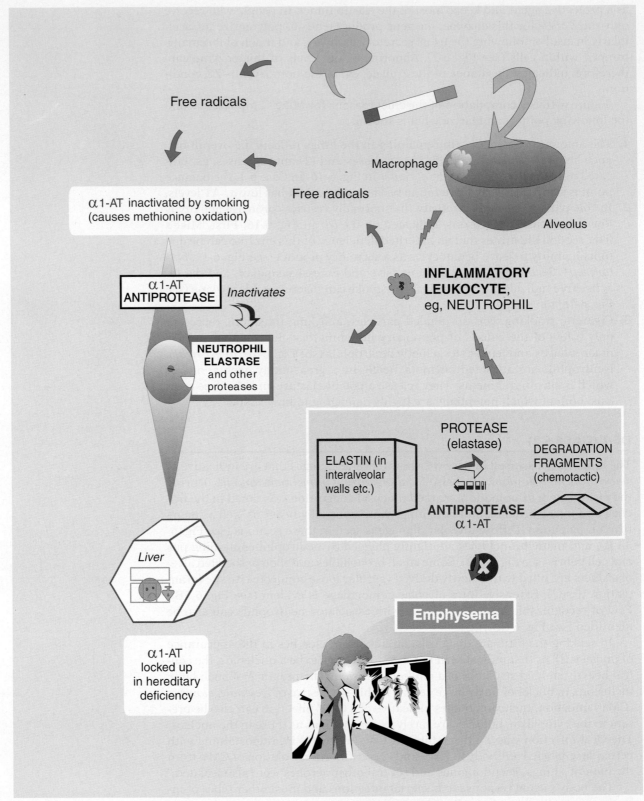

Free radicals

Macrophage

Free radicals

Alveolus

α1-AT inactivated by smoking
(causes methionine oxidation)

α1-AT
ANTIPROTEASE

Inactivates

**INFLAMMATORY
LEUKOCYTE,
eg, NEUTROPHIL**

**NEUTROPHIL
ELASTASE**
and other
proteases

ELASTIN (in
interalveolar
walls etc.)

PROTEASE
(elastase)

DEGRADATION
FRAGMENTS
(chemotactic)

ANTIPROTEASE
α1-AT

Liver

Emphysema

α1-AT
locked up
in hereditary
deficiency

FIGURE 6-16 Synopsis of key factors leading to the development of emphysema in patients with α_1-antitrypsin (α_1-AT) deficiency (Case 6-1). The α_1-AT produced by their hepatocytes fails to follow the normal secretory pathway and therefore remains trapped in the rER. Cigarette smoking is doubly damaging in these patients because it accelerates neutrophil-mediated destruction of their pulmonary elastin and it further diminishes their low α_1-AT antiprotease activity. This ultimately results in critical loss of pulmonary elastin.

The second mechanism involves the lipopolysaccharide (*LPS*) in the outer membrane of these bacteria. Known also as bacterial *endotoxin*, LPS is a major inducer of *interleukin-1* (*IL-1, endogenous pyrogen*) release by macrophages and other cells. It also causes these cells to release another cytokine, *tumor necrosis factor* α (TNF-α), that in turn elicits additional release of IL-1 from macrophages and other cells. An important effect of IL-1, and one that is thought to be amplified by involvement of other cytokines, is that it brings about an increase in prostaglandin synthesis. In the hypothalamus, stimulation of prostaglandin synthesis has an important effect on thermoregulation. When it occurs in the temperature regulating center, it raises the set-point for body temperature and thereby produces a fever. Aspirin (acetylsalicylic acid) and other inhibitors of the cyclooxygenase pathway counteract this stimulatory effect on prostaglandin synthesis; hence, non-steroidal anti-inflammatory drugs (NSAIDs) are generally of benefit in reducing a fever.

Another important effect of endotoxin is that it causes a shift to the left. This action is described, in connection with Case 3-3, in part D3-4 of the Discussion section of Chapter 3.

D6-3 (CASE 6-3)

This case is a fairly typical presentation of *bronchial carcinoma*. Part of the wall structure of a bronchus is discernible on the right in Fig. 6-5A. Hyaline cartilage (which is not seen in Fig. 6-5A), if associated with a glandular mucosa containing mucous glands, is a distinctive combination found in large airways. Encroaching into the lumen of this bronchus is a malignant tumor mass (seen on the left) that appears to have arisen from overlying dysplastic bronchial epithelium. It is likely that the patient's profuse cigarette smoking was involved etiologically in emergence of the tumor. Although this tumor is not highly differentiated, it shows evidence of focal squamous differentiation and keratinization and is, therefore, a *squamous cell carcinoma*. To a certain extent, the tumor cells (see Fig. 6-5B) resemble epidermal squamous epithelial cells (keratinocytes), and whorls of them may bear a certain resemblance to thymic (Hassal's) corpuscles. Also present are solid nests and anastomosing trabeculae of tumor cells; and at the periphery of the tumor, an invasive growth pattern may be recognized.

In addition, the pathologist found indications of obstructive pneumonia, and noticed small epithelioid granulomata in the lung tissue surrounding the tumor. Similar granulomata were found in the enlarged peribronchial lymph nodes, but no signs of malignant growth were seen in these nodes. The most likely explanation for the presence of such granulomata in the lung parenchyma and peribronchial nodes is that it represents a sarcoid-like reaction to the tumor. In cases of lung cancer, it is more common for enlarged regional draining nodes to contain foci of secondary tumor growth. Such a finding is associated with a poorer prognosis because it indicates that lymphatic dissemination of the tumor cells has already occurred.

D6-4 (FIG. 6-6)

This patient's condition is called *bronchiectasis* (Gk. *ektasis*, dilatation), a term denoting permanent (chronic) dilatation of bronchi. Numerous bronchial inflammatory reactions to pulmonary infections have resulted in hyperplasia of the mucus-secreting cells in the bronchial glands (see Fig. 6-6A), with consequent excessive production of mucus. Some focal thickening has occurred in the basement membrane under the pseudostratified ciliated columnar epithelium, and a patchy infiltrate of lymphocytes and plasma cells is present in the submucosa. In other bronchi, the smooth muscle and mucous glands have become replaced by vascular fibrous tissue. Many of this patient's bronchi show evidence of both acute and chronic inflammation and are filled with purulent exudate. There is also chronic inflammation of bronchioles.

BIBLIOGRAPHY

Alton E, Caplen N, Geddes D, Williamson R. New treatments for cystic fibrosis. Br Med Bull 48:785, 1992.

Bachofen H, Schürch S, Weibel ER. Experimental hydrostatic pulmonary edema in rabbit lungs. II. Barrier lesions. Am Rev Respir Dis 147:997, 1993.

Colby TV, Lombard C, Yousem SA, Kitaichi M. Atlas of Pulmonary Surgical Pathology. Philadelphia, W.B. Saunders, 1991.

Crapo JD. New concepts in the formation of pulmonary edema. Editorial. Am Rev Respir Dis 147:790, 1993.

Crystal RG, West JB, eds. Lung Injury. New York, Raven Press, 1992.

Dobbs LG. Pulmonary surfactant. Annu Rev Med 40:431, 1989.

Grippi MA. Pulmonary Pathophysiology. Philadelphia, J.B. Lippincott, 1995.

Higgins CF. Cystic fibrosis transmembrane conductance regulator (CFTR). Br Med Bull 48:754, 1992.

Parent RA. Comprehensive Treatise on Pulmonary Toxicology, vol 1: Comparative Biology of the Normal Lung. Boca Raton, Fla., CRC Press, 1991.

Polak JM, Becker KL, Cutz E, Gail DB, Goniakowska-Witalinska L, Gosney JR, Lauweryns JM, Linnoila I, McDowell EM, et al. Lung endocrine cell markers, peptides, and amines. Anat Rec 236:169, 1993.

Rodger IW. Airway smooth muscle. Br Med Bull 48:97, 1992.

Ryrfeldt Å, Bannenberg G, Moldéus P. Free radicals and lung disease. Br Med Bull 49:588, 1993.

Sferra TJ, Collins FS. The molecular biology of cystic fibrosis. Annu Rev Med 44:133, 1993.

Sherman CB. The health consequences of cigarette smoking. Med Clin North Am 76:355, 1992.

Stern L, ed. Hyaline Membrane Disease: Pathogenesis and Pathophysiology. Orlando, Fla., Grune & Stratton, 1984.

Sturgess JM, Turner JAP. The immotile cilia syndrome. In: Chernick V, Kendig EL, eds. Kendig's Disorders of the Respiratory Tract in Children, ed 5. Philadelphia, W.B. Saunders, 1990, p 675.

Tattersfield AE. Bronchodilators: New developments. Br Med Bull 48:190, 1992.

Thepen T, Kraal G, Holt PG. The role of alveolar macrophages in regulation of lung inflammation. Ann N Y Acad Sci 725:200, 1994.

Weibel ER. Lung cell biology. In: Fishman AP, ed. Handbook of Physiology, sect 3: The Respiratory System, vol 1. Circulation and Nonrespiratory Functions. Bethesda, Md, American Physiological Society, 1985, p 47.

Welsh MJ, Smith AE. Cystic fibrosis. Sci Am 273:52, 1995.

West JB. Pulmonary Pathophysiology: The Essentials, ed 4. Baltimore, Md, Williams & Wilkins, 1992.

Review Items: Cross References

Information relevant to the Review Item included in this chapter may be found in the following pages of Cormack, DH. Essential Histology. Philadelphia, J.B. Lippincott, 1993:

REVIEW ITEM	PAGES
6-1	75–77

CHAPTER 7

Kidneys

CASE 7-1

Carlos Santos, aged 43 years, began to feel unwell about 3 months ago. His legs started to swell up and he experienced cramps in his feet. Then his legs began to itch.

When Carlos is seen in the nephrology clinic, his legs are so swollen that the skin shows signs of breaking down and appears wet. His appetite is good, yet his energy level remains low. His bowel habits are unchanged but occasionally he has nonspecific abdominal pain. He has not noticed frothing of his urine or the presence in it of any blood.

During his physical examination, massive edema is found in the legs, abdominal wall, scrotum, and right arm. The abdominal examination also shows accumulation of excess fluid (ascites) within the abdominal cavity. The serum albumin level is decreased, and the 24-hour urinary protein concentration is greatly increased. The serum creatinine level is normal. Numerous hyaline casts and some granular and fatty casts are present in the urinary sediment. A needle biopsy from the right kidney confirms the provisional diagnosis. Representative areas of the kidney biopsy are shown in Fig. 7-1A through 7-1C.

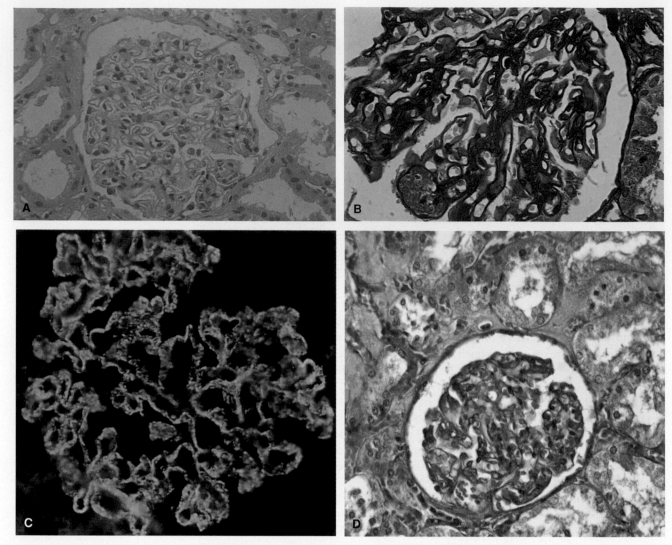

FIGURE 7-1 Renal corpuscles from Case 7-1, seen (**A**) in an H&E section (medium power), (**B**) in a PAS section (medium power), and (**C**) after immunofluorescence staining for IgG (medium power). (**D**) Normal renal corpuscle for comparison (H&E section, medium power).

ANALYSIS
Case 7-1

A What is the large ovoid structure in the middle of Fig. 7-1A?

B How does its appearance differ from normal?

C How do such changes affect its function?

D What are hyaline, granular, and fatty casts, and what do they indicate?

E Why does this patient have such widespread edema? What term is used for his overall clinical condition?

F What is the prognosis for this condition?

(The answers are considered in part D7-1 of the Discussion section of this chapter.)

CASE 7-2

When Brandon Searles, aged 26 years, is seen in the Emergency Room, his blood pressure is 150/85, his pulse is 110/min, and his respiratory rate is 40/min. His body temperature is 38.5°C. He is agitated, disoriented, and has urinary incontinence. His speech is slurred and incoherent.

He was brought to the hospital after staggering about, falling down from time to time, vomiting, and then falling out of bed. No odor of alcohol and no evidence of trauma are noted during his physical examination. The electrocardiogram and chest x-ray are both normal. Urinalysis discloses proteinuria, erythrocytes in the urinary sediment, and an increased urinary oxalate level. Preliminary toxicological screening indicates the presence of cocaine, salicylates, and nicotine in his urine.

Evidence of bilateral abducens (cranial nerve VI) paralysis is noted on the day of admission, after which stupor sets in. On the following day, the patient becomes anuric and has seizures. Hemodialysis is begun but the blood urea nitrogen continues to rise each day. Death ensues 3 days later, apparently as a result of multiple drug intoxication and substance abuse. The sediment obtained postmortem from irrigating the bladder contains calcium oxalate crystals.

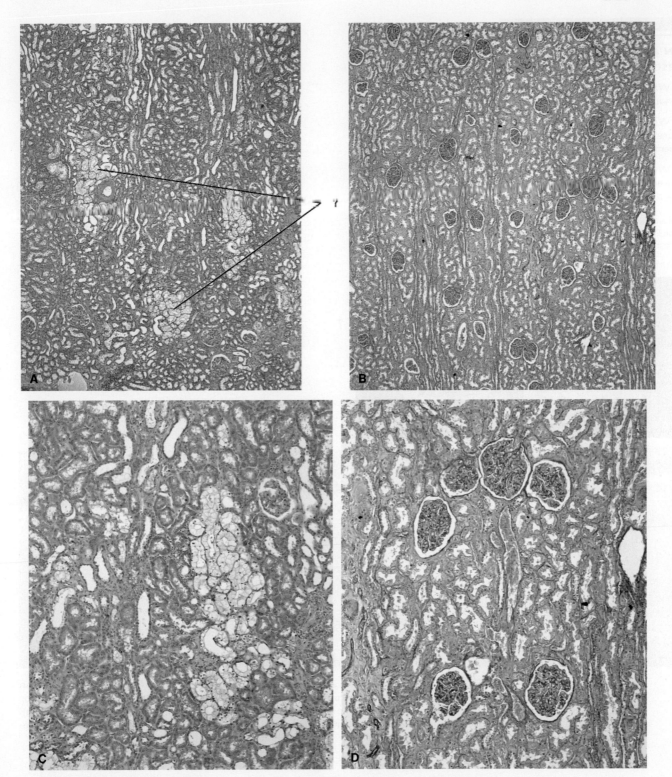

FIGURE 7-2 (**A**) Kidney cortex from Case 7-2 (low power; the features labeled (?) are potentially informative). (**B**) Normal kidney cortex (low power). (**C**) Kidney cortex from Case 7-2 (medium power). (**D**) Normal kidney cortex (medium power).

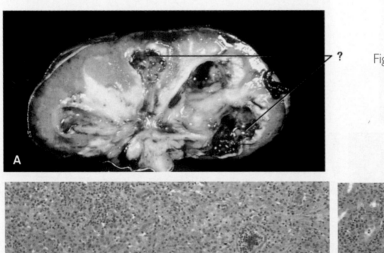

?

Figure 7-3 is an additional pictorial item for analysis.

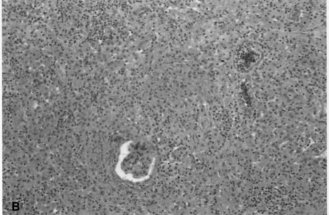

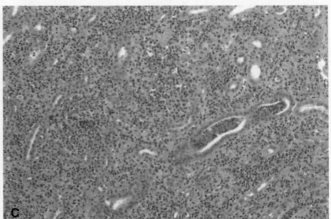

FIGURE 7-3 Photograph (**A**) and histological sections (**B,C**) of a kidney from a middle-aged woman with a history of hematuria, recurring fever, and severe flank pain who underwent a nephrectomy for an impacted renal calculus. (The features indicated with the label (?) in **A** are potentially informative). Bacteria and pus were present in her urine. (**D**) Normal renal cortex for comparison. (**E**) Normal renal medulla for comparison.

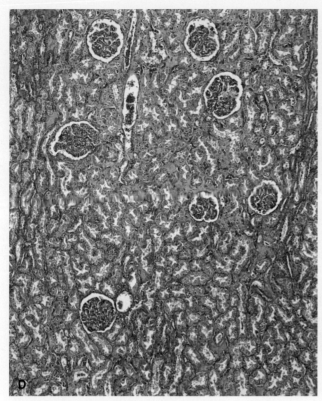
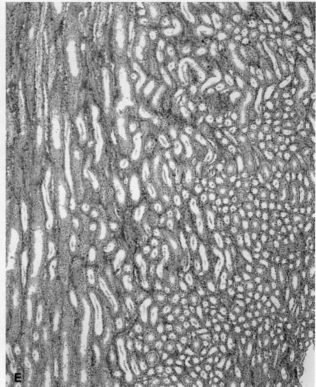

FIGURE 7-3 (Continued)

ESSENTIAL FEATURES OF THE KIDNEYS

The unique design and arrangement of epithelial tubules and associated blood vessels in the renal parenchyma enables these tubules (1) to eliminate a variety of waste products (notably, metabolic byproducts, toxic exogenous molecules, and breakdown products of such molecules) from the bloodstream, and (2) to keep the body's extracellular water content and ionic composition almost constant, even though the dietary intake of water and salts may vary. The fundamental importance of the kidneys in maintaining the stability of the body's internal environment may be surmised from the fact that, in the absence of therapeutic intervention, complete bilateral renal failure can lead to death within 1 month.

The term *renal (kidney) tubule* is sometimes used to denote the *nephron*, which is the blind-ending epithelial tubule responsible for filtration and most of the secretion and resorption in the kidneys. However, the same term can be used in a more comprehensive sense to denote *collecting tubules* (alternatively known as *collecting ducts*) as well as the *nephrons* that drain into them. Each kidney is provided with approximately one million nephrons. Each cortical collecting duct drains approximately ten nephrons.

General Organization of the Renal Parenchyma

The outer part of the kidney, where its filtration units are situated, is known as the *renal cortex*. The inner part, which contains collecting ducts opening onto a papilla, is called the *renal medulla*.

The kidney is also a *multilobed* organ, consisting of up to 14 lobes (generally seven to nine), each with a cortex and a pyramidal medulla (Fig. 7-4).

Renal Cortex

Most of the *renal cortex* is made up of filtration units known as *renal corpuscles* and the convoluted segments of nephrons (Fig. 7-5). This major component of the renal cortex, often referred to as the *cortical labyrinth*, is readily distinguishable from a second component of the cortex that is known as the *medullary ray* because its striated appearance resembles that of the medulla. Medullary rays contain straight segments of nephrons and cortical collecting tubules (ducts) into which these nephrons empty (Fig. 7-5).

Renal Medulla

The *renal medulla* contains straight segments of nephrons (thin-walled and thick-walled portions of loops of Henle) and medullary collecting ducts. Superficial nephrons (shown on the left in Fig. 7-5) have a comparatively short loop of Henle that only reaches the outer medulla. Deeper-lying nephrons (shown on the right) have a longer loop of Henle that extends into the inner medulla. The apex of each conical *pyramid* of medullary tissue, known as its *papilla*, projects into the renal pelvis (see Fig. 7-4).

Lobes and Lobules

Although the essentially lobar arrangement of the kidney parenchyma is not as evident postnatally as in fetal life, each lobe remains represented by a conical mass of medullary tissue, called a renal *pyramid*, and its surrounding associated

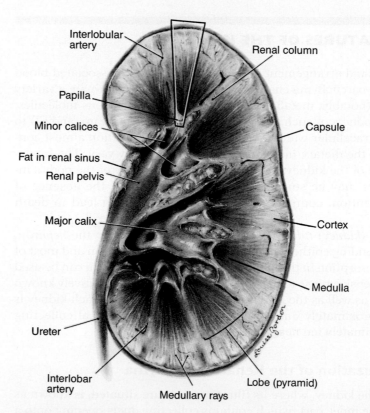

FIGURE 7-4 Main features seen on a cut surface of a kidney (coronal section).

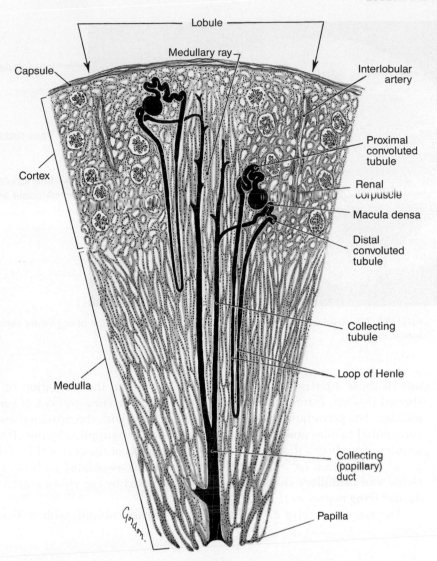

FIGURE 7-5 Lobule of the kidney, showing (superimposed) the course of two of its nephrons and their collecting ducts (indicated in black).

mass of cortical tissue. The cortex can be thicker at the base of the pyramid than between pyramids, where it constitutes partitions called *renal columns (of Bertin)*, indicated in Fig. 7-5. As in other compound glands, each lobe is made up of a number of lobules. Although the lateral margins of the kidney lobule are not distinctly delineated, their position is indicated in sections by the presence of *interlobular blood vessels* (see Fig. 7-5). The middle of the lobule is easier to recognize because it is a medullary ray. A kidney lobule is made up of a main medullary collecting duct (papillary duct) and all the cortical collecting ducts and associated nephrons that empty into it.

Renal Blood Supply

Lobes and lobules are easier to recognize in histological preparations of kidneys that have been injected to demonstrate their blood supply (Fig. 7-6). The chief blood vessels discernible in kidney sections (or on a cut surface of the kidney) are shown in Fig. 7-7. *Arcuate arteries* (L. *arcuatus*, arched), which arise from the *interlobar arteries*, extend along the corticomedullary border. There are no anastomoses between interlobar arteries or between arcuate arteries. Occlusion of

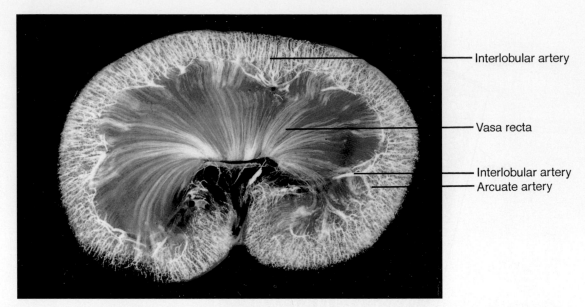

FIGURE 7-6 Renal vasculature (microangiograph, 1-mm-thick section of dog kidney perfused with barium sulfate).

one of these arteries, therefore, commonly leads to the formation of wedge-shaped *infarcts*. *Intralobular arteries* supply the *afferent arterioles* of renal corpuscles. The peritubular capillary beds associated with the proximal and distal convoluted tubules and cortical collecting ducts are supplied by the efferent arterioles of nephrons that lie in the outer two-thirds of the cortex (Fig. 7-7, levels 1 and 2). The vasa recta and peritubular plexuses associated with the loops of Henle and medullary collecting ducts are supplied by the efferent arterioles of deeper-lying nephrons (Fig. 7-7, levels 3 and 4).

The kidneys receive 23% of the resting cardiac output, with >90% of this

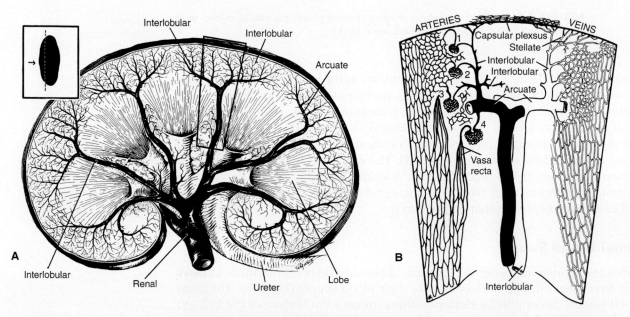

FIGURE 7-7 Renal blood supply. (**A**) Chief arteries in plane shown in inset at top left. (**B**) Detailed vascular organization of the renal cortex and medulla, showing their capillary blood supply (equivalent to the area indicated in **A**).

going to the cortex. Since the renal medulla lacks a direct arterial blood supply, all the blood that reaches the medulla has already passed through the cortex.

Tubular Organization of the Kidneys

Each *nephron* consists of a renal corpuscle, proximal convoluted tubule, descending portion of the loop of Henle (proximally thick walled and distally thin walled), ascending portion of the loop of Henle (proximally thin walled and distally thick walled), and distal convoluted tubule (Fig. 7-8).

The nephron is widely cited as the basic functional unit of the kidney. However, such an assertion ignores the established roles of collecting ducts and vasa recta, without which the kidneys would accomplish far less. A more comprehensive definition of the functional unit would be the nephron, its collecting ducts, and the associated blood supply.

Renal Corpuscle

The main histological features of the *renal corpuscle*, also known as *Bowman's capsule*, are outlined in Fig. 7-9. This structure represents the expanded blind

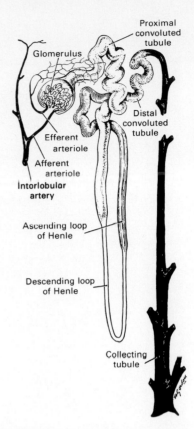

FIGURE 7-8 The parts of a nephron and its collecting duct. The distal tubule comes into close apposition with the root of the glomerulus, fitting into the small space shown here between the afferent and efferent arterioles. The macula densa is found at this site (see Fig. 7-9).

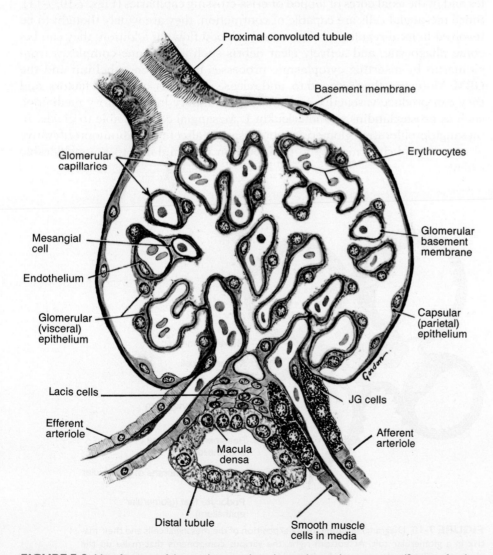

FIGURE 7-9 Main features of the renal corpuscle and juxtaglomerular apparatus. (See text for details.)

end of the nephron, with a tuft of blood capillaries termed the *glomerulus* invaginated into it. The *glomerular (visceral) layer* of epithelial cells (ie, the epithelium intimately associated with the basement membrane of the glomerular capillaries) is made up of *podocytes* (Gk. *podos*, foot), which are cells that have foot processes. The *capsular (parietal) layer* is a simple squamous epithelium. Urinary filtrate enters the *capsular (Bowman's) space*, so this is also known as the *urinary space*.

The glomerular capillaries lie interposed between an *afferent arteriole* and an *efferent arteriole*. This unique vascular arrangement produces a relatively high filtration pressure in the renal corpuscle. Also, the glomerular capillary endothelium possesses open fenestrae that promote ultrafiltration by providing free access of the blood plasma to the glomerular basement membrane (GBM). Estimates of the mean hydrostatic pressure in the glomerular capillaries vary between 45 mm Hg and 60 mm Hg. The normal mean filtration pressure of the glomerulus is approximately 10 mm Hg.

Irregularly shaped, modified smooth muscle cells known as *mesangial cells* (Gk. *mesos*, middle; *angeion*, vessel), together with extracellular matrix that they produce, provide axial support for the anastomosing glomerular capillaries. They are found in the stalk regions of lobular networks of glomerular capillaries and in the axial cores of looped or criss-crossing capillaries (Figs. 7-10, 7-11). Since mesangial cells are capable of contraction, they are widely thought to be involved in local regulation of glomerular blood flow. In addition, they can become phagocytic, and actively clear debris such as immune complexes from glomeruli by inserting cytoplasmic processes between endothelium and the GBM. Moreover, they respond to, and release, a number of growth factors, and they can produce vasoactive and immunoregulatory inflammatory mediators, such as prostaglandins and interleukin 1. Mesangial cells are able to divide. In mesangioproliferative glomerulonephritis, and also in membranoproliferative glomerulonephritis, mesangial proliferation is stimulated to a considerable extent.

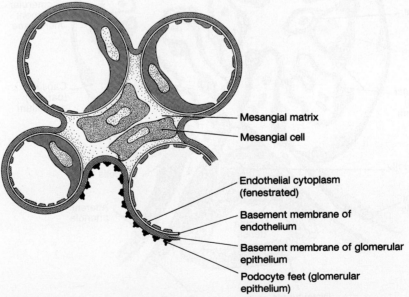

Mesangial matrix
Mesangial cell

Endothelial cytoplasm
(fenestrated)
Basement membrane of
endothelium
Basement membrane of glomerular
epithelium
Podocyte feet (glomerular
epithelium)

FIGURE 7-10 Diagram indicating the axial position of the mesangial cells and their matrix in a glomerular tuft. At bottom right, the various components that make up the glomerular filtration barrier are also included.

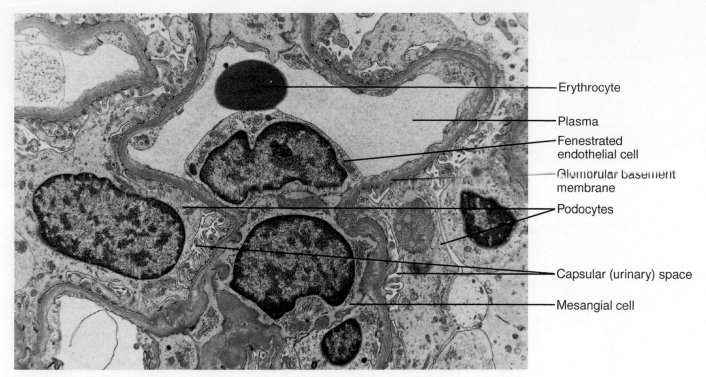

Erythrocyte

Plasma

Fenestrated endothelial cell

Glomerular basement membrane

Podocytes

Capsular (urinary) space

Mesangial cell

FIGURE 7-11 Glomerular capillary with associated podocytes and mesangial cells (electron micrograph, ×4,800).

Proximal Convoluted Tubule

The proximal convoluted tubule extends from the tubular pole of the renal corpuscle to a medullary ray, where it descends as the thick-walled descending portion of the loop of Henle, alternatively known as the pars recta of the proximal tubule. The convoluted and straight parts of the proximal tubule have essentially similar structure and functions. Up to 2.5 cm in length, the proximal tubule is the longest segment of the nephron. In LM sections, its simple columnar epithelial cells commonly appear wide and triangular. They are characterized by having a PAS-positive brush (striated) luminal border, made up of numerous long microvilli (Fig. 7-12), that possesses associated carbonic anhydrase activity. This feature, and the presence of abundant mitochondria and numerous basolateral interdigitating processes, is related to the intense resorptive activity of this segment of the nephron. The pars recta has fewer microvilli and mitochondria.

An important primary active transport enzyme, situated in the basolateral domain of the cell membrane of proximal tubular cells, is Na^+K^+-ATPase, which pumps Na^+ into the interstitial space. Na^+ accordingly moves from the lumen into the proximal tubular cells, down its concentration gradient. Water leaves the filtrate by osmosis. The proximal segment of the nephron withdraws between 60% and 70% of the total Na^+ and water present in the filtrate, and they rapidly pass into the bloodstream.

Loop of Henle

The thick-walled descending portion of the loop of Henle is the pars recta of the proximal tubule. Histologically, (1) it closely resembles the convoluted proximal tubule, except that there are not quite as many mitochondria or microvilli, (2) the microvilli are somewhat shorter, and (3) basolateral interdigitation is less conspicuous.

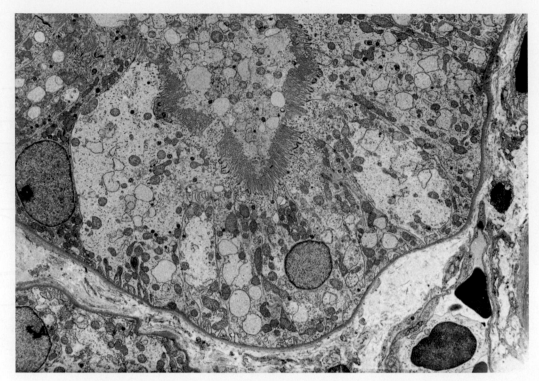

FIGURE 7-12 Proximal convoluted tubule (electron micrograph, ×2,000).

The *thin-walled portion* of the loop of Henle is made up of simple squamous epithelium, in most regions without basolateral interdigitation. In its entirety, this part of the loop is permeable to both NaCl and water. NaCl pumped from the thick-walled part of the loop, therefore, enters the thin-walled part, and water is osmotically withdrawn from it. This results in lateral recycling of NaCl from the ascending limb to the descending limb of the thin-walled loop. Water osmotically withdrawn from the thin-walled descending limb, and also from the descending vasa recta, is osmotically resorbed into returning blood in the ascending vasa recta and, hence, does not accumulate. The vasa recta, therefore, act as a passive *countercurrent exchanger*.

The *thick-walled portion* of the loop of Henle consists of a single layer of interdigitating low columnar epithelial cells that have abundant mitochondria but relatively few microvilli. Because these cells resemble those of the distal tubule, the thick-walled portion of the loop of Henle is alternatively known as the pars recta of the distal tubule. Na^+ is actively extruded from this part of the nephron by Na^+K^+-ATPase, but water is prevented from leaving.

The two parts of each loop of Henle act together as an active *countercurrent multiplier*. They produce a hypertonic longitudinal concentration gradient of NaCl within the renal medullary interstitium. This gradient is maximal in concentration at the renal papilla. Approximately 20% of the Na^+ and 15% of the water in the urinary filtrate are withdrawn by the loop of Henle.

Distal Convoluted Tubule

The distal convoluted tubule is significantly shorter than the proximal convoluted tubule. Also, its cells are low columnar and, hence, somewhat smaller. Their basolateral surfaces interdigitate and their mitochondria are plentiful (Fig. 7-13). The microvilli on these cells are sparse and short, so this segment lacks a luminal PAS-positive brush (striated) border. These are essentially the

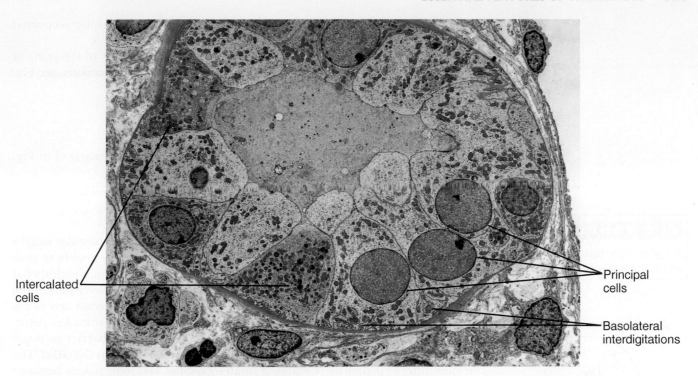

Intercalated cells

Principal cells

Basolateral interdigitations

FIGURE 7-13 Distal portion of distal convoluted tubule (electron micrograph, ×1,600).

same characteristics as those seen in the thick-walled ascending portion of the loop of Henle.

Scattered among the principal cells of the distal convoluted tubule and collecting duct are darker-staining cells known as *intercalated cells* (see Fig. 7-13) with the capacity to secrete H^+ into the filtrate.

The cells of the thick-walled ascending portion of the loop of Henle (ie, pars recta of the distal tubule), and the principal cells of the distal convoluted tubule, have Na^+K^+-ATPase on their basolateral surface. In addition, the luminal domain of their cell membrane has a symport transporter (cotransporter), driven by the inwardly directed Na^+ gradient, that couples inward Cl^- transport to Na^+ and K^+ transport. Almost all the remaining Na^+, and approximately 5% of the water in the filtrate, become resorbed in the distal convoluted tubule. Na^+ resorption in this segment of the nephron is promoted by mineralocorticoids, primarily aldosterone.

Collecting Ducts

Cortical collecting ducts are characterized by a simple cuboidal epithelium with distinct lateral borders. Their cells have a few stubby luminal microvilli and a corrugated basal surface, but do not interdigitate laterally.

Medullary collecting ducts are essentially similar, except that their epithelium is simple columnar. The epithelium of the papillary ducts is tall simple columnar.

Principal cells of the collecting ducts respond to antidiuretic hormone (ADH, known also as vasopressin) by becoming permeable to water. In the presence of aldosterone and ADH, most of the residual Na^+ (1% or so) is resorbed, primarily by cortical collecting ducts, together with approximately 10% of the water. The filtrate then enters medullary collecting ducts traversing the medullary interstitium, and drains through papillary ducts into a ureter. As the filtrate passes through the medullary interstitial hypertonic concentration gradient, a further

5–10% of the water in the filtrate is osmotically removed. The water recovered from the collecting ducts rapidly passes into ascending vasa recta.

For a comparison of the typical cross-sectional appearances of the parts of the renal tubule that are readily distinguishable in histological sections, see Fig. 7-14A through 7-14D.

Renal Functions

A number of key functions carried out by the kidneys are summarized in Fig. 7-15, and are discussed below.

Production of Urinary Filtrate

Macromolecular constituents of blood plasma that (1) have a molecular weight of more than 69,000 or (2) carry a high net negative charge are unable to pass through the GBM, even though they have free access to it through endothelial fenestrae. Thus albumin, with a molecular weight of 69,000, barely passes the GBM because of its net negative charge. The small traces that do get across are recovered almost entirely by the proximal convoluted tubule. A third key determinant in glomerular filtration is molecular shape. The chief barrier to negatively charged macromolecules is heparan sulfate proteoglycan in the GBM. The urinary filtrate, primarily containing small molecules and ions, passes between the foot processes (*pedicels*) of podocytes into the *capsular (urinary) space* (Fig. 7-16). Although a *filtration slit diaphragm* bridges the 25–60 nm gap between the interdigitating foot processes of adjacent podocytes, it does not alter the composition of the filtrate. Hence, the selective functional glomerular filter that retains plasma proteins is the GBM.

The GBM is thick, since it represents the fused basement membranes of podocytes and glomerular endothelial cells. Podocytes continue to produce basement membrane constituents; hence, there is progressive thickening (for 40 years or so) and a turnover of macromolecular constituents of the GBM. Vigilant phagocytic activity of mesangial cells helps to maintain the selective permeability of the GBM.

Urinary Sediment

During a routine examination of the urine, microscopic observation of the urinary sediment (ie, the deposit obtained on centrifugation) can provide useful supplementary information regarding diagnosis and prognosis.

Normally, the urine is almost free of erythrocytes and contains very few leukocytes. Occasional sloughed epithelial cells or hyaline casts may also be found. *Casts* are cylindrical plugs from renal tubules. They are made of protein if they appear hyaline (ie, clear and colorless).

Erythrocytes are much more plentiful in *microscopic hematuria* (microhemorrhage into the urine), which is associated with most renal and urinary tract disorders, including acute glomerulonephritis and malignancies ("from trauma to tumor"). Increased numbers of leukocytes, also typical of the great majority of renal disorders, can indicate pyelonephritis or urinary tract infection, especially when bacteria are also present. Other kinds of casts are also indicative of certain renal diseases. Examples include fatty casts (made of compacted oil droplets) in nephrotic syndrome, red cell casts in acute glomerulonephritis, white cell casts in pyelonephritis, and epithelial casts in tubular degeneration. An abundance of transparent hyaline casts may indicate glomerular damage with resulting proteinuria. Broad, refractile waxy casts (formed in the collecting ducts) can be indicative of chronic renal failure, and their presence has ominous

---

A Proximal convoluted tubule

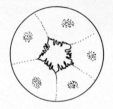

B Thin segment of loop of Henle

C Distal convoluted tubule

D Collecting tubule

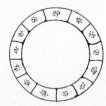

FIGURE 7-14 Diagrammatic representation of cross sections of different parts of the renal tubule.

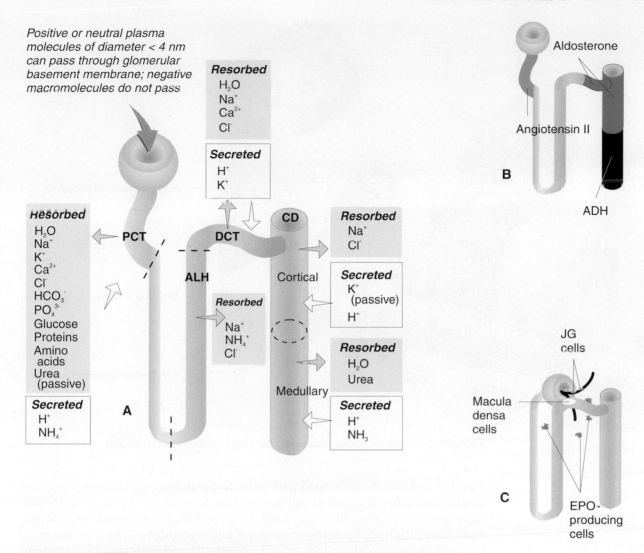

FIGURE 7-15 (**A**) Key resorptive and secretory activities of major segments of nephrons and collecting ducts. (PCT, proximal convoluted tubule; ALH, ascending portion of loop of Henle; DCT, distal convoluted tubule; CD, collecting duct.) (**B**) Major sites of regulated resorption in the kidney. Angiotensin II promotes Na^+ and HCO_3^- resorption in the proximal convoluted tubule. Aldosterone promotes Na^+ resorption in the cortical collecting duct and, to a lesser extent, both the distal portion of the distal convoluted tubule and the medullary collecting duct. (**C**) Monitoring components in the kidney. JG (juxtaglomerular) cells release renin if the effective circulating volume decreases. Macula densa cells respond if the concentrations of Na^+ and Cl^- decrease in the filtrate within the distal convoluted tubule. EPO-producing cells release erythropoietin (EPO) in response to hypoxia.

significance. The presence of epithelial cells with abnormal nuclei can be indicative of carcinoma.

Various kinds of crystals may also be found, depending on the pH of the urine. Only a few of these, eg, the amino acids leucine, tyrosine, or cystine (which can result from genetically defective tubular amino acid transport), or cholesterol, are considered abnormal.

Kidney Stones

Obstructive *renal calculi (kidney stones)* are a complication of certain biochemical abnormalities. Examples of *urolithiasis* (Gk. *lithos*, stone) include the presence of calcium stones, which are commonly associated with elevated urinary levels of calcium, oxalic acid, or uric acid, and uric acid stones, which can be id-

REVIEW ITEM 7-1

Which histological features of the ureters facilitate passage of renal calculi a few millimeters in diameter?

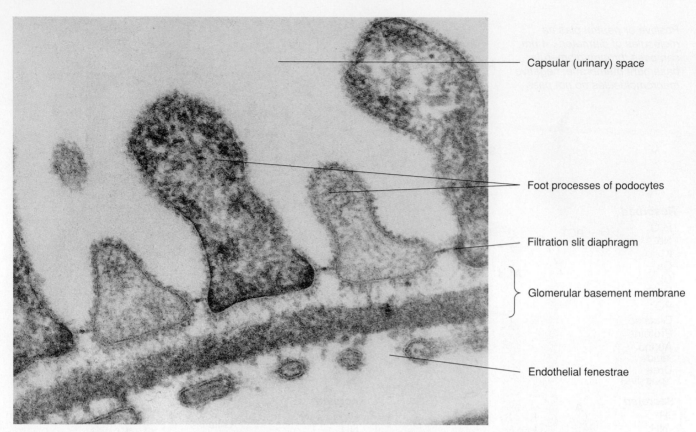

Capsular (urinary) space

Foot processes of podocytes

Filtration slit diaphragm

Glomerular basement membrane

Endothelial fenestrae

FIGURE 7-16 The glomerular filtration barrier (electron micrograph, ×60,000)

iopathic and may be associated with gout. In North America, kidney stones are most commonly composed of calcium oxalate. Struvite stones, made of magnesium ammonium phosphate and calcium carbonate, are a complication of urinary tract infections by urease-producing microorganisms. The breakdown of urea results in a combination of high urinary pH and high ammonia content, which in the presence of phosphate ions causes precipitation, producing struvite stones that grow rapidly and tend to harbor the infecting organism. Struvite stones that form in the renal pelvis and take on the shape of its major and minor calyces are often described as *staghorn calculi*. Cystine stones can form in patients with hereditary cystinuria.

Formation of Medullary Interstitial Gradient

Hypertonicity of the medullary interstitium is partly the result of countercurrent multiplication of the effects of Na^+ and Cl^- transport from the thick-walled ascending portion of the loop of Henle. In addition, urea (an end-product of protein metabolism) becomes trapped in the medullary interstitium. Thus, if ADH is present, water is withdrawn osmotically from the filtrate in collecting ducts. In the presence of ADH, urea also leaves the medullary collecting ducts, down its concentration gradient, and enters the medullary interstitium along with resorbed water. The concentration of interstitial urea gradually builds up as a consequence of repeated re-entry into thin-walled portions of loops of Henle and re-delivery to medullary collecting ducts. Recirculating urea accordingly accumulates in the medullary interstitium and contributes up to 50% of its total osmolarity.

Nephrotoxicity

The kidneys are susceptible to extensive damage by a number of toxins and drugs. Some injurious effects are attributable to intense metabolic activity of certain nephron segments, notably those in the cortex. Others are caused by increased concentrations of potentially damaging substances produced within specific segments of renal tubules through their local concentrating mechanisms. The renal papillae are especially vulnerable since their interstitial concentration gradient has the effect of further concentrating the toxic substances in the filtrate. An additional hazard is the looped arrangement of the vasa recta in the renal papillae. Lateral diffusion through the interstitium makes delivery of oxygen and elimination of carbon dioxide very inefficient. Ischemia or infarction of the papillae (eg, as a complication of severe pyelonephritis) can lead to acute papillary necrosis (necrotizing papillitis).

Some drugs, notably certain antibiotics and non-steroidal anti-inflammatory drugs [eg, phenacetin, a major metabolite of which is in acetaminophen (paracetamol)] can elicit an allergic type of renal inflammation called *acute tubulointerstitial nephritis*. The combination of aspirin and phenacetin is markedly damaging, especially when absorbed under conditions of water depletion. *Chronic tubulointerstitial nephritis*, with associated papillary necrosis, can result from the long-continued heavy use of certain combinations of analgesics. It is often referred to as *analgesic nephropathy*.

Renal Involvement in Blood Pressure Regulation

A major determinant of cardiac output and, hence, blood pressure, is the intravascular volume, which is regulated by the kidneys. Accordingly, (1) chronic parenchymal damage with resulting Na^+ and water retention, and (2) renal arterial stenosis (due, for example, to atherosclerosis) both have a potentially hypertensive effect. The cells that respond to a decrease in renal arterial blood flow are called *juxtaglomerular (JG) cells* (see Fig. 7-15C). These modified smooth muscle cells are present in the walls of afferent arterioles. They release renin (described below under the heading Juxtaglomerular Apparatus) when the effective circulating volume decreases. By initially causing angiotensin I to be produced from an inactive precursor (see below), renin elicits arteriolar vasoconstriction and sodium retention. Tubular segments that are characterized by regulated Na^+ resorption are indicated in blue in Fig. 7-15B; the site of regulated water resorption is indicated in black in this diagram.

Juxtaglomerular Apparatus

As shown in Figs. 7-5 and 7-15C, the distal convoluted tubule of each nephron comes into close apposition with the renal corpuscle of that nephron. At this site, the distal tubule passes through a crevice between the afferent and efferent arterioles (see Fig. 7-9), and the wall of the tubule is specialized as the *macula densa* (a dense spot where the nuclei are crowded together). An intimate structural association exists among the macula densa, JG cells, and a group of extraglomerular mesangial cells alternatively known as *lacis cells*. The macula densa, JG, and lacis cells comprise the *juxtaglomerular apparatus*, a functionally integrated regulatory unit that continuously adjusts the amount of renin being released from the JG cells.

The proteolytic enzyme *renin* (L. *renis*, kidney) is a constituent glycoprotein of the PAS-positive secretory granules in JG cells. This acid protease cleaves *angiotensin I* from the N-terminal end of *angiotensinogen*, which is a plasma α_2-globulin synthesized in the liver. A decrease in the effective circulating volume

TABLE 7-1
ROLE OF RENIN IN REGULATION OF INTRAVASCULAR VOLUME

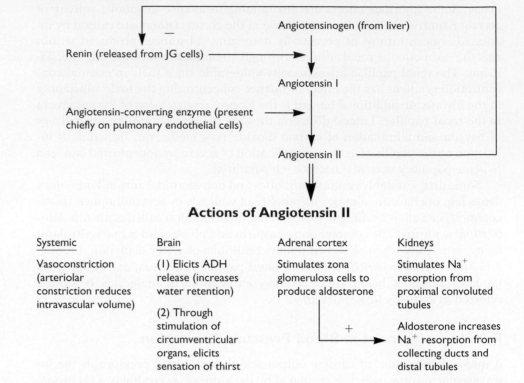

Angiotensinogen (from liver)

Renin (released from JG cells) $\longrightarrow$

Angiotensin I

Angiotensin-converting enzyme (present
chiefly on pulmonary endothelial cells) $\longrightarrow$

Angiotensin II

Actions of Angiotensin II

Systemic	Brain	Adrenal cortex	Kidneys
Vasoconstriction (arteriolar constriction reduces intravascular volume)	(1) Elicits ADH release (increases water retention)	Stimulates zona glomerulosa cells to produce aldosterone	Stimulates Na$^+$ resorption from proximal convoluted tubules
	(2) Through stimulation of circumventricular organs, elicits sensation of thirst	+	Aldosterone increases Na$^+$ resorption from collecting ducts and distal tubules

(eg, a hypovolemia caused by a fall in blood pressure, hemorrhage, or dehydration) elicits a release of renin from JG cells, presumably by reducing the degree of stretch in these cells. In addition, the macula densa cells are able to detect decreases in the concentrations of Na$^+$ and Cl$^-$ in the filtrate that passes along the distal convoluted tubule. Such a decrease also stimulates a release of renin. Lacis cells are believed to be involved in transmitting information from macula densa cells to JG cells, since lacis cells are coupled with one another and with JG cells by gap junctions. The macula densa, lacis, and JG cells seem to cooperate functionally in summating the amount of renin to be released. Some other stimuli that elicit renin secretion are noradrenergic sympathetic renal nerve impulses, Na$^+$ depletion, and prostacyclin.

The main compensatory mechanisms through which hypovolemia is rectified by renin are outlined in Table 7-1.

Regulatory Role in Erythropoiesis

Another type of monitoring cell in the kidneys is the *erythropoietin (EPO)-producing cell* (see Fig. 7-15C), which responds to hypoxia by releasing EPO. Although the precise cellular source of this hormone is not resolved, it is known that anemia induces EPO synthesis in some of the peritubular interstitial cells of the inner cortex and outer medulla. These are widely assumed to be capillary endothelial cells or fibroblasts. Different studies indicate that hypoxia-inducible EPO synthesis occurs in tubular epithelial cells of the inner cortex. Hepatic sources producing approximately 10% of the total EPO have also been identified.

Anemia in Chronic Renal Failure

A common complication of chronic renal failure is a normochromic, normocytic anemia that results primarily from underproduction of EPO by the diseased kidneys. The erythrocytes of uremic patients may also have a shorter lifespan. Recombinant EPO has been successfully produced from the cloned EPO gene, and is now available for treating kidney patients with anemia.

CASE DISCUSSIONS

D7 I (CASE 7-I)

The structure seen in the middle of Fig. 7-1A is a *renal corpuscle*. This is a highly distinctive structure made up of a tuft of capillaries, the *glomerulus*, a visceral layer of epithelium, and a parietal layer of epithelium. Only the parietal epithelium is discernible as a distinct layer. When this renal corpuscle is compared with a normal one (see Fig. 7-1D), its glomerular basement membrane seems to be more evident, a change broadly described as a *membranous nephropathy*. The total number of nucleated cells in the patient's renal corpuscle is, nevertheless, essentially normal; its glomerular capillaries are neither collapsed nor dilated. This particular case is an example of *membranous glomerulonephritis*. The basement membrane of the glomerular capillaries is somewhat more conspicuous because it is uniformly thickened, as becomes particularly evident after PAS staining (see Fig. 7-1B). Such marked thickening is commonly a consequence of the deposition of antigen–antibody complexes within the glomerular basement membrane, and with suitable immunofluorescent or immunochemical staining, the class of antibody involved may be identified (see Fig. 7-1C).

It may appear paradoxical that a thickening of the glomerular basement membrane could destroy its selective filtration properties. Such damage nevertheless explains why plasma proteins normally retained by the renal filtration barrier are present in high concentration in this patient's urine. Deposition of immune complexes within the glomerular filtration barrier compromises its selective filtration properties and can lead to severe proteinuria. The resulting hypoalbuminemia accounts for the massive bodywide edema (*anasarca*) that characterizes this patient's condition. Chronic daily loss of plasma albumin significantly decreases the intravascular colloid osmotic pressure, which under normal circumstances would draw much of the tissue fluid back into the blood. As a result, vast amounts of tissue fluid can accumulate interstitially, creating a severe peripheral *osmotic edema*. The contribution that hypoalbuminemia makes to the development of ascites is considered in connection with Case 8-3 in part D8-3 of the Discussion section of Chapter 8. The clinical condition characterized by severe proteinuria, often associated with generalized peripheral edema and hypoalbuminemia (without hematuria), is termed the *nephrotic syndrome*.

Casts found in the urinary sediment during urinalysis can provide useful diagnostic information. Colorless, refractile *hyaline casts* are produced when protein leaks from the glomerular capillaries. They are essentially plugs of precipitated protein that become released from distal and collecting tubules. *Granular casts* generally represent precipitated plasma proteins or impacted cell debris, and can be a further indication of glomerulonephritis. *Fatty casts* contain droplets of accumulated lipid from renal tubule cells and are indicative of the nephrotic syndrome.

The normal serum creatinine level in this patient indicates that his renal filtration function has not become significantly impaired. Patients in this age group who have membranous glomerulonephritis have a 50% chance of maintaining adequate renal function. Continuing urinary loss of plasma protein, nevertheless, may be expected, as complete remission of proteinuria occurs only in children.

D7-2 (CASE 7-2)

Careful observation and interpretation of the kidney section seen in Fig. 7-2 may lead to recognition of an atypical array of pale-stained tubules that appear to be associated with a medullary ray. Some cortical collecting tubules might be expected in such a position, but these pale-stained tubules are far too numerous for that to be the explanation. Moreover, when these tubules are observed at higher magnification (see Fig. 7-2C), it is evident that their cells are broad, not columnar as would be the case for collecting tubules. The lateral cell borders in proximal or distal convoluted tubules are rarely distinct because they interdigitate extensively; however, in these tubules, the lateral borders are quite distinct. If the small number of cells in each tubular cross section and their overall shape are taken into account, it becomes apparent that these are *proximal tubular cells* that show substantial ballooning. This is an example of *acute proximal tubular necrosis*.

From the few clues available in this patient's medical history and from the type of kidney damage that he sustained, it may be surmised that due to unusual circumstances, something potentially nephrotoxic was absorbed into his body. He did, in fact, intentionally ingest a massive amount of the antifreeze *ethylene glycol*. In certain European countries, this viscous nice-tasting sweet substance was at one time sadly misused to adulterate wine, but Brandon drank it right out of the bottle.

Rapid and aggressive treatment, including hemodialysis, generally results in a favorable outcome in such patients, unless severe brain damage or circulatory failure ensue or cardiopulmonary or other complications develop.

Patients intoxicated by ethylene glycol develop a primary metabolic acidosis, chiefly because of increased lactic acid production. They exhibit the rapid deep breathing (Kussmaul respiration) characteristic of marked acidosis. In addition, calcium oxalate crystals may appear in the renal tubular cells, the tubular lumen, or the urine. This is because alcohol dehydrogenase and a series of other other hepatocyte enzymes metabolize ethylene glycol to glyoxylate, which may then become metabolized in a number of ways. Oxalate, one of its metabolic end products, is known to be highly nephrotoxic. Most of the toxicity of ethylene glycol is therefore attributed to its metabolites.

In Brandon's case, the changed microscopic appearance of proximal convoluted tubules foreshadows *acute tubular necrosis*. This sign of cell damage is called *hydropic swelling* (Gk. *hydrops*, watery accumulation). The absorptive cells have a swollen appearance because the energy-dependent ion pump (Na^+K^+-ATPase) that normally pumps Na^+ from them has ceased to function. Together with Na^+, water accumulates in these cells, causing an obvious cell swelling that in this case precedes cell death. Crystals of calcium oxalate that also may be present are considered unlikely to be the cause of tubular damage, but their identification assists in differential diagnosis. Acute tubular necrosis can induce vasoconstriction in glomerular arterioles, and renal tubules can become obstructed by necrotic debris. Acute tubular necrosis can, therefore, lead to acute renal failure.

D7-3 (FIG. 7-3)

Red areas of inflammation may be recognized on the cut surface of the kidney shown in Fig. 7-3A. Figure 7-3B shows an affected part of the renal cortex. The presence of chronic as well as acute inflammatory cells indicates a *chronic in-*

terstitial nephritis as a response to recurring kidney infections. This late stage of suppurative (acute) *pyelonephritis* has now entered a chronic phase. Since extensive tissue destruction has occurred, the renal tubules are very hard to discern. However, the remains of a renal corpuscle are still recognizable. Collecting tubules, one with pus in its lumen, may also be recognized in this patient's renal medulla (see Fig. 7-3C). Numerous small lymphocytes are present in the interstitium. The adjacent region of the medulla contains numerous tubular spaces left by necrotic tubules in a hyalinized fibrous interstitium, with local accumulations of dead inflammatory leukocytes. This necrotic tissue from the tip of a renal papilla indicates that the patient has *necrotizing papillitis* or *acute papillary necrosis*. Tubular functions such as urinary concentration are accordingly greatly impaired.

Impacted kidney stones can cause urinary stasis because they are obstructive, and urinary obstruction predisposes patients to ascending infection with bacteria that may enter their urinary tract and infect their kidneys by way of papillary ducts. Such ascending infections are more common in women than in men.

BIBLIOGRAPHY

Brenner BM, Beeuwkes R. The renal circulations. Hosp Pract 13(7):35, 1978.

Brenner BM, Rector FC, eds. The Kidney, ed 4, vol 1. Philadelphia, W.B. Saunders, 1992.

Gosling JA, Dixon JS, Humpherson JR. Functional Anatomy of the Urinary Tract: An Integrated Text and Color Atlas. London, Gower Medical Publishing, 1983.

Kriz W, Elger M, Lemley K, Sakai T. Structure of the glomerular mesangium: A biomechanical interpretation. Kidney Int 38(suppl 30):S2, 1990.

Koury ST, Bondurant MC, Semenza GL, Koury MJ. The use of in situ hybridization to study erythropoietin gene expression in murine kidney and liver. Microsc Res Tech 25:29, 1993.

Koushanpour E, Kriz W. Renal Physiology: Principles, Structure, and Function, ed 2. New York, Springer-Verlag, 1986.

Lote CJ. Principles of Renal Physiology, ed 3. London, Chapman & Hall, 1994.

Ohno S, Baba T, Terada N, Fujii Y, Ueda H. Cell biology of kidney glomerulus. Int Rev Cytol 166:181, 1996.

Savage COS. The biology of the glomerulus: Endothelial cells. Kidney Int 45:314, 1994.

Sedor JR, Konieczkowski M, Huang S, Gronich JH, Nakazato Y, Gordon G, King CH. Cytokines, mesangial cell activation and glomerular injury. Kidney Int 43(suppl 39):S65, 1993.

Skott O, Jensen BL. Cellular and intrarenal control of renin secretion. Clin Sci 84:1, 1993.

Wardle EN. Cell biology and glomerulonephritis. Nephron 59:529, 1991.

Review Items: Cross References

Information relevant to the Review Item listed in this chapter may be found in the following page of Cormack, DH. Essential Histology. Philadelphia, J.B. Lippincott, 1993:

REVIEW ITEM	PAGES
7-1	334

CHAPTER 8

Gastrointestinal Tract and Liver

CASE 8-1

Martin Clements, a 37-year-old laboratory technician, is easily stressed when extra duties arise at work. At about 11 am, he experiences a gnawing epigastric pain, which can be much worse if he has recently taken an analgesic for a headache. The pain is just as severe if he puts cream in the coffee that he enjoys along with his mid-morning cigarette. A similar episode of acute pain generally occurs about 2 hours after lunch. His family doctor prescribes a histamine 2-receptor antagonist and advises him not to take aspirin, but the symptoms persist.

Figure 8-1 shows the histological and endoscopic appearance of the lesion that is involved.

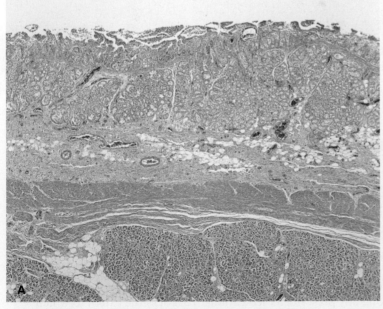
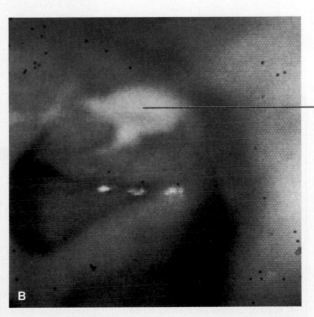

FIGURE 8-1 (**A**) Lesion in Case 8-1 (low power). (**B**) Endoscopic view of this lesion (the feature labeled (?) is potentially informative). (See questions for Case 8-1, the answers to which are discussed in part D8-1 of the Discussion section of this chapter.)

ANALYSIS
Case 8-1

A How might the histology seen in Fig. 8-1 account for the clinical history given in Case 8-1?

B Is there enough information in Fig. 8-1 for you to recognize which part of the gut is involved?

C Which tissue layers are the most affected? Why?

D Which microorganism is associated with the recurrence of peptic ulcers?

E Why is the pain epigastric?

F Which diagnostic procedure has most potential for revealing the precise site of the lesion?

G How long does resolution of this condition take if the patient's treatment is effective?

H Can you account for lack of effectiveness of the prescribed medication?

(The answers are considered in part D8-1 of the Discussion section of this chapter.)

CASE 8-2

Meg Hammond, aged 19 years, is brought to hospital in a wretched state, following an all-night party. She appears pale after an episode of weakness, nausea, and vomiting that was characterized by profuse sweating, abdominal cramps, and diarrhea. Before going to the party, she took a triple adult dose of a non-prescribed extra-strength pain-killer for a persistent migraine headache. After appropriate emergency care, Meg's acute symptoms subside but she is left with discomfort in the right upper abdominal quadrant. Significant elevation of her serum ALT (alanine aminotransferase) level indicates a need for further liver function tests and a percutaneous needle biopsy. The biopsy specimen referred for histological evaluation is illustrated in Fig. 8-2. Later it is found that Meg has not been coping well with loss of her boyfriend. He was killed two years previously in a motorcycle accident.

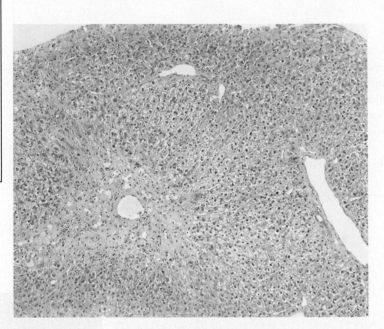

FIGURE 8-2 Liver biopsy in Case 8-2 (medium power). (For confirmation and a discussion of the findings, see part D8-2 of the Discussion section of this chapter.)

ANALYSIS
Case 8-2

A Does the histological appearance of the liver biopsy in Fig. 8-2 differ from normal?

B Does some aspect of the clinical history or the biopsy result suggest that acetaminophen (paracetamol) may have been involved?

C Which part of the liver acinus seems to be most affected?

D Is alcohol tolerance likely to be increased or reduced in this patient?

(The answers are considered in part D8-2 of the Discussion section of this chapter.)

CASE 8-3

Fred Harrison, aged 64 years, presents with a record of chronically poor health. On physical examination, his blood pressure is 170/110, and his pulse is 100/min and regular. His abdomen is distended but not tender, with a shifting dullness on percussion. Slight respiratory difficulty is also detected. The liver extends three fingerbreadths below the right costal margin and feels moderately firm. Bruises are noted on the arms and legs. The periphery of the sclerae is mildly discolored. The serum albumin level is decreased; the prothrombin time is prolonged. The patient is not taking any prescribed medications. To assess the extent to which the liver is affected and confirm the clinical diagnosis, a percutaneous biopsy is taken from the liver. Its microscopic appearance is shown in Fig. 8-3. Figure 8-4 contributes some additional information about this patient.

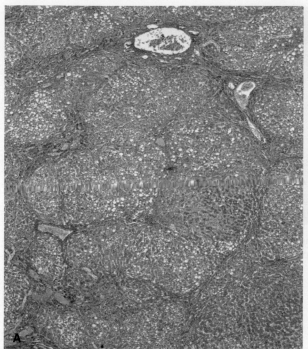

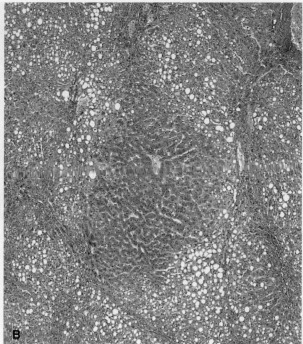

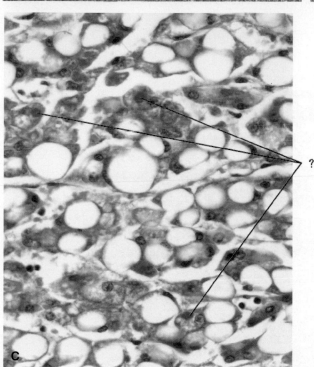

FIGURE 8-3 Histological features of liver biopsy in Case 8-3. (**A**) Medium power. (**B**) A region where there are some recognizable hepatocytes (low power). (**C**) What is the significance of the reddish-purple material indicated by the label (?) in these lipid-laden hepatocytes (medium power)? (The findings are considered in part D8-3 of the Discussion section of this chapter.)

ANALYSIS
Case 8-3

A Which features of the liver biopsy seen in Fig. 8-3 do not look normal?

B What caused the scleral discoloration?

C What caused the abdominal distention?

D What unusual feature is seen in Fig. 8-4? Does it have any clinical significance? Can you identify the precise location?

E What is the patient's condition and what is the prognosis?

(The answers are considered in part D8-3 of the Discussion.)

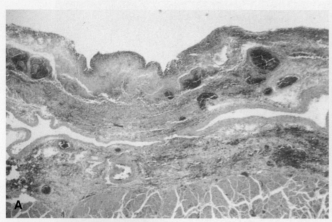

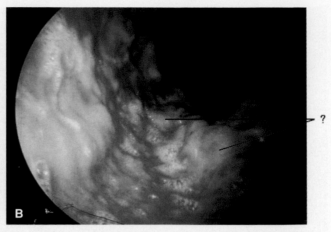

FIGURE 8-4 (A) A supplementary section that provides further information about the patient's condition in Case 8-3. (B) Endoscopic view of the luminal surface seen at the top of A.

Figures 8-5 and 8-6 are additional pictorial items for analysis (see the captions for these figures).

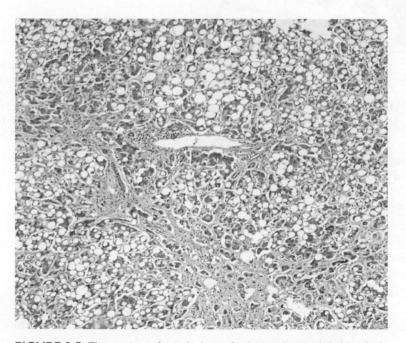

FIGURE 8-4 (Continued) (C) Barium contrast radiograph in Case 8-3. (See part D8-3 of the Discussion section of this chapter.)

FIGURE 8-5 This section is from the liver of a driver who was killed in a highway accident. It suggests a possible reason for his losing control of his car. (The findings are discussed in part D8-5 of the Discussion section of this chapter.)

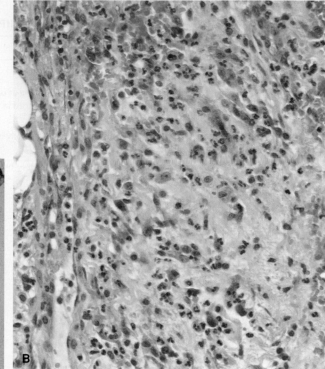

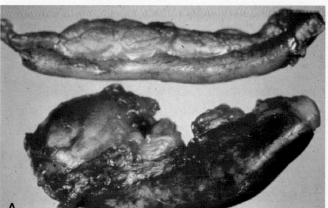

FIGURE 8-6 (**A**) Two surgical specimens from appendectomies. (**B**) Part of the wall (medium power). It should be possible to predict whether this section was obtained from the upper or lower specimen in **A**. (See discussion in part D8-6 of the Discussion section of this chapter.)

ESSENTIAL FEATURES OF THE GASTROINTESTINAL TRACT

The gastrointestinal tract is concerned chiefly with digestion, absorption, excretion, and self-protection. In order to fulfill these duties, various exocrine secretions must reach its lumen from associated accessory glands (eg, pancreas and liver). Regional specializations that facilitate such functions are compiled in Table 8-1. All these primary functions require the progression of food and its residues along the tract. Appropriate histological organization of the enteric wall, and local regulation of muscular contraction, are necessary for the peristalsis through which this is achieved.

Wall Structure of the Gastrointestinal Tract

The general wall plan of the gastrointestinal tract is outlined in Fig. 8-7. For a specific example of the appearance of the different layers, observed under very low power, see Fig. 8-8.

The term *mucous membrane (mucosa)*, used here and elsewhere, generally refers to the wet lining *epithelium*, its glandular invaginations (*mucosal glands*), and the intimate supporting layer of loose connective tissue (*lamina propria*). Also included with the mucosa of the gastrointestinal tract is the underlying layer of associated smooth muscle (*muscularis mucosae*). Villi are present only in the small intestine. The *submucosal* connective tissue also contains glands in certain parts of the tract. In regions where simple squamous epithelium (vis-

TABLE 8-1
PRINCIPAL STRUCTURAL–FUNCTIONAL RELATIONSHIPS IN THE GASTROINTESTINAL TRACT

Part of Tract	Structural Features	Functional Features
Esophagus	Stratified squamous non-keratinizing epithelium	Resists abrasion
	Mucous esophageal cardiac glands in lamina propria at upper and lower end; mucous esophageal glands scattered in submucosa	Provide lubrication
	Inferior constrictor muscle of pharynx and structurally indistinct gastroesophageal sphincter	Function as upper and lower esophageal sphincters
	Muscularis externa: skeletal in top third, smooth in bottom third, mixture of both in middle third	Dysphagia (difficulty in swallowing) associated with dysfunction and diseases of skeletal muscle; ineffective voluntary control of contraction; involuntary peristalsis
Stomach	Simple columnar mucus-secreting epithelium	Produces protective mucus
	Gastric pits (mucosal)	Openings for glands
	Rugae with submucosal cores	Flatten when stomach fills
	Cardiac glands (mucosal)	Provide protective mucus and gastrointestinal hormones
	Fundic glands with parietal cells (mucosal)	Provide HCl, intrinsic factor, enzymes, and hormones
	Pyloric glands (mucosal)	Provide protective mucus and hormones
	Pyloric sphincter (muscularis externa)	Regulates emptying of stomach
Small intestine	Plicae with submucosal cores	Plicae, villi, and microvilli increase absorptive area
	Villi with lamina propria cores	
	Microvilli on absorptive cells	
	Absorptive cells	Supply brush border enzymes, absorb products of digestion
	Goblet cells	Provide protective mucus
	Crypts	Renew epithelial cells and provide hormones
	Submucosal (Brunner's) glands in duodenum	Provide protective mucus
	Peyer's patches in ileum	Provide mucosal immunity
Large intestine	No villi	Less vigorous in absorptive activity
	Abundant goblet cells	Provide protective mucus
	Deep crypts	Renew epithelial cells and provide hormones
	Teniae coli in muscularis externa of colon	Produce sacculation
	Large, confluent lymphoid follicles in appendix	Provide mucosal immunity
Pancreas	Exocrine acini	Supply digestive enzymes
	Centroacinar cells and other duct cells	Supply bicarbonate
	Endocrine islets	Supply insulin, glucagon, somatostatin, and pancreatic polypeptide
	Thin, loose connective tissue sheath and septa	Provide fragile support
Liver	Hepatocytes (parenchymal) with bile canaliculi	Store glycogen, secrete plasma proteins, lipoprotein, bilirubin, bile salts, and IgA; metabolism of alcohol, hormones, drugs, and toxins
	Lipocytes (parenchymal)	Provide support for sinusoids and store fat; potential for fibrosis
	Portal tracts (stromal)	Convey hepatic artery, portal vein, and bile duct
	Acinar organization	Zone 1 well nourished; zone 3 less advantaged
	Sinusoids with space of Disse and Kupffer cells	Efficient exchanges between plasma and hepatocytes; phagocytosis

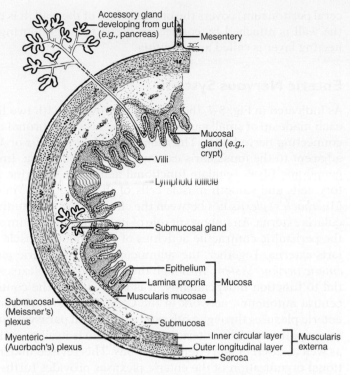

FIGURE 8-7 Tissue organization in the wall of the gastrointestinal tract.

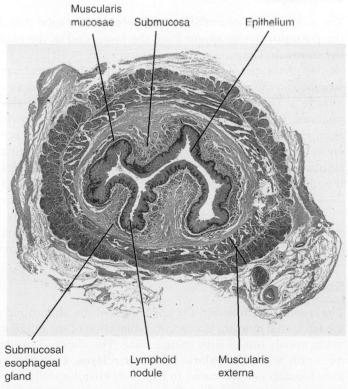

FIGURE 8-8 Constituent layers of the wall of the esophagus (middle third, very low power).

ceral peritoneum) covers the outer surface of the wall, it is called a *serosa*. Where the wall is attached by connective tissue to neighbouring structures, the connecting layer is called an *adventitia*.

Enteric Nervous System

As indicated in Fig. 8-7, the gut wall is provided with two linked nerve plexuses, each made up of small ganglia (ie, aggregates of neuronal cell bodies) and interconnecting nerve fibers. The *submucosal (submucous or Meissner's) plexus* lies adjacent to the muscularis externa, in the submucosa. Impulses from its postganglionic fibers regulate functional activity in exocrine and endocrine secretory cells and smooth muscle cells of the muscularis mucosae. The *myenteric (Auerbach's) plexus* lies between the circular and longitudinal layers of the muscularis externa. An important role of its postganglionic impulses is to coordinate the peristaltic contractile activities of the smooth muscle layers of the muscularis externa. Together, the submucosal and myenteric plexuses constitute the *enteric nervous system*. Although the intrinsic dual plexus system has the potential to function independently, it is partly under the control of a coordinating central autonomic network in the CNS. This network communicates with the enteric plexuses through both sympathetic and parasympathetic afferent and efferent pathways. The enteric nervous system is itself provided with interneurons as well as afferent and efferent neurons. This revised understanding of the functional organization of the enteric plexuses provides further insight into the basis of a number of gastrointestinal responses and motility disorders.

Esophagus

The *esophagus* is essentially a muscular-walled tube that descends vertically in the posterior mediastinum from the lower end of the pharynx to the cardia of the stomach. The *upper esophageal sphincter* (which lies at the level of the lower border of the cricoid cartilage) is the cricopharyngeal part of the inferior constrictor muscle of the pharynx (sometimes described as the "cricopharyngeus muscle"). Tonic contraction of this muscle closes off the esophagus from the pharynx. Relaxation occurs during deglutition (swallowing). The *lower esophageal sphincter*, which constricts the cardiac ostium, is not a distinct structural entity. It is considered to be a localized segment of the muscularis externa. Tonic contraction of this functional sphincter effectively closes the cardiac ostium, thereby preventing regurgitation of gastric contents. If significant regurgitation does occur, it causes *pyrosis* (heartburn; Gk. for burning) and *reflux esophagitis*.

The main histological features of the esophagus (Fig. 8-8) and their functional attributes are summarized in Table 8-1. Esophageal veins are discussed below in the context of the liver, under the heading Portal Circulation.

Stomach

The *stomach*, situated in the upper part of the abdominal cavity mostly behind the left costal margin, is a saccular dilatation of the gut in which swallowed food is vigorously mixed with gastric juice. The churned product enters the duodenum only when the pyloric sphincter relaxes. The chief anatomical regions of the stomach are indicated in Fig. 8-9. Histologically, three merging mucosal zones are distinguishable. The *cardiac region*, which extends 1–2 cm from the cardiac ostium, contains mucus-secreting glands (*cardiac glands*). The *body (fundus)* of the stomach is characterized by having glands that produce pepsin, acid, and mucus (*fundic glands*). The *pyloric region*, which begins 3–5 cm proximal to the pylorus, is provided with mucus-secreting glands (*pyloric glands*). The

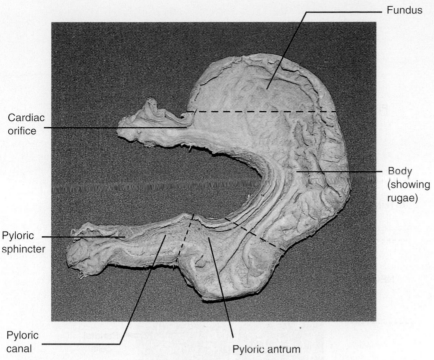

FIGURE 8-9 Anatomical and histological regions of the stomach.

squamocolumnar junction at the esophageal–gastric junction generally lies 0.5–2 cm proximal to the distal anatomical end of the esophagus.

Cardiac Region

The mucous glands of the cardiac region are essentially similar to the *cardiac glands* of the esophagus (see Table 8-1). Besides containing mucus-secreting cells, some of these glands have variable numbers of acid-producing parietal cells (described below).

Fundic Region

The *fundic (zymogenic) glands*, several of which open into each *gastric pit* (Figs. 8-10, 8-11), contain mucus-secreting *mucous neck cells*, hydrochloric acid (HCl)-producing *parietal (oxyntic) cells*, which also produce the *intrinsic factor* required for intestinal absorption of vitamin B_{12}, and pepsinogen-producing *chief (zymogenic) cells*, along with *gastrointestinal endocrine (enteroendocrine) cells* that secrete hormones or hormone-like substances, eg, serotonin, glucagon, and somatostatin. Additional secretory products of the chief cells are the enzymes rennin and lipase.

> **REVIEW ITEM 8-1**
>
> What is the difference between a gastric gland and a gastric pit?

HCl Production by Parietal Cells

When observed in the EM, *parietal (oxyntic) cells* have a highly distinctive appearance. An H^+K^+-ATPase proton pump is present in the luminal domain of the cell membrane. This pump actively transports protons (ie, H^+ ions) into extensive cytoplasmic *canaliculi* (tubular luminal invaginations), the secretory surfaces of which bear protruding long *microvilli* (Fig. 8-12). Abundant *mitochondria* provide requisite amounts of ATP. Protons are produced through the intracellular dissociation of carbonic acid (H_2CO_3), which is derived from CO_2

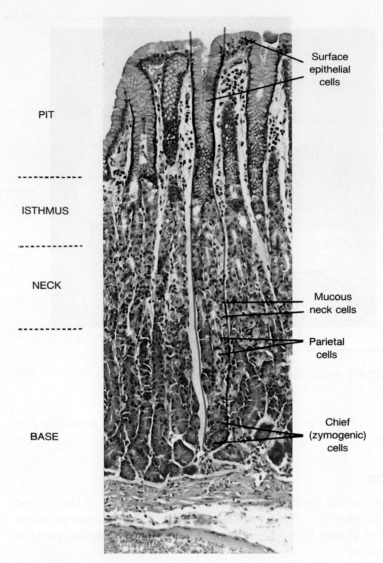

PIT

ISTHMUS

NECK

BASE

Surface epithelial cells

Mucous neck cells

Parietal cells

Chief (zymogenic) cells

FIGURE 8-10 Gastric pits and fundic glands of the fundic region of the stomach. The blue outline indicates a gland that has been cut longitudinally.

REVIEW ITEM 8-2

What role does mucus play in protecting the gastric mucosa from acid-mediated damage?

and H_2O (ie, in the same manner as in osteoclasts, see Fig. 4-16). The dissociation is brought about by a high intracellular activity of *carbonic anhydrase* in parietal cells. In addition, Cl becomes transported into the cell by a $Cl^--HCO_3^-$ antiport exchanger in the basolateral membrane, and then passes through Cl^- channels in the canalicular membrane. HCO_3^- extruded from the basolateral surface of the cell enters the interstitial space, where it protects locally against inwardly diffusing H^+ and even raises the pH of gastric venous blood.

The drug *omeprazole* is a highly effective inhibitor of the H^+K^+-ATPase proton pump in parietal cells. It can therefore be used to reduce the production of gastric HCl in patients with peptic ulcer disease.

Pyloric Region

The *pyloric glands*, which open into comparatively deep pits, are mucus secreting. However, additional HCl is also produced at the proximal border of this region. Gastrointestinal amines and peptide hormones secreted by the enteroendocrine cells present in the pylorus and pyloric antrum include serotonin,

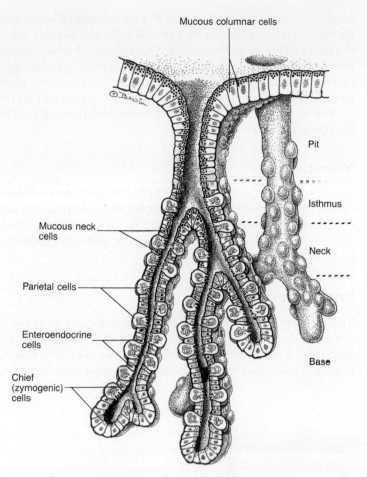

Mucous columnar cells

Pit

Isthmus

Mucous neck cells

Neck

Parietal cells

Enteroendocrine cells

Base

Chief (zymogenic) cells

FIGURE 8-11 Component regions and cells of gastric pits and fundic glands.

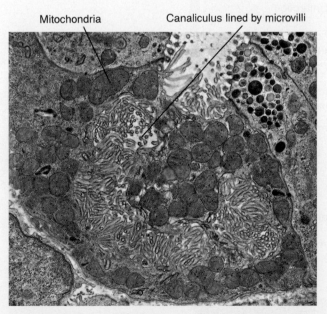

Mitochondria

Canaliculus lined by microvilli

FIGURE 8-12 Parietal cell in a fundic gland (electron micrograph, ×9,500). The cells at upper right are mucous neck cells.

gastrin, somatostatin, substance P, and vasoactive intestinal polypeptide (VIP). *Gastrin*, produced mainly by antral *G cells*, is a peptide that stimulates the production of HCl by parietal cells. The *pyloric sphincter* represents the thickened circular layer of the muscularis externa, which in the stomach consists of three layers instead of two. The innermost layer is oblique, the middle layer (thickened at the pyloric sphincter) is circular, and the outermost layer is longitudinal.

For an overview of histological characteristics and functional features of the stomach, see Table 8-1.

Vomiting

Besides being responsible for the initial stages of food digestion, the stomach becomes actively involved in the complex physiological response known as *emesis* (vomiting). Its participation, and the various factors that contribute to this stereotypic reaction to toxins, pain, stress, and other unpleasant stimuli, are outlined in Figs. 8-13 and 8-14.

Small Intestine

The primary functions of the small intestine are to complete the digestion of food, to absorb the useful products of digestion, and to produce additional amounts of gastrointestinal hormones. The area over which absorption occurs is greatly increased by the presence of circular mucosal folds (*plicae circulares*),

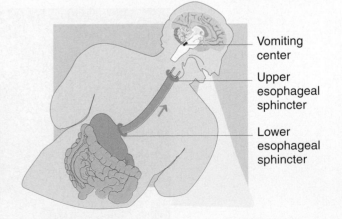

EMETIC RESPONSE

CAUSES

- Acute abdominal organ inflammation
- Acute myocardial infarction
- Gut obstruction
- Gut distention
- Gut mucosal inflammation or irritation

- Food poisoning
- Drug toxicity or side effect
- Chemotherapy toxicity
- Ionizing radiation
- Toxins
- Uremia
- Hypoxemia

- Liver disease
- Alcoholic binges
- Increased intracranial pressure
- Pregnancy
- Vestibular overstimulation (motion sickness)

Vomiting center

Upper esophageal sphincter

Lower esophageal sphincter

FIGURE 8-13 The emetic response: some common causes and major structures involved.

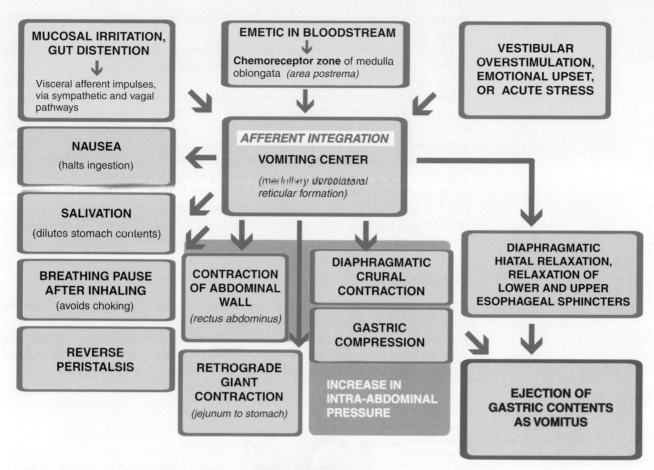

FIGURE 8-14 The emetic response: contributing and coordinating factors.

intestinal *villi*, and *microvilli* on the luminal surface of the absorptive cells. Geographic variation in villus height reflects differences of diet and bacterial flora. Both the villus height and the crypt depth:villus height ratio are relevant in diagnosis. Villus atrophy results in malabsorption.

The process of digestion essentially starts with addition of gastric HCl and enzymes. Following subsequent addition of pancreatic enzymes, it is completed in the small intestine. Terminal digestion of carbohydrates and proteins occurs in association with the striated (brush) border of the absorptive columnar cells, the luminal integral membrane glycoproteins of which include enterokinase (which activates trypsinogen) and a variety of disaccharidases and peptidases (*brush border enzymes*).

These cells then absorb the monosaccharides and amino acids that are produced. In the presence of bile salts from the liver, pancreatic lipase hydrolyzes neutral fats (triglycerides) in the luminal contents to free fatty acids, monoglycerides, and glycerol. Absorbed free fatty acids and monoglycerides are then recombined with newly synthesized glycerophosphate by the absorptive columnar cells, which synthesize triglycerides in their sER (smooth-surfaced endoplasmic reticulum). The newly synthesized triglycerides pass to the Golgi region and, in intimate association with lipoproteins, leave it in secretory vesicles that subsequently fuse with lateral regions of the cell membrane. The discharged lipoprotein-covered fat globules range in diameter from 75 nm to 1 μm. Known as *chylomicrons* (Gk. *chylos*, juice; *micros*, small), they are made up of triglycerides, phospholipids, cholesterol, cholesteryl ester, and lipoprotein. They pass with interstitial fluid into the central *lacteal* of villi and other *lymphatic capillaries* of the

the lamina propria, and reach the bloodstream indirectly by way of the lymphatic ducts.

Intestinal epithelial cells are produced deep in the crypts from stem cells called *crypt base columnar cells*. Absorptive and goblet cells become progressively displaced from the crypts to the villi, and are then shed as degenerating cells from an extrusion zone on the tip of each villus. Their lifespan (5–6 days) is similar to that of gastric epithelial cells (4–6 days). Other crypt cells include *Paneth cells*, which contain large acidophilic granules and secrete antibacterial peptides (cryptdins), phospholipase A_2, the antibacterial enzyme *lysozyme*, and a guanylyl cyclase-binding gastrointestinal polypeptide called *guanylin*. Also present is a great variety of *gastrointestinal endocrine (enteroendocrine) cells*, including those mentioned above and other ones that secrete cholecystokinin (CCK), secretin, gastric inhibitory polypeptide (glucose-dependent insulinotropic polypeptide, GIP), motilin (which elicits smooth muscle contraction), enkephalins, gut-type glucagon, and its related hormone, glicentin.

Duodenum

The *duodenum* is largely retroperitoneal. Its most distinctive histological feature is the presence of large mucus-secreting *submucosal glands* called *Brunner's glands* (Fig. 8-15). These secrete a viscid, alkaline mucus that helps to protect the mucosa from the acidity of incoming gastric contents. Under conditions of local hyperacidity, these submucosal glands may undergo hyperplasia.

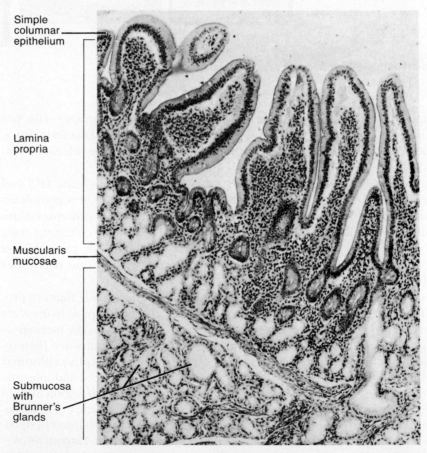

Simple columnar epithelium

Lamina propria

Muscularis mucosae

Submucosa with Brunner's glands

FIGURE 8-15 Duodenum. Submucosal (Brunner's) glands extend through the muscularis mucosae into the lamina propria. This region of the small intestine has broad, flattened villi.

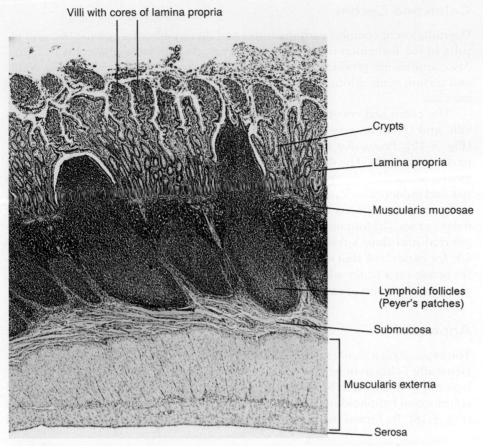

Villi with cores of lamina propria

Crypts

Lamina propria

Muscularis mucosae

Lymphoid follicles (Peyer's patches)

Submucosa

Muscularis externa

Serosa

FIGURE 8-16 Ileum. Peyer's patches extend through the muscularis mucosae, from the lamina propria to the submucosa.

Jejunum

The *jejunum*, which lies mostly in the upper part of the abdominal cavity, has narrower villi than the duodenum and is covered by a serosa, but it is otherwise lacking in distinctive histological features. Plicae circulares are numerous in this region.

Ileum

The *ileum* lies mostly in the lower part of the abdominal cavity and pelvis, covered by a serosa. Goblet cells are numerous, and the villi are shorter. This segment of the small intestine is characterized by the presence of numerous *lymphoid follicles (nodules)* that include large permanent follicular aggregates known as *Peyer's patches* (Fig. 8-16). Distributed along the antimesenteric border, these confluent follicles lie in the lamina propria but generally extend into the submucosa.

Large Intestine

Major functions of the large intestine include water and Na^+ retrieval and temporary storage of the consolidating residue. K^+ and HCO_3^- are secreted into its lumen, hence chronic diarrhea can lead to severe K^+ depletion.

Colon and Cecum

Degradation of complex carbohydrates and dietary fiber by colonic bacteria results in the formation of short-chain fatty acids and some of the gas in flatus. Also, amines are produced through the decarboxylation of amino acids. Water and certain medications are readily absorbed if administered in suppositories or enemas.

The colon and cecum are histologically characterized by (1) an absence of villi, and (2) an increased proportion of goblet cells relative to absorptive cells (Fig. 8-17). Protective mucus becomes increasingly necessary as fecal compaction proceeds. The deep crypts contain stem cells, differentiating cells, and gastrointestinal endocrine cells (described above), as well as absorptive columnar and goblet cells. Paneth cells may also be present in the crypts of the cecum and proximal colon. As in the small intestine, epithelial cells are renewed every 6 days or so. The longitudinal outer layer of the muscularis externa is chiefly organized into three substantial longitudinal bundles called *teniae* (L., from the Gk. for bands) *coli* that maintain tonus and cause sacculations called *haustra* (L. for scoop on a water wheel) to form. Since the ascending and descending segments of the colon are retroperitoneal, their outermost layer is an adventitia.

Appendix

The *appendix* is a slender, blind-ended tubular extension of the proximal cecum. Generally 7–10 cm in length, it is located near the ileocecal junction. It is histologically characterized by the presence of numerous large, persisting organized submucosal lymphoid follicles (nodules) that extend up into the lamina propria (Fig. 8-18). Its lumen is generally restricted. The appendix is a site of mucosal

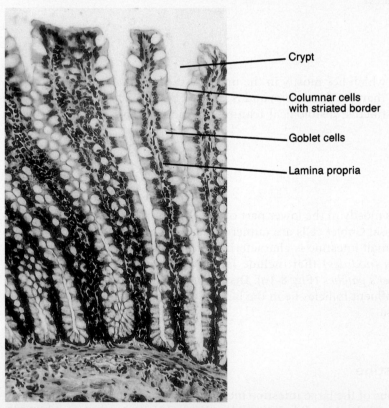

Crypt

Columnar cells with striated border

Goblet cells

Lamina propria

FIGURE 8-17 Large intestine. Crypts are seen, but villi are not present. Goblet cells are numerous in this part of the intestine.

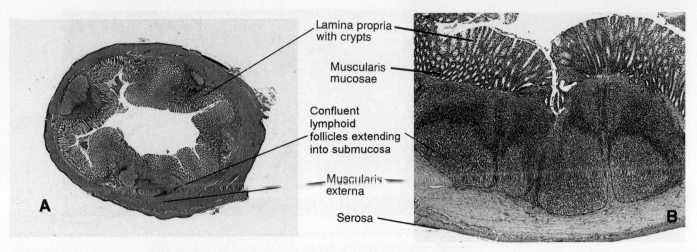

FIGURE 8-18 Appendix. (**A**) Very low power. (**B**) Low power. Large confluent lymphoid follicles (lymphatic nodules) extend down through the muscularis mucosae into the submucosa.

immune responses, primarily IgA-mediated, to microbial and parasite antigens in the luminal contents of the gut. Bacterial infection of the walls of the appendix causes *acute appendicitis*, and perforations of the inflamed appendix can lead to potentially dangerous *bacterial peritonitis* (inflammation that is elicited by the presence of bacteria in the peritoneal cavity).

For a summary of the main histological and associated functional features of the various parts of the small and large intestines, see Table 8-1.

ESSENTIAL FEATURES OF THE PANCREAS

The *pancreas* is the main enzyme-producing gland of the gastrointestinal tract. Its exocrine secretion, pancreatic juice, contains trypsin, elastase, chymotrypsins, and carboxypeptidases (which are all proteolytic), lipase and colipase (which are lipolytic), α amylase (which hydrolyzes starch), phospholipase A_2, cholesteryl ester hydrolase, deoxyribonuclease, and ribonuclease. It is also alkaline due to a substantial HCO_3^- concentration. The release of pancreatic enzymes is elicited by CCK; production of the HCO_3^--containing watery duct secretion in which they are dissolved is triggered by secretin. Vagal cholinergic (parasympathetic) stimulation also promotes the release of pancreatic enzymes. In addition, the pancreas produces insulin and glucagon, two hormones that regulate carbohydrate metabolism. Hence, the pancreas is regarded as both exocrine and endocrine. In addition to insulin and glucagon, somatostatin and pancreatic polypeptide are produced in the pancreatic endocrine functional units, which are known as the *pancreatic islets* or *islets of Langerhans* (described in Chapter 9).

Except for the presence of islets, the main histological organization of the pancreas is that of a typical compound exocrine gland. However, one or two unusual features permit its specific recognition. Instead of having a typical substantial fibrous capsule and strong supporting septa, it is provided with only a thin sheath, and thin, frail septa, of loose connective tissue (Fig. 8-19). Hence, it is vulnerable to trauma in crushing-type injuries. Another distinctive feature of the pancreas is the presence of a *centroacinar cell* (Fig. 8-20) in the middle of many of the acini. The term *acinus* is used to describe the spherical secretory unit of the pancreas that represents its exocrine functional unit. These cells represent proximal duct cells inserted into the acinus (Fig. 8-21). Pancreatic in-

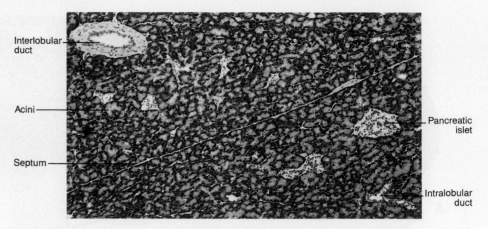

FIGURE 8-19 Pancreas (low power), showing its general features. Islets and interlobular ducts are generally somewhat easier to discern than septa and intralobular ducts.

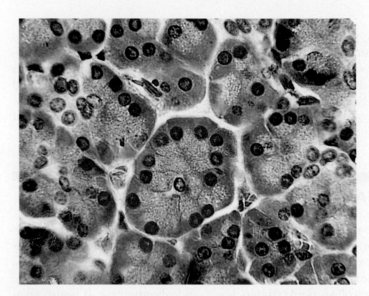

FIGURE 8-20 The nucleus seen in the middle of this pancreatic acinus is that of a centro-acinar cell.

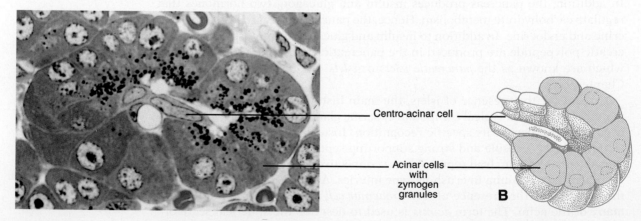

FIGURE 8-21 (**A**) Pancreatic islet with a centro-acinar cell cut longitudinally. (**B**) Explanatory diagram.

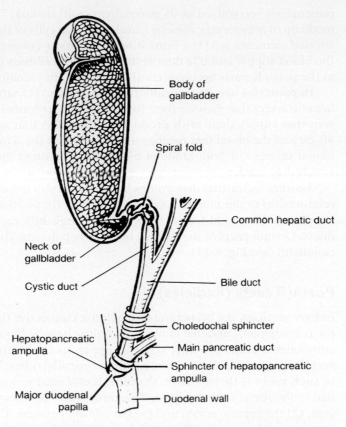

Body of
gallbladder

Spiral fold

Common hepatic duct

Neck of
gallbladder

Bile duct

Cystic duct

Hepatopancreatic
ampulla

Choledochal sphincter

Main pancreatic duct

Sphincter of hepatopancreatic
ampulla

Major duodenal
papilla

Duodenal wall

FIGURE 8-22 Anatomical relationship between the gallbladder, cystic duct, common hepatic duct, bile duct, and hepatopancreatic ampulla.

tralobular ducts are less conspicuous than the interlobular ducts. In contrast, the *main pancreatic duct* and *accessory pancreatic duct* are readily recognizable in sections because they are surrounded by a substantial sheath of dense ordinary connective tissue. The junction between the main pancreatic duct and the bile duct lies distal to the choledochal sphincter but proximal to the sphincter of the hepatopancreatic ampulla (Fig. 8-22).

ESSENTIAL FEATURES OF THE LIVER

Weighing approximately 1.5 kg, the *liver* is the body's largest compound gland and chief metabolic organ. Without essential hepatic function, patients usually die within 12 hours. Secretory activities of the liver that relate to gastrointestinal functions are (1) production of *bile salts* that facilitate fat digestion and absorption, and (2) secretion of *bilirubin*, an excretory product that reaches the duodenum by way of bile canaliculi and the bile duct once it becomes conjugated in hepatocytes (see below).

Other key functions of hepatocytes include the following: (1) secretion of *plasma proteins* (eg, albumin, fibrinogen, and prothrombin), *very low density lipoprotein* (VLDL), and *IgA* (a component of bile); (2) storage of absorbed glucose as *glycogen*; (3) storage of *lipids* and the lipid-soluble *vitamins A, D, E, K,* and B_{12} (which are stored to an even greater extent in lipid-storing cells called lipocytes, described below); and (4) *detoxification* of steroids, alcohol, and toxic exogenous chemicals that have entered the bloodstream.

Consistent with the basic glandular organization of the liver, its major components are recognized as its parenchyma and stroma. The *liver parenchyma* is made up of *hepatocytes*, *lipocytes*, and epithelial cells of the *bile duct* system. The *stromal* elements are (1) a branching tree of *loose connective tissue* that follows the blood supply and bile duct system, and (2) a fibrous (Glisson's) *capsule* that at the porta hepatis becomes continuous with the remainder of the stroma.

Hepatocytes are strategically positioned near (1) terminal branches of the hepatic artery that provide their oxygen, and (2) terminal branches of the portal vein that supply them with products of digestion that need to be stored. Only 40–50% of the blood that reaches them is arterial; the remainder is portal. A regulated mixture of both kinds of blood flows through the venous sinusoids on which they border.

Another factor that determines how hepatocytes are arranged is their spatial relationship to the bile duct system. Efficient elimination of bilirubin depends on the unobstructed free flow of bile through bile canaliculi, ductules, and ducts. Certain parts of the surface of every hepatocyte, therefore, border on bile canaliculi (see Fig. 8-24).

Portal Tracts (Radicles)

In liver sections, the branching tree of loose connective tissue that extends from the porta hepatis, and that conveys incoming hepatic blood vessels and the main components of the bile duct system, appears as connective tissue islands called *portal tracts (areas)* that contain a number parallel tubes. The minimum number of such tubes is three; hence, the term *portal triad* is sometimes used an alternative for *portal tract (radicle)*. The three tubes are branches of (1) the *portal vein*, (2) the *hepatic artery*, and (3) the *bile duct* system. Commonly, a *lymphatic* is also present as a fourth component. The widest of these tubes is the portal vein (see Fig. 8-23). The main functions of the portal tracts are to deliver blood to the parenchyma and to drain bile from it.

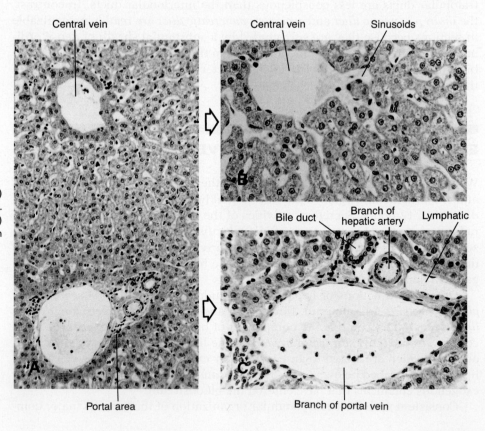

FIGURE 8-23 (**A**) Portal tract (area) and central vein of the liver (low power). (**B**) Central vein (medium power). (**C**) Components of a portal tract (medium power).

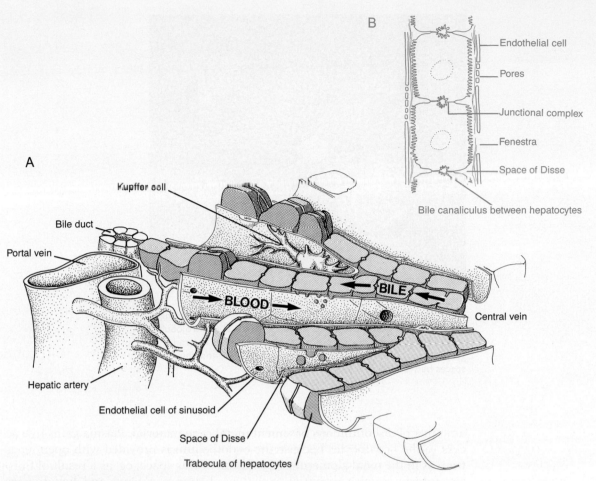

FIGURE 8-24 The components associated with a hepatic sinusoid. (**A**) Arrangement of sinusoids and associated hepatocytes in a classic lobule. The directions indicated for blood flow and bile flow relate to the components in the portal tract at left. (**B**) Diagram showing the relationship between the fenestrated sinusoidal endothelium, space of Disse, and bile canaliculi. Plasma constituents have free access to the microvillus-covered absorptive border of hepatocytes by way of endothelial fenestrae and the perisinusoidal space of Disse.

Hepatic Sinusoids

Blood arriving from the terminal branches of the portal vein and hepatic artery in portal tracts enters the venous sinusoids (*hepatic sinusoids*) that border on hepatocytes. Hepatic sinusoids are relatively wide, thin-walled, low pressure vessels lined with a fenestrated endothelium. Entry of portal blood from portal venules is regulated by inlet sphincters. Arterial blood is admitted by branched hepatic arterioles. The blood leaving hepatic sinusoids enters terminal hepatic venules (alternatively known as central or centrolobular veins), and leaves the liver by way of hepatic veins that open into the inferior vena cava (see Fig. 8-29).

As shown in Fig. 8-24A, a narrow extravascular space called the *perisinusoidal space* or *space of Disse* exists between the fenestrated endothelium of the sinusoid and the adjacent borders of hepatocytes. The part of the hepatocyte surface that is in contact with the space of Disse bears microvilli and is, accordingly, absorptive (Fig. 8-24B*B*). Other sinusoid-associated components are (1) *Kupffer cells*, which are intensely phagocytic, monocyte-derived resident macrophages, and (2) *lipocytes (fat-storing cells of Ito)*, which are believed to have a supporting function. Whereas the Kupffer cells are intraluminal or insinuated into the vessel lining, lipocytes are situated in the space of Disse. This perisinusoidal space also contains a scaffolding of reticular fibers and minimal

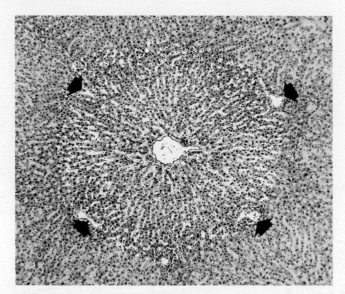

FIGURE 8-25 Section of liver, showing an example of a classic liver lobule. Arrows point to four portal tracts that appear to be arranged in a circle. The white space in its middle is a central (centrolobular) vein, which corresponds to a terminal hepatic venule. The radiating grey structures are rows or plates of hepatocytes, and the white spaces between them are sinusoids.

amounts of discontinuous basement membrane material. Plasma gains free access to the hepatocytes because the endothelium is provided with open fenestrae, as in the renal glomerulus. Occlusion of this space, eg, as a result of fibrosis, interferes with essential exchanges between plasma and hepatocytes. Lipocytes respond to hepatic injury by undergoing a phenotypic change in which they become contractile and produce collagen types I and III instead of the type IV collagen that they normally produce.

Hepatocyte Arrangement

Two main concepts exist concerning the organization of liver parenchyma. The long-entrenched concept of the classic *liver lobule* is becoming displaced and largely superseded by that of the *liver acinus*.

To visualize the boundaries of a classic *liver lobule*, it is necessary to find two to four portal tracts that appear to be arranged in a ring (Fig. 8-25). If rows of hepatocytes appear to be radially oriented with respect to the center of the ring, and a thin-walled vessel is present at the center, the parenchymal area within the ring is considered to be a liver lobule in transverse section, and the central vessel is referred to as a *central (centrolobular) vein* (see Figs. 8-23, 8-24). Blood flows from portal tracts at the periphery of the lobule to its middle, and bile flows in the reverse direction (Fig. 8-24A).

A more useful concept is that of the *liver acinus* (Fig. 8-26). This is a novel usage of the term *acinus* (L. for berry or grape). It corresponds to a roughly egg-shaped mass of hepatic parenchyma that has as its central axis its *blood supply* (arterial and portal) instead of its venous drainage. However, the axial vessels are very difficult to find in uninjected routine sections, and the only morphological landmark that in any way marks the outer limits of an acinus is a central vein, which is now more commonly known as a *terminal hepatic venule*. Figure 8-26 shows the spatial relationship between liver acini and liver lobules. Hence, the liver acinus is essentially a *functional unit* (or concept) based on the hepatic

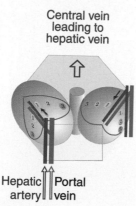

Central vein leading to hepatic vein

Hepatic artery | Portal vein

FIGURE 8-26 The concept of the liver acinus. Two acini, with their respective dual blood supplies coming from portal tracts, are shown in relation to a hexagonal classic lobule. The numbers indicate zonation of the acinus. In each acinus, zone 3 lies closest to the central vein, and zone 1 lies closest to the axial vessels extending along the lobular periphery.

blood supply, rather than a morphological concept derived from simple microscopic observation.

Zone 1 of the liver acinus lies closest to the vascular backbone of the structure. *Zone 3* lies farthest away, and its hepatocytes are more vulnerable to anoxia and are in a less favorable position to obtain nutrients. Toxic and reactive metabolites also pass into Zone 3, hence microscopic evidence of cell death is sometimes seen in Zone 3 (which is generally situated in the vicinity of terminal hepatic venules; see Fig. 8-26). Under normal circumstances, cell renewal compensates for any cell death, since hepatocytes represent a potentially renewable population. To a certain extent, the liver is therefore a self-regenerating organ.

For a summary of the main histological and associated functional features of the liver, see Table 8-1.

Hemoglobin Degradation and the Role of Hepatocytes in Bilirubin Excretion

As outlined in Fig. 8-27, the somewhat detailed process of hemoglobin degradation and bilirubin elimination begins with the phagocytosis of erythrocytes by macrophages, particularly those of the spleen. The principal breakdown products of hemoglobin that enter the blood plasma are (1) *iron* in the ferric state (Fe^{3+}) released from heme, and (2) *unconjugated bilirubin* derived from the intermediate compound, biliverdin. Some of the cells that take up Fe^{3+}, eg, macrophages, have the capacity to store it reversibly as an iron-containing protein called *ferritin*. Excessive amounts of iron may accumulate in such cells as an unusable yellowish-brown pigment called *hemosiderin*, which is a partly denatured form of ferritin. Under conditions of iron overload, eg, primary (hereditary) hemochromatosis, hemosiderin accumulates in cells, causing *hemosiderosis*. Free Fe^{3+} is recycled for hemoprotein synthesis.

Fenestrations in the endothelium of hepatic sinusoids allow free access of albumin-bound unconjugated bilirubin in the plasma to the space of Disse, from which it is taken up through facilitated transport across the absorptive hepatocyte surface that bears microvilli (Fig. 8-27, *middle left*). The hepatocytes conjugate bilirubin, the water solubility of which is relatively low, to glucuronic acid, producing *bilirubin diglucuronide*, which is freely water soluble and is known as *conjugated bilirubin*. Glucuronyl transferases, the enzymes responsible for this conjugation reaction, are associated with the sER. Conjugated bilirubin is actively transported across another structurally and functionally delimited domain of the cell membrane that borders on a sealed-off intercellular space known as a *bile canaliculus*. These groove-shaped canalicular domains are precisely apposed in adjacent cells. Continuous tight junctions in junctional complexes seal off the canalicular lumen from the remainder of the interstitial space (Fig. 8-24B). Hence, conjugated bilirubin passes with the other constituents of bile (which include bile salts, ie, sodium and potassium salts of cholic and chenodeoxycholic acid and their derivatives, along with cholesterol, lecithin, fatty acids, IgA, ions, and water) into the *bile canaliculi* and not into the main interstitial space. The bile produced by the liver is stored in the *gallbladder*. When discharged through CCK-elicited contraction of the gallbladder, bile reaches the duodenum by way of the *common bile duct* (Figs. 8-22, 8-27).

Once admitted by the *choledochal sphincter*, conjugated bilirubin and its derivatives recirculate, following an *enterohepatic circulation*. The principal bilirubin-derived urobilinoids are *urobilinogens* (also known as *stercobilinogens*) produced through the action of fecal bacteria. Urobilinoid absorbed from the intestine enters the portal blood and become re-excreted by hepatocytes into the bile. Unabsorbed urobilinoid remains in the feces. Only small amounts of absorbed urobilinogen (which is colorless) are removed from the circulation (ie, excreted) by the kidneys. An elevated level of urinary bilinogen can indicate

---

REVIEW ITEM 8-3

What are (1) canals of Hering and (2) bile preductules?

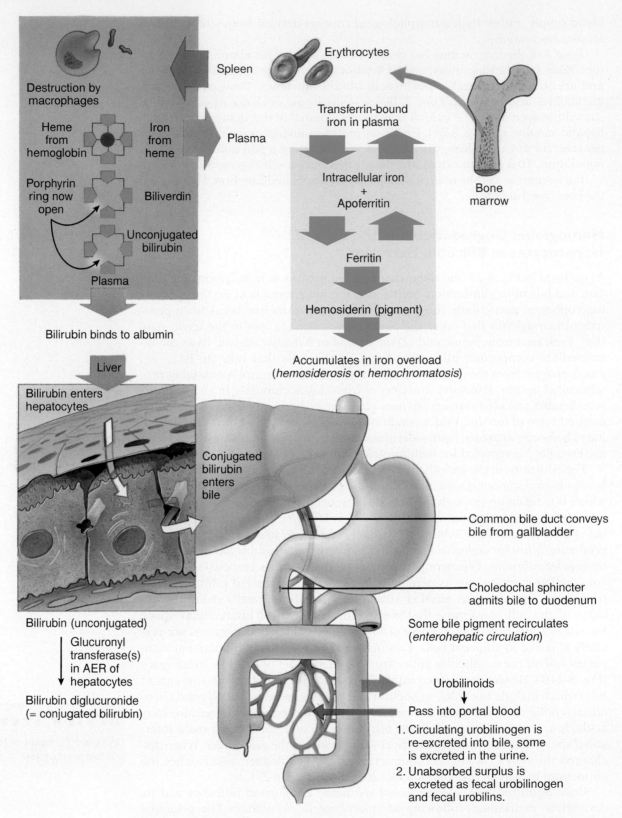

Spleen

Destruction by macrophages

Heme from hemoglobin

Iron from heme

Porphyrin ring now open

Biliverdin

Unconjugated bilirubin

Plasma

Plasma

Bilirubin binds to albumin

Erythrocytes

Transferrin-bound iron in plasma

Intracellular iron + Apoferritin

Bone marrow

Ferritin

Hemosiderin (pigment)

Accumulates in iron overload (*hemosiderosis* or *hemochromatosis*)

Liver

Bilirubin enters hepatocytes

Conjugated bilirubin enters bile

Common bile duct conveys bile from gallbladder

Choledochal sphincter admits bile to duodenum

Some bile pigment recirculates (*enterohepatic circulation*)

Bilirubin (unconjugated)

Glucuronyl transferase(s) in AER of hepatocytes

Bilirubin diglucuronide (= conjugated bilirubin)

Urobilinoids

Pass into portal blood

1. Circulating urobilinogen is re-excreted into bile, some is excreted in the urine.
2. Unabsorbed surplus is excreted as fecal urobilinogen and fecal urobilins.

FIGURE 8-27 Key stages of hemoglobin breakdown and elimination of bilirubin from the body. (See text for details.)

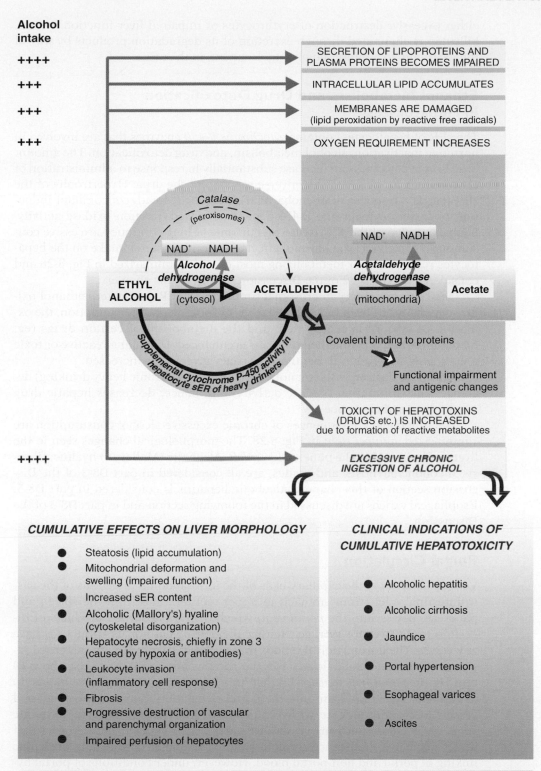

Alcohol
intake

++++ → SECRETION OF LIPOPROTEINS AND PLASMA PROTEINS BECOMES IMPAIRED

+++ → INTRACELLULAR LIPID ACCUMULATES

+++ → MEMBRANES ARE DAMAGED (lipid peroxidation by reactive free radicals)

+++ → OXYGEN REQUIREMENT INCREASES

Catalase (peroxisomes)

NAD⁺ NADH
Alcohol dehydrogenase

NAD⁺ NADH
Acetaldehyde dehydrogenase

ETHYL ALCOHOL (cytosol) → ACETALDEHYDE (mitochondria) → Acetate

Supplemental cytochrome P-450 activity in hepatocyte sER of heavy drinkers

Covalent binding to proteins

Functional impairment and antigenic changes

TOXICITY OF HEPATOTOXINS (DRUGS etc.) IS INCREASED due to formation of reactive metabolites

++++ → EXCESSIVE CHRONIC INGESTION OF ALCOHOL

CUMULATIVE EFFECTS ON LIVER MORPHOLOGY

- Steatosis (lipid accumulation)
- Mitochondrial deformation and swelling (impaired function)
- Increased sER content
- Alcoholic (Mallory's) hyaline (cytoskeletal disorganization)
- Hepatocyte necrosis, chiefly in zone 3 (caused by hypoxia or antibodies)
- Leukocyte invasion (inflammatory cell response)
- Fibrosis
- Progressive destruction of vascular and parenchymal organization
- Impaired perfusion of hepatocytes

CLINICAL INDICATIONS OF CUMULATIVE HEPATOTOXICITY

- Alcoholic hepatitis
- Alcoholic cirrhosis
- Jaundice
- Portal hypertension
- Esophageal varices
- Ascites

The specific cytochrome P-450 that chiefly metabolizes ethyl alcohol is also known as the microsomal ethanol oxidizing system (MEOS)
NAD⁺ = nicotinamide adenine dinucleotide

FIGURE 8-28 Oxidative elimination of ethyl alcohol from the body. This metabolism occurs primarily in hepatocytes of zone 3 of liver acini. Important medical consequences of excessive alcohol consumption are emphasized.

either excessive destruction of erythrocytes or impaired liver function. Hence, bilirubin is eliminated through excretion of its degradation products by way of the feces and, to a minor, augmentable extent, in the urine.

Ethanol Metabolism and Drug Detoxification in Hepatocytes

The sER of hepatocytes contains *cytochrome P-450* enzymes that are involved in hormone inactivation, alcohol metabolism, and drug detoxification. The amount of sER in hepatocytes can increase substantially in response to administration of certain drugs or if there is an adverse reaction to the drug. Hypertrophy of the sER (eg, as a response to phenobarbital) is associated with concomitant induction of further cytochrome P-450-dependent mixed-function oxidase activity. Such expansion of the sER is also an outcome of long-continued, excessive consumption of alcohol. The harmful effects of chronic ethanol intake on the hepatocytes responsible for metabolizing most of it are summarized in Fig. 8-28 and considered in part D8-2 of the Discussion section of this chapter.

Once supplementary microsomal (in this case, sER-associated) ethanol-oxidizing activity has been induced by heavy, chronic alcohol consumption, the oxidation of ethanol is accelerated, and the metabolism of certain drugs (eg, methadone) and potential hepatotoxins is enhanced. Damaging reactive or toxic metabolites are produced. Synthesis of triacylglycerols is increased.

Acute intoxication with ethanol (as distinct from chronic heavy drinking) decreases mixed-function oxidase activity and, hence, decreases hepatic drug metabolism and clearance.

The functional consequences of chronic excessive alcohol consumption are summarized at *upper right* in Fig. 8-28. The morphological changes seen in the liver are indicated in the panel at *lower left*. Alcoholic (Mallory's) hyaline, fibrosis, alcoholic cirrhosis, and ascites, are all considered in part D8-3 of the Discussion section of this chapter. Alcoholic hepatitis is considered in part D8-5. Esophageal varices are discussed in the following section and in part D8-3 of the Discussion.

Portal Circulation

Venous blood from the capillary beds of the intra-abdominal regions of the gastrointestinal tract (from stomach to upper rectum), and from the spleen and pancreas, passes into the *portal vein*, which delivers absorbed products of digestion to the liver for storage. Neither the portal vein nor its tributaries have any valves. The normal portal venous pressure is 5–10 mm Hg. An increased resistance to hepatic blood flow causes the portal venous pressure to rise above 10 mm Hg (ie, *portal hypertension*). When this happens, a backpressure builds up in capillary beds that drain into the portal circulation. Some of the congested vessels also communicate with venules that drain into non-portal systemic veins. Such communicating vessels are latent *portal–systemic anastomoses* that under normal circumstances remain small in diameter permit only negligible mixing of portal and non-portal blood. However, under conditions of portal hypertension, these anastomotic vessels dilate and permit portal blood to spill over into the general systemic circulation.

Four sites where veins that drain into the portal circulation lie in comparatively close proximity to veins that drain into the general systemic circulation are indicated in Fig. 8-29. These sites are predisposed for the development of *portal collateral vessels* from the pre-existing vasculature. A clinically important site in this respect is the submucosa of the lower end of the esophagus (*1* in Fig. 8-29). In contrast to the veins of (1) the middle third of the esophagus, which open into the azygos (or, in a few cases, the hemiazygos) vein, and (2) the upper

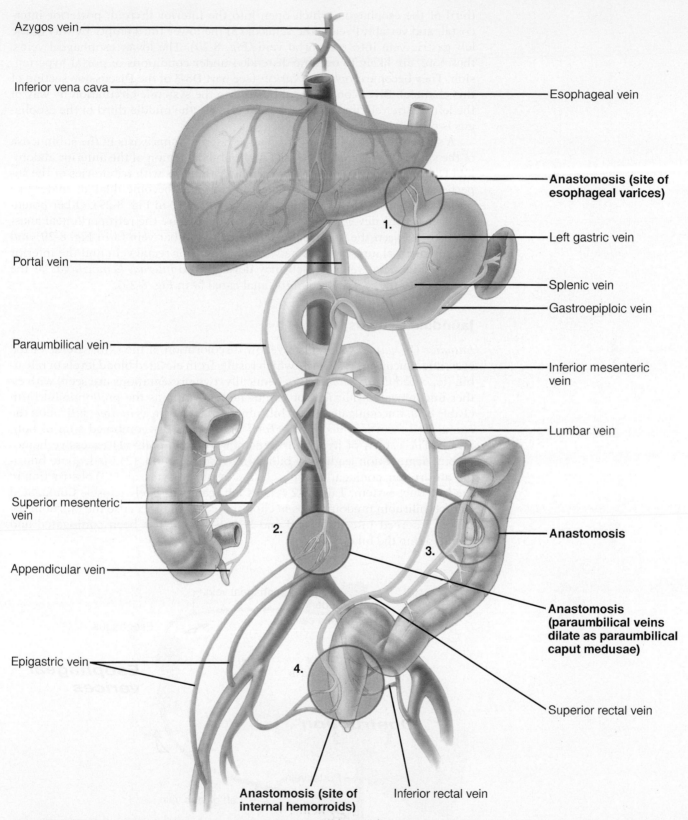

Azygos vein

Inferior vena cava

Portal vein

Paraumbilical vein

Superior mesenteric vein

Appendicular vein

Epigastric vein

Esophageal vein

Anastomosis (site of esophageal varices)

Left gastric vein

Splenic vein

Gastroepiploic vein

Inferior mesenteric vein

Lumbar vein

Anastomosis

Anastomosis (paraumbilical veins dilate as paraumbilical caput medusae)

Superior rectal vein

1.

2.

3.

4.

Anastomosis (site of internal hemorrhoids)

Inferior rectal vein

FIGURE 8-29 Some major portal–systemic venous anastomoses: (1) left gastric–esophageal; (2) paraumbilical–superficial epigastric; (3) colic–lumbar; (4) superior rectal–middle and inferior rectal.

third of the esophagus, which open into the inferior thyroid, posterior intercostal, and vertebral veins, the veins of (3) the lower third empty by way of the left gastric vein into the portal vein (Fig. 8-29). The lower esophageal veins, therefore, are likely to become distended under conditions of portal hypertension. They become *esophageal varices* (see part D8-3 of the Discussion section of this chapter). Diversion of portal blood into the systemic circulation by way of the left gastric vein and the esophageal veins in the middle third of the esophagus is outlined in Fig. 8-30.

A similar juxtaposition of portal and systemic veins exists in the submucosa of the stomach. A second site is the periumbilical region of the anterior abdominal wall, where the paraumbilical vein anastomoses with tributaries of the superficial epigastric veins. These anastomoses may become dilated, spider-like portal collateral vessels known as *caput medusae* (*2* in Fig. 8-29). Other potential sites for the development of portal collaterals are the retroperitoneal anastomoses between the superior rectal vein and lumbar vein (*3* in Fig. 8-29) and the submucosal anastomoses between the superior rectal vein and the inferior and middle rectal veins, which may develop into *internal hemorrhoids* at the lower end of the rectum and in the anal canal (*4* in Fig. 8-29).

Jaundice (Icterus)

Jaundice (Fr. *jaune*, yellow) is a yellow discoloration of the skin, sclerae of the eyes, and mucous membranes, which results from elevated blood levels of bilirubin (ie, *hyperbilirubinemia*). Biochemically, two presentations are seen, with either unconjugated bilirubin or conjugated bilirubin as the predominant form (Table 8-2). Unconjugated (free) bilirubin also is known as *indirect* bilirubin; the conjugated form is called *direct*. *Total* bilirubin is the combined sum of both forms. The causes of hyperbilirubinemia are essentially (1) excessive hemoglobin, degradation leading to bilirubin overproduction, (2) inadequate bilirubin absorption, conjugation, or secretion by hepatocytes, and (3) obstruction to the bile duct system. Table 8-2 relates lab results to likely causes. Conjugated (direct) bilirubin predominates in cholestatic jaundice because the bilirubin becomes resorbed into the blood and lymph after it has been conjugated and secreted into the bile.

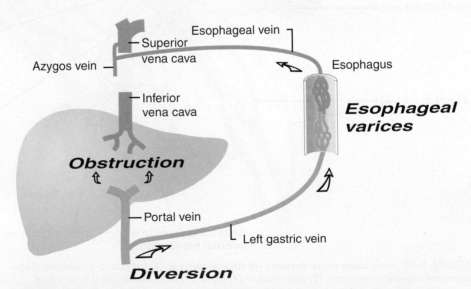

FIGURE 8-30 In portal hypertension, obstruction of intrahepatic portal blood flow (eg, as a result of fibrosis) shunts venous blood from the portal vein to the superior vena cava by way of the left gastric, esophageal, and azygos veins. The increased portal pressure in submucosal esophageal veins may result in their dilatation and lead to the formation of *esophageal varices*.

TABLE 8-2
CAUSES OF JAUNDICE

UNCONJUGATED HYPERBILIRUBINEMIA (INDIRECT BILIRUBIN PREDOMINATES)
Bilirubin overloading, eg, due to hemolysis

Insufficient bilirubin uptake by hepatocytes

Insufficient bilirubin conjugation by hepatocytes

CONJUGATED HYPERBILIRUBINEMIA (WITH BILIRUBINURIA; DIRECT BILIRUBIN PREDOMINATES)
Insufficient transport of conjugated bilirubin into canaliculi

Hepatotoxic damage, eg, hepatitis, drugs (hepatocellular)

Bile duct obstruction (cholestatic)

CASE DISCUSSIONS

D8-1 (CASE 8-1)

In Fig. 8-1, a mucosal lesion—either a *peptic ulcer* or an *acute gastric erosion*—can be recognized at the level of the *duodenum*. The site may be inferred from the presence of (1) submucosal mucous glands (Brunner's glands) and (2) a part of the pancreas in the same section. At this magnification, it is difficult to decide whether the lesion is an ulcer penetrating the muscularis mucosae or an erosion that does not. Since peptic ulcers occur at insufficiently protected sites that are exposed to gastric hydrochloric acid and pepsin, the mucosa is the layer that is most severely damaged. Under normal conditions, partial neutralization of the acid by both alkaline pancreatic juice and local interstitial bicarbonate ions, the protective effect of overlying mucus, and rapid turnover of mucosal epithelial cells minimize or compensate for mucosal damage in the duodenum. It has been suggested that insufficient production of bicarbonate by the duodenal mucosa predisposes to development of duodenal ulcers. Also implicated in the etiology of peptic ulcer disease, along with hydrochloric acid and pepsin, is the gram-negative bacterium *Helicobacter pylori*. This species of bacteria colonizes the gastric epithelium of most patients who have chronic gastritis. The antibiotics to which it is susceptible not only promote the healing of peptic ulcers but also decrease their recurrence.

The patient experiences epigastric pain because any pain from the upper GI tract is referred to the epigastric area (see Chap. 4, section D4-9, for a discussion of referred pain). Endoscopic observation is more likely than an upper GI barium-contrast x-ray series to reveal a mucosal erosion. When luminal acidity is sufficiently reduced, the damaged tissues are able to repair themselves in 1 to 2 months. However, cigarette smoking and alcohol have both been found to delay effective healing, and coffee acts as a stimulus for gastrin secretion, promoting acid formation in the stomach. Yet another stimulus for acid secretion by the parietal cells is calcium, which is a major constituent of milk. Two possible reasons for the medication's lack of effectiveness in this case are (1) patient noncompliance and (2) the fact that approximately 10% of peptic ulcers fail to respond to H_2-receptor blocking agents. A more effective way of treating resistant peptic ulcers is to use the drug omeprazole to inhibit H^+K^+-ATPase, which is the proton pump in the parietal cells. Aspirin can injure the gastric mucosa and elicit gastrointestinal bleeding. Particularly if taken in conjunction with smoking and alcohol, aspirin and other non-steroidal anti-inflammatory agents may even incite an erosive (acute) gastritis.

D8-2 (CASE 8-2)

Figure 8-2 shows histological evidence of *acute toxic hepatitis*. This condition has the potential to progress to acute liver failure. Elevated serum aminotransferase levels indicate hepatocyte damage. The so-called centrilobular, pericentral, or perivenular zone 3 necrosis evident in this biopsy is consistent with extreme susceptibility of this patient to frequent large doses of acetaminophen. Such extreme hepatotoxicity is equally consistent with earlier attempts to overdose with the drug, resulting in permanent toxic damage to hepatocytes that may reach a critical level.

Extensive liver damage leaves a diminished reserve of cytosolic alcohol dehydrogenase and sER-associated cytochrome P-450 to metabolize alcohol in large quantities. Furthermore, alcohol-mediated induction of cytochrome P-450 activity in the surviving hepatocytes can augment the hepatotoxicity of acetaminophen. Reserves of glutathione, required for urinary excretion of a toxic metabolite of acetaminophen, may become critically depleted. Necrosis of zone 3 in the pericentral areas results if this reactive metabolite becomes covalently bound to essential hepatocyte macromolecules instead of being eliminated by way of the urine after conjugation to glutathione. (Alcohol catabolism and harmful cumulative effects of ethanol are summarized in Fig. 8-28.)

D8-3 (CASE 8-3)

A distinctive feature of the liver biopsy shown in Fig. 8-3 is its content of small (ie, microscopic) nodules (*micronodules*). Micronodules resembling lobules are often referred to as *pseudolobules*. Most of the parenchymal cells seen in this biopsy have very large lipid droplets in their cytoplasm and are scarcely recognizable as hepatocytes. The liver has lost its normal so-called lobular and acinar organization. Micronodules and pseudolobules (see Fig. 8-3B, central area) result from a chronic reparative process that is unsuccessful in regenerating normal lobular organization from surviving regions of acini (zone 1). The resulting micronodules may lack a terminal hepatic venule (central vein) in their middle, or they may be inadequately supplied by portal areas because they are only the regenerated portions of lobules. Also noticeable are wide bands of *fibrous scar tissue* that extend from the portal areas (see Fig. 8-3A). Such fibrous regions around the micronodules and pseudolobules commonly connect portal areas either to each other or to terminal hepatic venules (central veins). When numerous parenchymal cells die, they become replaced by stromal fibrous connective tissue and the liver's normal lobular, vascular, and acinar organization is not restored. In this type of cirrhosis (*alcoholic cirrhosis*) the liver is generally also enlarged. Another distinctive feature seen in many of the hepatocytes is the presence of large irregular cytoplasmic inclusions that stain a reddish-purple (see Fig. 8-3C). Termed *alcoholic (Mallory's) hyaline* or *Mallory bodies*, these inclusions contain condensations of keratin filaments, a type of intermediate filament. They are presumed to be a consequence of cytoskeletal disorganization. Also found in a variety of other liver disorders, Mallory bodies are considered a hallmark of *alcoholic hepatitis*, which is the condition that precedes alcoholic cirrhosis, the late end-stage disease of the chronic alcoholic. (For an overview and summary of morphological changes found in the liver as a consequence of long-term heavy alcohol consumption, see Fig. 8-28.)

The mild scleral discoloration indicates that this patient also has *hyperbilirubinemia*. Conspicuous yellowing of the sclerae, nailbeds, or skin by the hemoglobin-derived pigment *bilirubin* is described as *jaundice* (Fr. *jaune*, yellow) or *icterus* (Gk. *ikteros*, jaundice). The hyperbilirubinemia associated with cirrhosis is a result of extensive hepatocellular damage that permits leakage of bile from canaliculi into the bloodstream.

The abdominal distention and slight difficulty with breathing are caused by the presence of free fluid in the abdominal cavity, ie, *ascites*. Normally, the balance of forces is such that approximately 85% of the tissue fluid reaching the interstitial space from the blood plasma is taken back into the blood; the remainder returns as lymph. This efficient resorption of the fluid is due to the fact that, at sites other than the renal cortex, the osmotic pressure of the blood at the venular end of capillaries is generally higher than the hydrostatic pressure, and as a consequence, tissue fluid is drawn back in. The volume of extravascular fluid that accumulates depends on the hydrostatic pressure along the length of the capillaries (filtration pressure), the osmotic pressure of the plasma proteins (oncotic pressure), the interstitial concentration of proteins, and a number of other parameters. Accumulation of extravascular *ascitic fluid* within the abdominal cavity is essentially a result of an imbalance created by (1) elevated portal blood pressure (portal hypertension) and (2) diminished intravascular oncotic pressure (a consequence of the decreased albumin content of plasma). Hypoalbuminemia resulting from liver damage commonly also results in peripheral edema. Another factor that contributes to formation of ascitic fluid is backpressure in the liver sinusoids. This increases the amount of interstitial fluid entering the perisinusoidal space of Disse. Under normal conditions, all this fluid drains from the liver as hepatic lymph, but a large excess of it can pass directly from the liver surface into the peritoneal cavity. The "shifting dullness" heard on percussion is a dullness over the flanks that shifts laterally when the patient turns over on one side. In addition, a "fluid wave," a further indication of ascites, can often be felt over one flank when the other flank is tapped. A routine procedure for establishing or confirming the cause of ascites is diagnostic *paracentesis* (percutaneous aspiration of a sample of ascitic fluid). Prognosis is poorer once alcoholics with cirrhosis develop ascites.

A further indication of the prognosis is provided in Fig. 8-4A. In this section, it is possible to recognize a stratified squamous non-keratinizing epithelium and some skeletal muscle at the lower border; these are two characteristics of the lower third of the esophagus. An enlarged blood vessel lies in the submucosa. Its size and wall structure indicate that it is an esophageal vein, ie, a tributary of the azygos vein (see Fig. 8-30). This vessel has become widely dilated as a result of portal hypertension. Normally, much of the blood that it is now carrying would leave by way of esophageal tributaries of the left gastric vein, which opens into the portal vein and is part of the portal circulation (see Figs. 8-29, 8-30). However, any backpressure due to portal obstruction can divert more blood into leaving by the alternate route—the systemic vessels (veins) that return blood from this and other sites of portal–systemic anastomosis (see Fig. 8-29). *Esophageal varices* that commonly develop in the lower third of the esophagus in patients with cirrhosis may be detected by endoscopy (see Fig. 8-4B) or demonstrated by barium swallow, ie, barium-contrast esophagography (see Fig. 8-4C). Their clinical significance is that they and other dilated thin-walled esophageal vessels are easily ruptured, eg, during the swallowing of food. Unless brought under control, the vigorous bleeding that ensues may almost exsanguinate the patient. The situation is worse if the production of clotting factors has also been impaired as a result of hepatocyte damage. Ruptured esophageal varices require immediate emergency attention and prompt management.

D8-5 (FIG. 8-5)

Under certain circumstances, the condition illustrated in Fig. 8-5, *alcoholic hepatitis*, may deteriorate and lead to the severe scarring and distortion that characterize alcoholic cirrhosis (see Fig. 8-3). There are several indications that this driver overindulged in alcoholic beverages or enjoyed bouts of heavy drinking. A large proportion of hepatocytes are filled with lipid, resulting in a *fatty liver (fatty infiltration* or *steatosis)*. Some of the hepatocytes have degenerated, and the resulting necrosis has led to parenchymal invasion by neutrophils and lymphocytes. *Alcoholic* or *Mallory's hyaline (Mallory bodies)*, described above (see section D8-3), is present in damaged zones (chiefly zone 3 in the pericentral areas) and in periportal areas. Under conditions of total abstinence from alcohol, this type of hepatitis may be prevented from progressing and, in some cases, slow resolution ensues because of the liver's remarkable capacity for regeneration.

Excessive alcohol consumption over a long period may also result in *chronic pancreatitis*, with associated steatorrhea (presence of fat in the feces) due to decreased lipase secretion. Insulin levels may also be reduced. In *acute alcoholic pancreatitis*, occlusive plugs form in the small ducts of the pancreas as a result of precipitation of highly concentrated pancreatic enzymes. Resulting damage by prematurely activated digestive enzymes causes necrosis, hemorrhage, enzyme leakage into the retroperitoneum, and painful inflammation.

D8-6 (FIG. 8-6)

Figure 8-6A shows a normal appendix above, and an acutely inflamed appendix below. Figure 8-6B reveals the presence of a large population of *neutrophils*, which are diagnostic for *acute appendicitis*.

BIBLIOGRAPHY

Burwen SJ, Schmucker DL, Jones AL. Subcellular and molecular mechanisms of bile secretion. Int Rev Cytol 135:269, 1992.

Delvalle J, Yamada T. The gut as an endocrine organ. Annu Rev Med 41:447, 1990.

Doe WF. The intestinal immune system. Gut 30:1679, 1989.

Erlinger S. Bile secretion. Br Med Bull 48:860, 1992.

Goyal RK, Hirano I. The enteric nervous system. N Engl J Med 334:1106, 1996.

Gumucio JJ. Hepatocyte heterogeneity: The coming of age from the description of a biological curiosity to a partial understanding of its physiological meaning and regulation. Hepatology 9:154, 1989.

Henderson JM. Gastrointestinal Pathophysiology, Philadelphia, Lippincott-Raven, 1996.

Ito S, Lacy ER. Morphology of gastric mucosal damage, defenses and restitution in the presence of luminal ethanol. Gastroenterology 88:250, 1985.

Komuro T, Seki K. Fine structural study of interstitial cells associated with the deep muscular plexus of the rat small intestine, with special reference to the intestinal pacemaker cells. Cell Tissue Res 282:129, 1995.

Lieber CS. The metabolism of alcohol and its implications for the pathogenesis of disease. In: Preedy VR, Watson RR, eds. Alcohol and the Gastrointestinal Tract, Boca Raton, Fla., CRC Press, 1996, p 19.

Littlewood JM. Gastrointestinal complications. Br Med Bull 48:847, 1992.

Miyai K. Structure-function relationship of the liver in health and disease. In: Gitnick G, Hollander D, Kaplowitz N, Samloff IM, Schoenfield LJ, eds. Principles and Practice of Gastroenterology and Hepatology. New York, Elsevier, 1988, p 1051.

Motta PM. Three-dimensional architecture of the mammalian liver. A scanning electron microscopic review. In: Allen DJ, Motta PM, DiDio JA, eds. Three Dimensional Microanatomy of Cells and Tissue Surfaces. New York, Elsevier/North Holland, 1981.

Motta PM, ed. Biopathology of the Liver: An Ultrastructural Approach. Boston, Kluwer Academic Publishers, 1988.

Motta P, Muto M, Fujita T. The Liver. An Atlas of Scanning Electron Microscopy. Tokyo, Igaku-Shoin, 1978.

Owen D. Normal histology of the stomach. Am J Surg Pathol 10:48, 1986.

Rappaport AM, MacPhee PJ, Fisher MM, Phillips MJ. The scarring of the liver acini (cirrhosis): Tridimensional and microcirculatory considerations. Virchows Arch A 402:107, 1983.

Riva A, Motta PM, eds. Ultrastructure of the Extraparietal Glands of the Digestive Tract. Boston, Kluwer Academic Publishers, 1990.

Rumessen JJ, Thuneberg L. Pacemaker cells in the gastrointestinal tract: Interstitial cells of Cajal. Scand J Gastroenterol 31(suppl 216):82, 1996.

Sanders KM. A case for interstitial cells of Cajal as pacemakers and mediators of neuro-transmission in the gastrointestinal tract. Gastroenterology 111:492, 1996.

Sherman DIN, Williams R. Liver damage: Mechanisms and management. Br Med Bull 50:124, 1994.

Silen W, Ito S. Mechanisms for rapid epithelialization of the gastric mucosal surface. Annu Rev Physiol 47:217, 1985.

Taché Y, Wingate D. Brain-Gut Interactions. Boca Raton, Fla., CRC Press, 1991.

Terblanche J, Krige JEJ, Bornman PC. The treatment of esophageal varices. Annu Rev Med 43:69, 1992.

Wake K, Decker K, Kirn A, et al. Cell biology and kinetics of Kupffer cells in the liver. Int Rev Cytol 118:173, 1989.

Williams SGJ, Westaby D, Tanner MS, Mowat AP. Liver and biliary problems in cystic fibrosis. Br Med Bull 48:877, 1992.

Wolfe MM, Soll AH. The physiology of gastric acid secretion. N Engl J Med 319:1707, 1988.

Review Items: Cross References

Information relevant to the Review Items listed in this chapter may be found in the following pages of Cormack, DH. Essential Histology. Philadelphia, J.B. Lippincott, 1993:

REVIEW ITEM	PAGES
8-1	284–285
8-2	286
8-3	300

CHAPTER 9

Endocrine and Reproductive Systems

CASE 9-1

Susan Brown, a university student in her mid-twenties, is becoming increasingly concerned about a painless anterolateral neck lump that shifts slightly when she swallows. During the last 4 months, it has enlarged to a diameter of approximately 2 cm. Except for having this palpable nodular mass, Susan is asymptomatic. Her serum T4 and T3 levels are normal. Her appetite is good and her body weight is normal. A "cold" (hypofunctioning) nodule is found on the thyroid scan obtained using (^{99m}Tc)pertechnetate. Subsequent investigation by needle biopsy indicates the need for total thyroidectomy. During the operation, a cervical lymph node is also excised. It confirms the provisional diagnosis. Representative histological features of the resected thyroid nodule and Susan's thyroid scan are shown in Fig. 9-1.

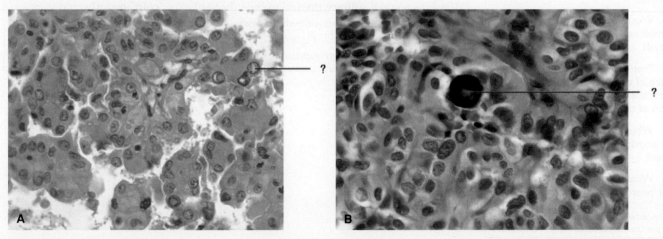

FIGURE 9-1 (**A**) and (**B**) Medium-power views of the surgical specimen in Case 9-1. (The features labeled (?) are potentially informative.)

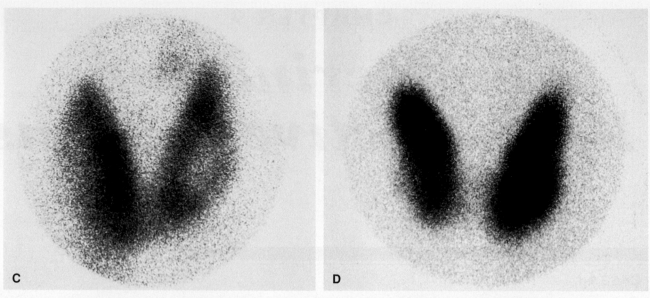

FIGURE 9-1 (Continued) (**C**) Thyroid scan in Case 9-1. (**D**) Normal thyroid scan for comparison. (For confirmation of your observations, see part D9-1 of the Discussion section of this chapter.)

ANALYSIS
Case 9-1

A Which, if any, of the histological features seen in Fig. 9-1A,B suggests that this nodule comes from the thyroid?

B Are there any histological features in Fig. 9-1A,B that differ from normal?

C Would you expect the resected lymph node to contain anything unusual?

D From the microscopic appearance of this tissue, would you expect that total or near-total resection of the thyroid was required?

E Which radionuclide is least likely to provide a misleading thyroid scan?

F What suggestions do you have for postoperative management?

(The answers are considered in part D9-1 of the Discussion section of this chapter.)

CASE 9-2

In her 40th year, Melissa Green is diagnosed as hypothyroid, and told that she has an enlarged thyroid. She is subsequently supplemented with L-thyroxine, and becomes asymptomatic and biochemically euthyroid. At the age of 50, she develops a small solitary thyroid nodule that appears "cold" on a thyroid scan. For further investigation a needle biopsy is obtained, after which a hemithyroidectomy is performed. Figure 9-2 shows the microscopic appearance of the resected nodule and surrounding tissues.

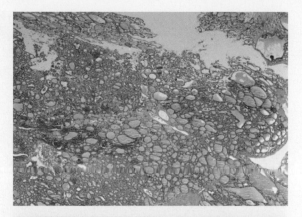

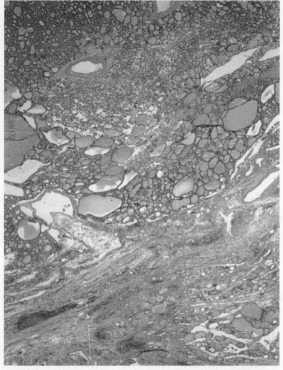

FIGURE 9-2 Thyroid biopsy in Case 9-2. (The findings are discussed in part D9-2 of the Discussion section of this chapter.)

ANALYSIS
Case 9-2

A Does the nodule in Fig. 9-2 differ in appearance from the rest of the gland?

B Does its tissue arrangement resemble that of the normal thyroid?

C What forms the boundaries of the nodule?

D Can you recognize anything outside the boundaries of the nodule that might suggest a cause for this patient's hypothyroidism?

E What constituents of her thyroid might have been causally related to her hypothyroidism?

(The answers are considered in part D9-2 of the Discussion section of this chapter.)

Figure 9-3, another example of an enlarged thyroid, was obtained from a different patient (see caption for details).

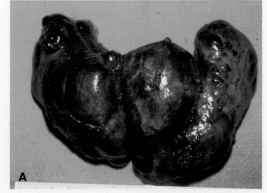

FIGURE 9-3 (A) This greatly enlarged thyroid gland was surgically removed chiefly for cosmetic reasons.

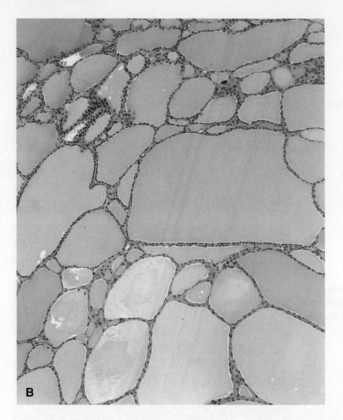

FIGURE 9-3 (Continued) (**B**) Is there anything unusual about its microscopic appearance? Is it likely that the thyroidectomy patient was clinically hyperthyroid at the time of surgery? (For confirmation of your answers, see part D9-4 of the Discussion section of this chapter.)

B

CASE 9-3

Jack McCarthy, decidedly overweight at the age of 66, hardly ever feels well. He has sporadic episodes of becoming nauseated and sweaty, often with throbbing headaches, heart palpitations, or abdominal cramps. His blood pressure fluctuates from being moderately increased to being markedly elevated. A need for frequent micturition makes trips from his house difficult. His condition is diagnosed as diabetes mellitus, and with appropriate management his blood sugar level normalizes. However, most of his symptoms continue. His output of urinary metanephrine is found to be elevated. Investigative ultrasound and CT scans of his abdomen reveal the presence of an abnormal mass at the level of L1 (Figs. 9-4, 9-5). Total excision of this mass is recommended following exploration by needle biopsy. The remaining symptoms dissipate after surgery. The resected tissue referred for histological evaluation is shown in Fig. 9-6.

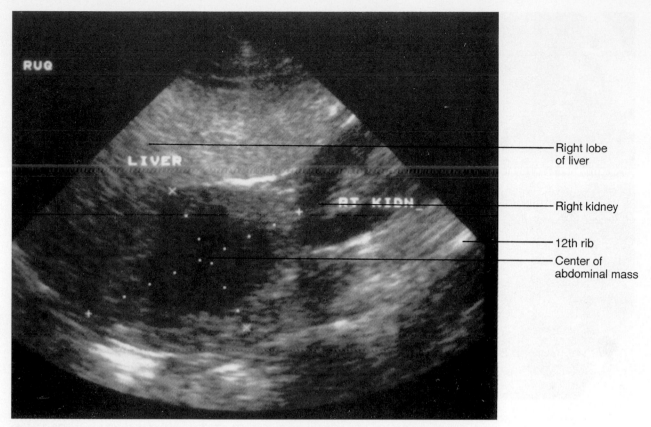

FIGURE 9-4 Abdominal ultrasound scan in Case 9-3. This is an extreme right sagittal scan of the right upper quadrant of the abdomen. The patient is in a prone position (ie, lying down), with his head at the left. Anterior is at the top. (The findings are discussed in part D9-3 of the Discussion section of this chapter.)

Labels on Figure 9-4:
- Right lobe of liver
- Right kidney
- 12th rib
- Center of abdominal mass

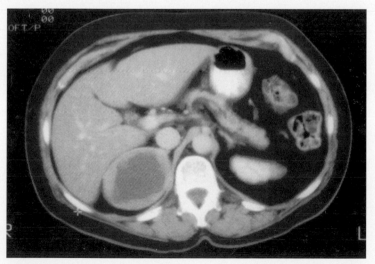

FIGURE 9-5 Abdominal axial CT scan in Case 9-3. (See part D9-3 of the Discussion section of this chapter.)

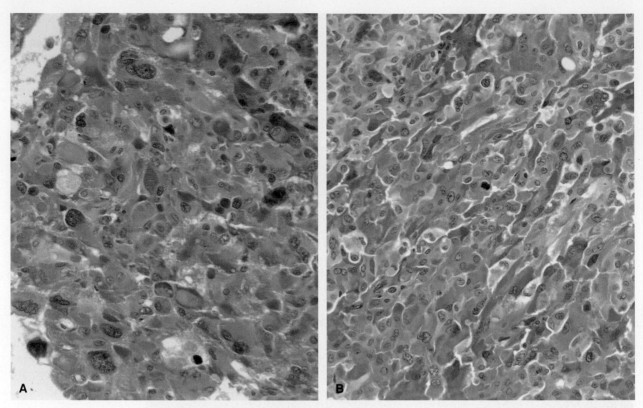

FIGURE 9-6 (**A**) Histological section of resected abdominal mass in Case 9-3. (**B**) Section of the same tissue after use of a dichromate fixative. (The findings are considered in part D9-3 of the Discussion section of this chapter.)

A N A L Y S I S
Case 9-3

A Which organs would you expect to find at the level of L1? (For assistance or confirmation, see the labeled version of the same axial CT scan, shown in Fig. 9-7.)

B Could the presence of a large abdominal mass in this position account for those symptoms that are not related to diabetes mellitus?

C What is the most likely cause of each of Jack's non-diabetic symptoms?

D Why have some of the cells in Fig. 9-6B stained a yellowish brown?

E How common are this patient's medical conditions?

F Do any features of the cells seen in Fig. 9-6 indicate that these cells are abnormal?

(The answers are considered in part D9-3 of the Discussion section of this chapter.)

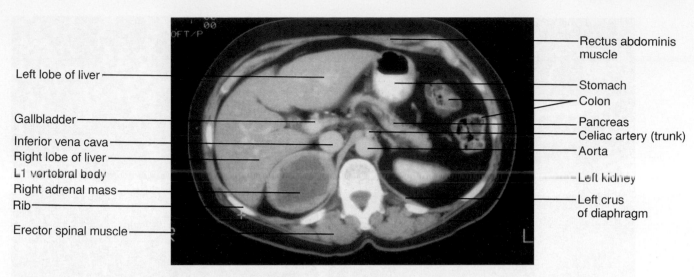

Left lobe of liver —
Gallbladder —
Inferior vena cava —
Right lobe of liver —
L1 vertobral body
Right adrenal mass —
Rib —
Erector spinal muscle —

— Rectus abdominis muscle
— Stomach
— Colon
— Pancreas
— Celiac artery (trunk)
— Aorta
— Left kidney
— Left crus of diaphragm

FIGURE 9-7 Abdominal axial CT scan in Case 9-3, labeled for comparison with Fig. 9-4.

CASE 9-4

Mary Banks, aged 29 years, is referred to an endocrinologist because she has not succeeded in becoming pregnant. About 18 months before referral, she began experiencing menstrual irregularities and then ceased menstruating. She is otherwise asymptomatic. She takes no oral contraceptives or tranquilizers, rarely gets headaches, and has not experienced any visual field disturbances. In the course of her physical examination, beads of white fluid exude from each nipple when the adjoining subareolar area is pressed. The other physical findings are normal. Although Mary's prolactin level is markedly elevated, normal values are returned for other endocrine tests. A CT scan reveals that there is an abnormal mass on the left side of the pituitary. Transphenoidal exploration enables this mass to be located and excised. The histological appearance of the resected tissue is illustrated in Fig. 9-8. Immunostaining and electron microscopy confirm that the abnormal mass is the source of excess prolactin and substantiate the provisional diagnosis (Fig. 9-8B,C).

ANALYSIS
Case 9-4

A Are there any features in Fig. 9-8 that suggest the surgical specimen in Case 9-4 came from the anterior lobe of the pituitary?

B What term is used for this patient's condition?

C Which hormones normally are required for the secretion and expression of breast milk?

D Would you expect Mary's estrogen levels to be higher or lower than normal?

E Why may the visual field become impaired in some patients with pituitary tumors?

(The answers are considered in part D9-5 of the Discussion section of this chapter.)

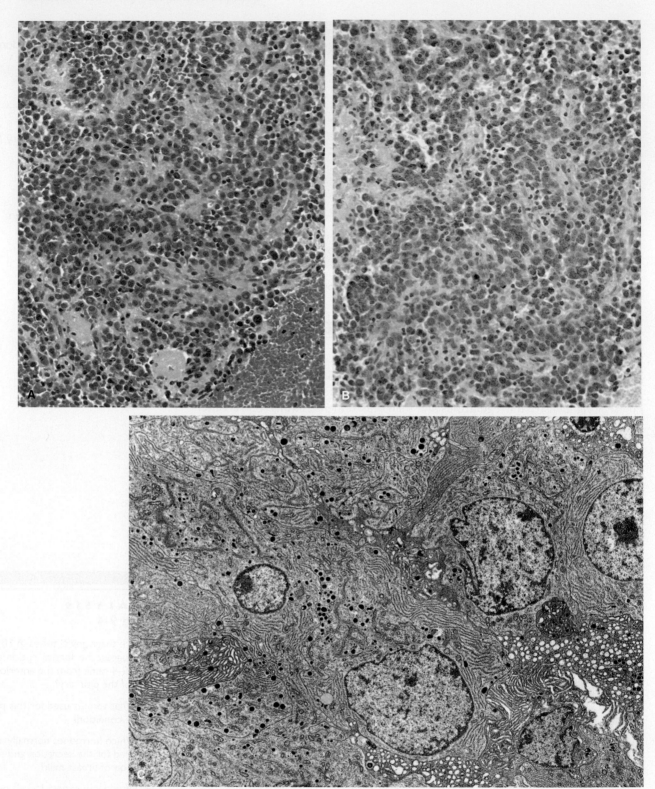

FIGURE 9-8 Histological sections (medium power) and electron micrographs of the surgical specimen in Case 9-4. (**A**) H&E section. (**B**) Immunostained section. (**C**) Electron micrograph (×3,000). (The findings are discussed in part D9-5 of the Discussion section of this chapter.)

CASE 9-5

Barely recognizable from a graduation photograph in which she looks pale and thin, Pamela Foster, now 34 years of age, has a round face, ruddy complexion, and too much facial hair. Marked abdominal obesity makes her fast movements awkward. Despite almost total elimination of dietary cholesterol, her body weight has risen quite alarmingly over the last 6 months. This patient complains of frequent headaches, shortness of breath, and undue tiring. Besides lacking energy, she seems miserable. Although she has no urinary problems or bowel symptoms, her menses have become irregular.

On physical examination, purple striae are seen on the abdomen. On her back, a non-tender mass of excess subcutaneous fat is evident at the base of the neck. Blood pressure is 180/100. Muscle wasting and weakness are evident, chiefly in the legs.

Laboratory findings include a mild hyperglycemia, some insulin resistance, and a decreased serum potassium level. The plasma cortisol level is elevated and remains steady, without diurnal variations, and the urinary output of cortisol metabolites is increased. A coronal MR image reveals a tiny abnormality in the central region of the pituitary. Using the transphenoidal approach, the abnormal tissue is resected following surgical exploration. Pamela's physical appearance subsequently shows a gradual return to normal. LM and EM sections of the excised pituitary tissue may be seen in Fig. 9-9. They show the cells that caused the problem.

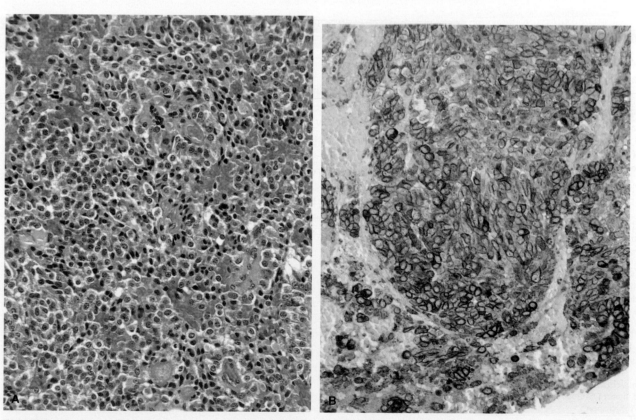

FIGURE 9-9 Surgical specimen in Case 9-5. (**A**). H&E-stained section; (**B**) Immunostained section;

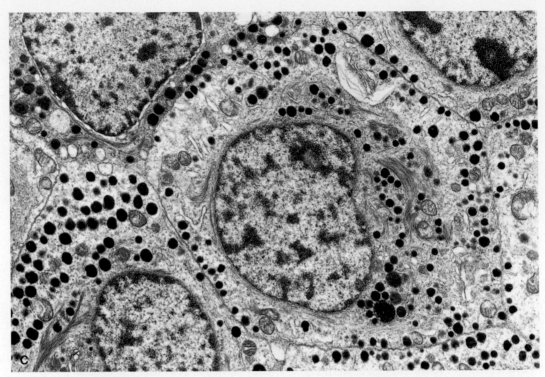

FIGURE 9-9 (Continued) (**C**) Electron micrograph (×7,000). (Considered in part D9-6 of the Discussion section of this chapter.)

ANALYSIS
Case 9-5

A What useful information does Fig. 9-9 provide about the cause of Pamela's condition? What may be inferred about the chemical composition of the pituitary hormone that is involved?

B What normally regulates cortisol secretion?

C What effects does the pituitary hormone overproduced in this patient have on her adrenals?

D Would you expect this patient's responsiveness to corticotropin-releasing hormone (CRH) to be higher or lower than normal?

E Why may patients with this condition be unduly susceptible to bacterial infections?

(The answers to these questions are considered in part D9-6 of the Discussion section of this chapter.)

CASE 9-6

When Millie Shaw hears that she is pregnant again at the age of 44, she has a vague sort of premonition. Her former pregnancies were without complications, and her other three babies all turned out to be healthy and normal. On this occasion, however, her family physician seems quite adamant about her undergoing prenatal screening for detectable genetic abnormalities.

In the 16th week of gestation, an amniocentesis is performed. The α_1-fetoprotein (AFP) concentration of the amniotic fluid is found to be decreased. A cell culture is started from fetal cells in the amniotic fluid in preparation for chromosomal analysis. The fetal karyotype that is obtained is shown in Fig. 9-10A.

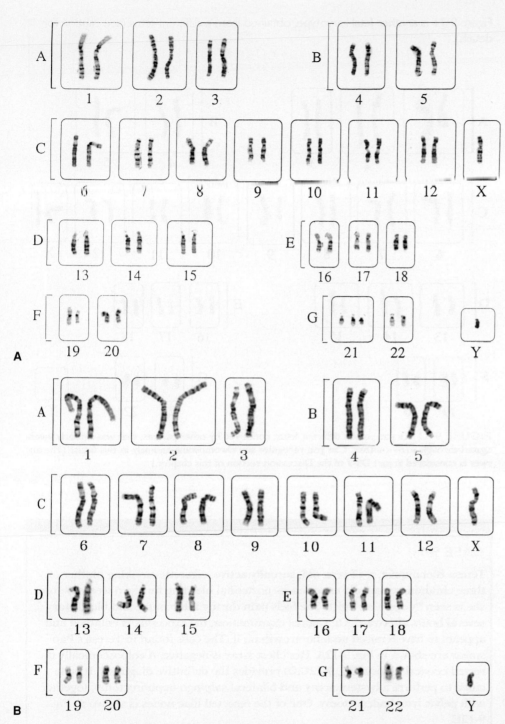

FIGURE 9-10 (**A**) Fetal karyotype obtained in Case 9-6. (**B**) Normal karyotype for comparison with part A.

ANALYSIS
Case 9-6

A What is the sex of the fetus whose karyotype is shown in Fig. 9-10A?

B Does Fig. 9-10A reveal any recognizable anomaly of the fetal chromosomes? If so, what is most likely causing the anomaly?

C How is the chromosome constitution of the fetus whose karyotype is shown in Fig. 9-10A recorded?

(To confirm your answers, see part D9-7 of the Discussion section of this chapter.)

Figure 9-11 is another fetal karyotype, obtained from a different fetus (see caption for details).

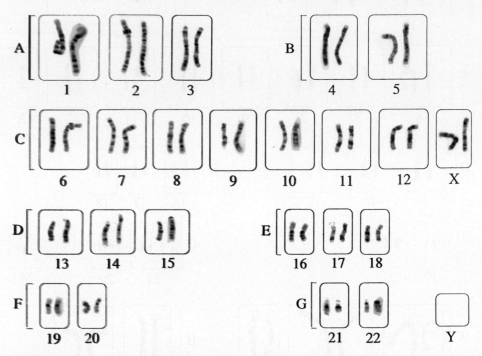

FIGURE 9-11 Karyotype of a different fetus, conceived by other parents, that was similarly investigated through amniocentesis. Can you recognize any chromosome anomaly in this fetus? (The answer is considered in part D9-7 of the Discussion section of this chapter.)

CASE 9-7

Teresa Bloomquist, a 42-year-old, sexually active, cigarette-smoking mother of three children, repeatedly experiences postcoital bleeding for the 6 weeks before she is seen by a gynecologist. She feels pain during intercourse and bleeds for several hours afterward. On vaginal examination, the exocervix is enlarged and appears to have a raised nodular growth on it. The cells found in Teresa's Pap smear are shown in Fig. 9-12A. Her chest x-ray is negative. A colposcopically directed cervical biopsy (Fig. 9-12C,D) provides the definitive diagnosis. It is decided to perform a hysterectomy and bilateral salpingo-oophorectomy, together with pelvic lymphadenectomy. One of the resected iliac nodes is shown in Fig. 9-12E.

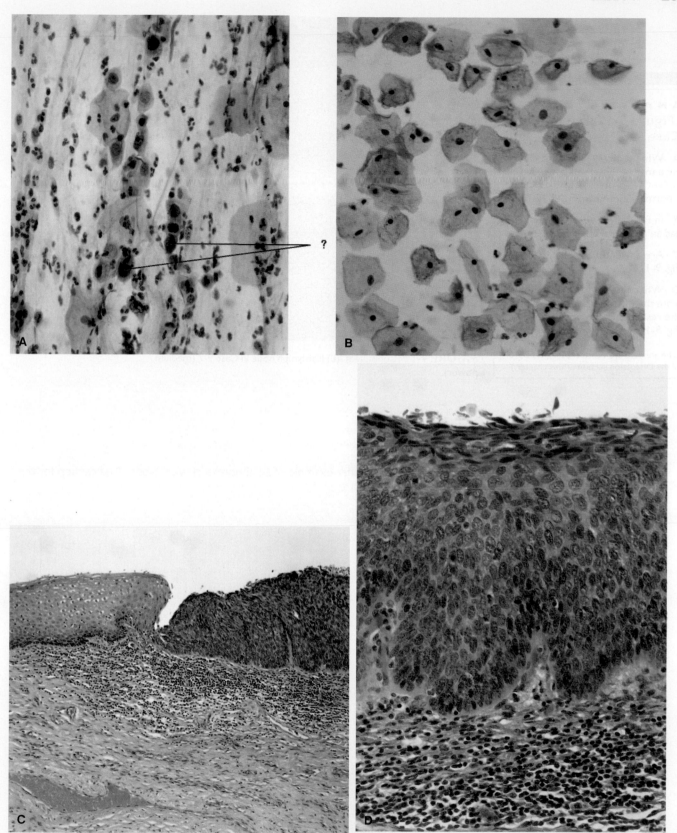

FIGURE 9-12 (**A**) Cells found in a Pap smear in Case 9-7. (The items labeled (?) are potentially informative.) (**B**) Normal Pap smear, for comparison with **A**. (**C**) Perimeter of cervical lesion in Case 9-7 (low power). (**D**) Epithelium lying to the right of the field in C (medium power).

ANALYSIS
(Figure 9-12 in relation to Case 9-7)

A What clinically significant difference may be observed between this patient's Pap smear (Fig. 9-12A) and a normal Pap smear (Fig. 9-12B)?

B In Fig. 9-12C, which component has an abnormal appearance?

C Are any unusual features seen in Fig. 9-12D?

D What information may be gained from the histological appearance of the resected lymph node shown in Fig. 9-12E?

(The answers are considered in part D9-8 of the Discussion section of this chapter.)

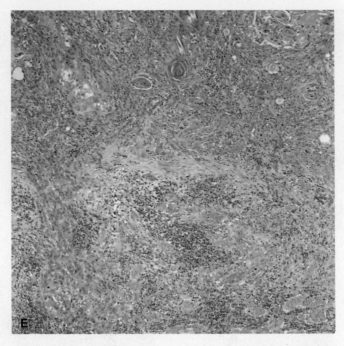

FIGURE 9-12 (Continued) (E) Iliac lymph node in Case 9-7 (medium power).

Figure 9-13 shows another example of an abnormal cervical biopsy (see caption for details).

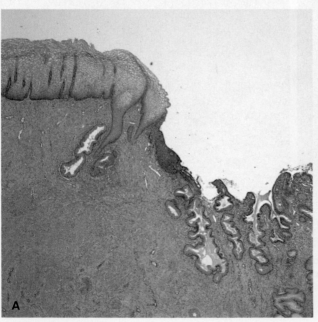

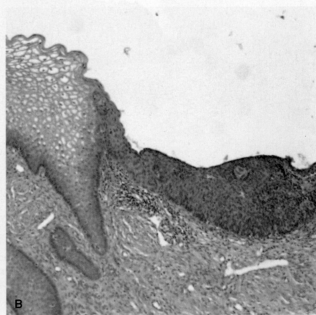

CASE 9-8

Acting on advice received at an information session for senior citizens, Jocelyn MacKinnon, aged 65 years, performs a breast self-examination. She discovers a non-tender lump in her right breast and makes an appointment to see a doctor. The breast mass appears firm and immobile on physical examination. No enlarged axillary lymph nodes are noted. Chest x-rays and bilateral mammograms are obtained. The lung parenchyma is clear, with no mass lesions. However, a spiculated irregular mass with an estimated diameter of 4.5 cm is noted in the upper outer quadrant of the right breast. The left breast reveals no mass lesions, architectural distortion, or clustered microcalcifications. A right modified radical mastectomy is subsequently performed. The histological appearance of the resected mass may be seen in Fig. 9-14. The estrogen receptor report returned for the tissue is ER−. Sinus hyperplasia and benign adipose infiltration are noted in the 11 resected axillary lymph nodes, but all appear to be free of malignant cells. The mastectomy specimen and the patient's mammogram are shown in Fig. 9-15.

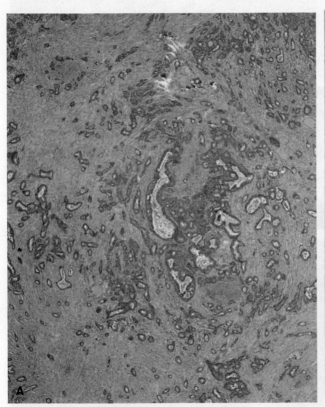 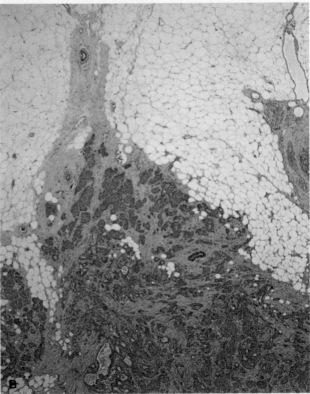

FIGURE 9-14 (**A**) and (**B**) Histological features of the excised mass in Case 9-8 (low power).

◄ **FIGURE 9-13** A Pap smear obtained from a 32-year-old woman indicates that she has CIN II (moderate cervical dysplasia). Colposcopic examination of her cervix shows an aceto-white lesion involving the anterior cervix and extending into the endocervical canal. A cone biopsy obtained from the cervix is seen here under (**A**) low power and (**B**) medium power. A small patch of CIN III with underlying lymphocytes may be recognized along the border of the normal vaginal stratified squamous non-keratinizing epithelium. The resection margins were found to be clear, and the patient was considered to be cured of dysplasia.

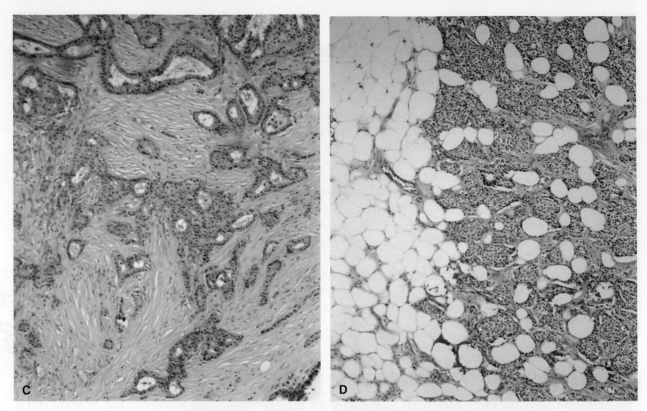

FIGURE 9-14 (Continued) (**C**) and (**D**) Details of this mass (medium power).

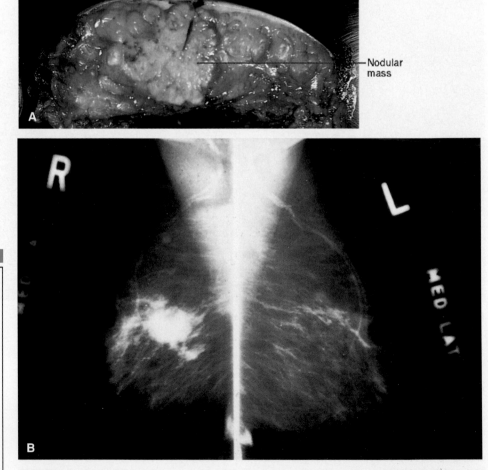

— Nodular mass

ANALYSIS
Case 9-8

A Are there any features in Fig. 9-14 that suggest this is breast tissue?

B Which features of Figs. 9-14 and 9-15 would confirm a clinical diagnosis of breast carcinoma?

C What is an estrogen receptor assay, and what is the significance of the result that was obtained?

(The answers are considered in part D9-9 of the Discussion section of this chapter.)

FIGURE 9-15 (**A**) Resected tissue in Case 9-8 (mastectomy specimen). (**B**) Mammogram in Case 9-8.

CASE 9-9

Endicott Thomas, aged 62 years, is admitted to hospital for a thorough investigation because of continuing problems with the voiding of urine. His history indicates a gradual progression of urinary retention. Rectal examination discloses that the prostate is enlarged, with a firm palpable nodule. A hypoechoic mass is noted in this position on the transrectal ultrasound scan. The radionuclide bone scan is essentially negative. Serum levels of prostate-specific antigen (PSA) and prostatic acid phosphatase (PAP) are both increased. An ultrasonographically directed transrectal needle biopsy is taken from the prostate. Based on the report, a decision is made to perform a radical prostatectomy. The biopsied prostate tissue is shown in Fig. 9-16.

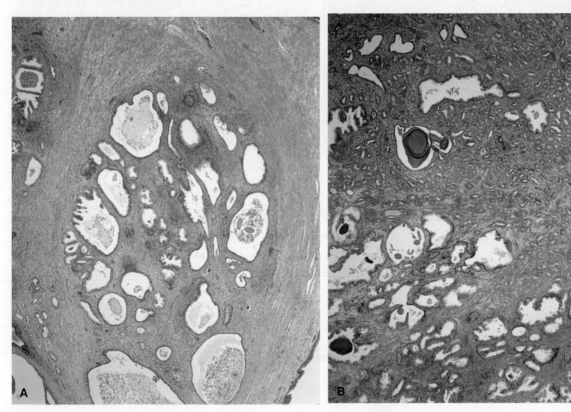

FIGURE 9-16 Prostate biopsy in Case 9-9. (**A**) and (**B**) Low power.

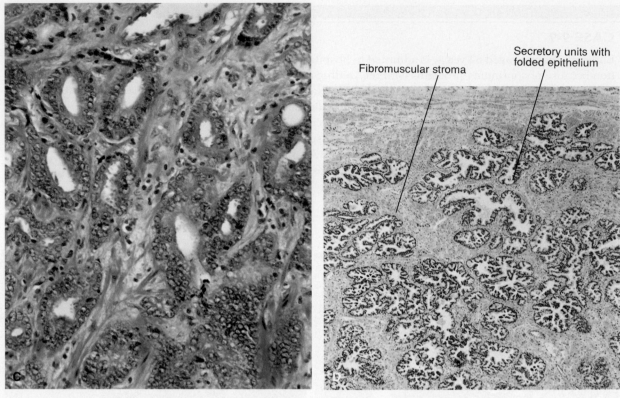

Fibromuscular stroma

Secretory units with folded epithelium

FIGURE 9-16 (Continued) **(C)** Medium power. **(D)** Normal prostate (low power) for comparison with A through C.

ANALYSIS
Case 9-9

A Does the biopsy obtained in Case 9-9 disclose only benign overgrowth of the gland? If not, which parts of Fig. 9-16 show any evidence of a malignancy?

B How common is benign overgrowth of the prostate? Is anything known about its cause?

C What complication is most frequently associated with urinary retention?

D Why was it important for the clinical investigation to include a bone scan?

(To confirm your answers, see part D9-10 of the Discussion section of this chapter.)

Figure 9-17 is a representative bone scan from a patient with advanced prostatic adenocarcinoma (see caption for details).

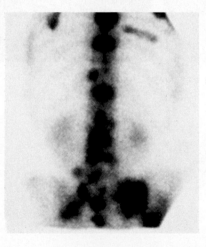

FIGURE 9-17 Bone scan, obtained using technetium (^{99m}Tc)-tagged biphosphonate and a γ camera. Because this tracer is taken up by actively secreting osteoblasts, bone scans reveal "hot spots" of intense osteoblastic activity. This scan of a patient with advanced prostatic adenocarcinoma indicates that he has multiple skeletal metastases, chiefly in the vertebrae and pelvis. Compact bone produced as a result of an intense osteoblastic reaction to metastatic cancer is known as reactive bone.

ESSENTIAL FEATURES OF THE ENDOCRINE SYSTEM

Unlike exocrine glands, which release their secretions onto body surfaces, *endocrine glands* release *hormones* into the bloodstream. The majority of endocrine glands store their hormones in some form, but steroid-secreting glands store the hormone precursor, cholesterol, as cholesteryl ester. Hormones are classically regarded as long-range, bodywide signaling molecules that provide a comparatively slow means of communication between cells. As part of an integrated neuroendocrine system, they represent a functional extension by which functional responses in cells are coordinated, broadened, and fine-tuned.

With the single exception of the thyroid hormone receptor, the *receptors* for all amino acid-derived hormones (ie, the peptide, protein, glycoprotein, and catecholamine hormones) are present in the *cell membrane* of the target cells. Cholesterol-derived hormones (ie, steroids) and thyroid hormone diffuse through the cell membrane, because they are lipid-soluble, and then bind to *intracellular hormone receptor proteins* in the target cells.

Endocrine disorders can arise from (1) hyperfunction or hypofunction of endocrine organs, and (2) excessive or inadequate responsiveness of target cells to hormones that are produced. Overstimulation or dysregulation of endocrine secretory responses generally result in hypersecretion. Damaging effects of inflammation or autoimmune responses generally result in hyposecretion.

> **KEY CONCEPT**
>
> Hormones act on target cells.

Thyroid

The *thyroid* is a comparatively large, bilobed gland that lies at the base of the larynx, lateral and anterior to the trachea. An unusual feature of this gland is that it stores its hormone *extracellularly*, in the form of an iodinated macromolecular precursor. The secreted glycoprotein precursor is called *thyroglobulin*. As soon as thyroglobulin has been secreted, it becomes iodinated. Thyroid hormone is then produced from iodinated precursor that has been taken up by endocytosis.

The structural and functional unit of the thyroid is the *thyroid follicle* (Fig. 9-18). Thyroid follicles are essentially spherical storage compartments with walls made up of simple cuboidal *follicular epithelial cells* that are derived from endoderm. These are actively secreting cells with an extensive rER (rough-surfaced endoplastic reticulum) and a large Golgi region. Their luminal surface is characterized by the presence of microvilli. Internal to the follicular basement membrane, yet not in contact with the follicular lumen, are small numbers of scattered *parafollicular (C) cells*, which are derived from neural crest and secrete the hormone *calcitonin* (see below). These cells lie beside follicles (Gk. *para*, beside) rather than being a part of them (Fig. 9-18), and do not secrete into the follicular lumen. Supporting the parenchymal follicles is a loose connective tissue stroma with abundant fenestrated capillaries.

Production of Thyroid Hormone

As outlined in Fig. 9-19, thyroglobulin is released from thyroid follicular epithelial cells by exocytosis through the microvillus-bearing luminal domain of the cell membrane. Iodide (I^-) is actively transported into these cells from the circulation and diffuses from the cells into the lumen. The intraluminal I^- becomes oxidized to I, which binds to tyrosine groups of the thyroglobulin molecule. Oxidation and binding are both promoted by the enzyme *thyroid peroxidase* (*thyroperoxidase*), delivered to the lumen in the same secretory vesicles as thyroglobulin.

The macromolecular intraluminal content of the follicles, widely known as

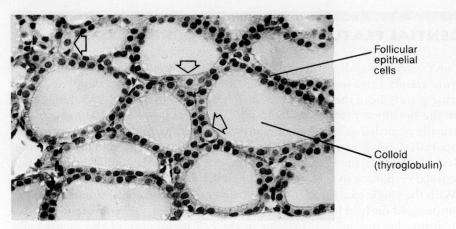

FIGURE 9-18 Thyroid follicles (dog thyroid). The follicular epithelial cells secrete thyroglobulin, the precursor from which they produce T_3 and T_4. The large pale-staining parafollicular (**C**) cells (*arrows*) produce calcitonin.

thyroid *colloid,* is continually ingested by the cells that secrete it. Following its phagocytosis, it is submitted to degradation by lysosomal enzymes in secondary lysosomes. Two products liberated as a result of intracellular proteolysis are *tetraiodothyronine* (T_4) and *triiodothyronine* (T_3), the circulating forms of *thyroid hormone*. These iodinated amino acid derivatives are able to diffuse out of the cells and pass readily into the bloodstream. Much of the circulating T_4 becomes converted into T_3. Both forms of the hormone bind to the intracellular receptor proteins, but T_3 has more potency than T_4.

As shown in Fig. 9-19, the entire process of thyroglobulin synthesis and se-

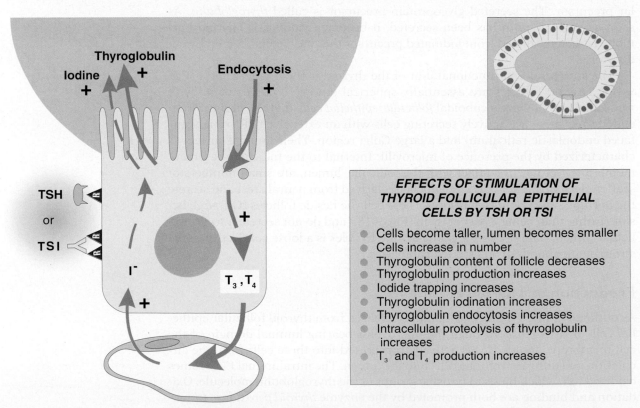

EFFECTS OF STIMULATION OF THYROID FOLLICULAR EPITHELIAL CELLS BY TSH OR TSI

- Cells become taller, lumen becomes smaller
- Cells increase in number
- Thyroglobulin content of follicle decreases
- Thyroglobulin production increases
- Iodide trapping increases
- Thyroglobulin iodination increases
- Thyroglobulin endocytosis increases
- Intracellular proteolysis of thyroglobulin increases
- T_3 and T_4 production increases

FIGURE 9-19 Synthesis of thyroglobulin, T_3, and T_4 by follicular epithelial cells. All the stages shown are promoted by TSH or TSI (thyroid-stimulating immunoglobulin). The effects of such stimulation are summarized in the panel. (See text for details.)

cretion, I⁻ trapping, and intracellular proteolysis is promoted by thyroid-stimulating hormone (TSH). The process is similarly stimulated by *thyroid-stimulating immunoglobulins* (TSI) produced in many patients with *Graves' disease* (Fig. 9-20). These autoimmune IgG antibodies are directed against parts of the TSH receptor, and when they bind to it they mimic the effects of TSH. The various effects of stimulation by TSH or TSI are summarized in the lower right panel of Fig. 9-20.

Goiter

The histological appearance of thyroid follicles and their component cells can be helpful in establishing reasons for thyroid enlargement after thyroid hormone levels have been determined. An enlarged thyroid is known as a *goiter* (from L. *guttur*, throat). If enlargement is due chiefly to hyperplasia and hypertrophy of follicular epithelial cells, the goiter may be described as a "parenchymatous goiter." If the main cause of enlargement is accumulation of large amounts of colloid, the goiter may be described as a "colloid goiter." As shown in Fig. 9-20, the hyperplastic, hypertrophic type of follicle may go on to become very large and evenly filled with accumulated colloid.

Three different etiologies of goiter are represented in Fig. 9-20. The panel on the left shows *endemic goiter*, which is now widely circumvented by adding I⁻ to table salt. Since normal levels of thyroid activity are not sustained when there is insufficient iodine, TSH levels rise and a *diffuse* (ie, non-localized) *nontoxic goiter* develops. Because TSH also stimulates colloid production, the goiter may

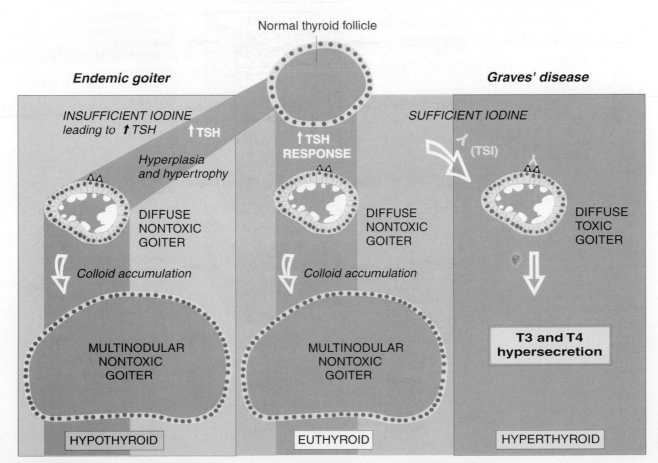

FIGURE 9-20 The changed histological appearance of thyroid follicles in some representative presentations of goiter. (See text for details.)

subsequently become *multinodular,* but it remains *nontoxic* (ie, shows no hypersecretory, inflammatory, or neoplastic changes). However, unless the iodine deficit is remedied, the patient remains hypothyroid, even though the TSH level is elevated.

In the middle panel, increased responsiveness to TSH results in similar histological changes, but in the absence of an iodine deficiency, a normal (euthyroid) state may be maintained.

In Graves disease, shown on the right, TSI chronically stimulates the follicular epithelial cells into making more thyroglobulin, iodinating it, ingesting it, and degrading it intracellularly. As a result, T_3 and T_4 are overproduced and intraluminal colloid is removed so rapidly that it does not accumulate. This type of goiter is termed a *diffuse toxic goiter.*

Adrenals

The *adrenals* (*suprarenals*) are bilateral endocrine glands situated at the superomedial border of each kidney. They are made up of a cortex and medulla characterized by different developmental origins, histological features, and secretory products. These two concentric regions are interlinked by an essentially mutual blood supply. Most of the blood entering the medullary venules has passed

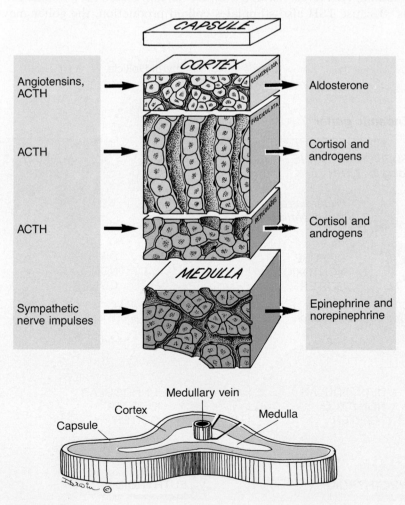

FIGURE 9-21 Functions carried out by the constituent histological regions of an adrenal gland.

through cortical capillaries before reaching the medullary capillaries. Supplementary arteriolar branches extend into the medulla and provide its cells with oxygen.

Adrenal Cortex

The *adrenal cortex,* which is derived from mesoderm, is the steroid-secreting part of the gland. It is conventionally regarded as having three zones, each of which is abundantly supplied with fenestrated capillaries. In the *zona glomerulosa* (L. *glomerulus,* little ball), the secretory cells are arranged in roughly spherical groups. They are the source of *aldosterone,* the secretion of which is stimulated by the angiotensins and, as a transient effect, by stress-related increases in adrenocorticotrophic hormone levels (Fig. 9-21). The secretory cells of the *zona fasciculata,* which is generally the thickest zone, are arranged in columns that border on radial fenestrated capillaries (Figs. 9-21, 9-22). These actively secretory cells produce *cortisol* and other glucocorticoids, eg, corticosterone and deoxycorticosterone, and a few comparatively weak androgens, eg, androstenedione and dehydroepiandrosterone. In the *zona reticularis,* the secretory cells are arranged as irregularly anastomosing cords. They produce the same hormones as the fasciculata cells, but in smaller amounts.

Adrenocorticotrophic hormone (ACTH, corticotropin), secreted by corticotrophs of the anterior pituitary, maintains the necessary mass and secretory activity of the adrenal cortex.

Adrenal corticosteroids are essential to life because they play a fundamental role in regulating key metabolic activities in the body. Adrenal cortical insufficiency requires compensatory substitution therapy. *Cortisol (hydrocortisone)* in particular has a number of important actions; eg, it promotes protein catabolism and raises the blood sugar level. The liver converts it to cortisone, a potent glucocorticoid that is used pharmacologically to alleviate inflammation and acute histamine-mediated allergic symptoms in a nonspecific manner. Cortisol and its synthetic analogs also reduce scarring and, if present in sufficient concentration, are immunosuppressive. Negative feedback by cortisol suppresses the secretion of both ACTH and its releasing hormone, CRH.

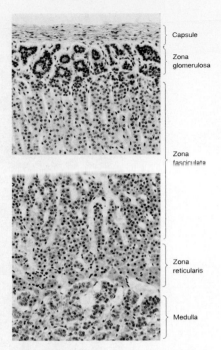

Capsule
Zona glomerulosa
Zona fasciculata
Zona reticularis
Medulla

FIGURE 9-22 Histological organization of an adrenal gland.

> **KEY CONCEPT**
>
> The required level of cortisol secretion by the adrenal cortex is maintained by ACTH.

Adrenal Medulla

The *adrenal medulla,* which is derived from neural crest, produces the catecholamine hormones *epinephrine* and *norepinephrine* (alternatively known as *adrenaline* and *noradrenaline*). The secretory cells are irregularly arranged as anastomosing cords that border on fenestrated capillaries (see Figs. 9-21, 9-22). They are known as *chromaffin cells* because their stored hormones stain with chromium salts. One type of chromaffin cell secretes *epinephrine,* and the other type secretes *norepinephrine.* At the EM level, the two different types may be distinguished on the basis of their granular morphology (Fig. 9-23).

Chromaffin cells are homologous with sympathetic ganglion cells and secrete their catecholamines in response to preganglionic cholinergic impulses. Their secretory activity increases under hypoglycemic or hypoxic conditions, in strenuous exercise, or in stressful emergency situations. Important physiological responses elicited by the adrenal medullary hormones, the chief one of which is *epinephrine,* include greater strength of cardiac contraction, acceleration of heart rate, redirection of blood flow toward muscles and the liver, a general increase in blood pressure, and a variety of metabolic effects. Dopamine and opioid peptides (enkephalins) appear to be additional secretory products of the adrenal medulla.

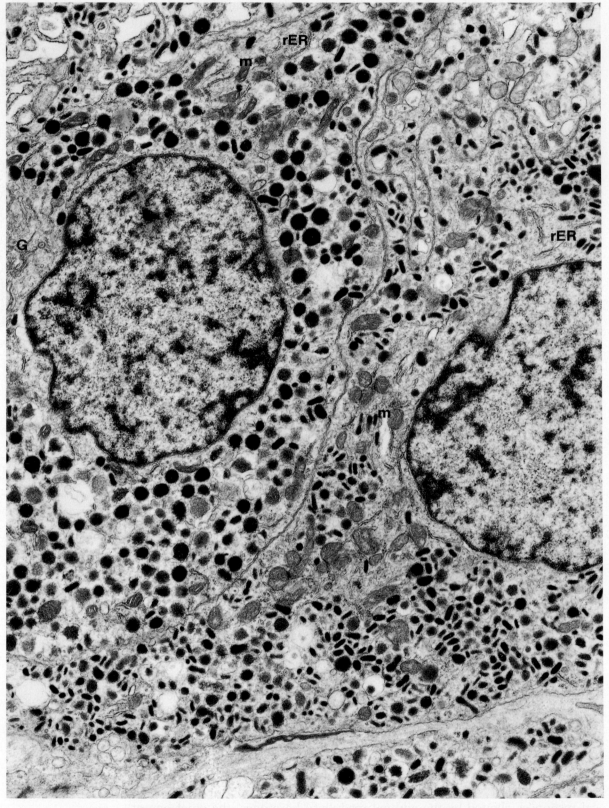

FIGURE 9-23 Two types of secretory cells of the adrenal medulla (electron micrograph). The cell seen at left secretes epinephrine; the cell at right secretes norepinephrine. Along with each cell's nucleus and secretory granules, mitochondria (m), rough-surfaced endoplasmic reticulum (rER), and Golgi region (G) may be discerned.

Pituitary

The *pituitary*, which is alternatively known as the *hypophysis*, is an ovoid endocrine gland attached to the inferior aspect of the brain. Measuring approximately 1 cm × 1.3 cm, the pituitary is connected by its *infundibular stalk* to the median eminence of the tuber cinereum (a part of the hypothalamus). It lies protected within the *sella turcica*, which is a concavity on the upper surface of the sphenoid bone. The pituitary is made up of two lobes (Fig. 9-24). The *anterior lobe*, derived from oral ectoderm, is an epithelial endocrine gland. The smaller, *posterior lobe*, which is a down-growth of the base of the brain, consists entirely of nervous tissue. Detailed descriptions of the pituitary run the risk of becoming obscured by a plethora of competing terminologies, but a broad subdivision into *anterior pituitary* and *posterior pituitary* often suffices. Other perpetuated synonyms for the *anterior lobe* are *pars distalis, pars anterior,* and *adenohypophysis;* although, strictly speaking, the adenohypophysis includes all parts of the pituitary that develop from oral ectoderm, including a collar-shaped extension called the *pars tuberalis* and an ill-defined intermediary zone called the *pars intermedia*. Alternative names for the *posterior lobe* are *pars nervosa* and *pars posterior*.

Above and anterior to the anterior lobe of the pituitary lies the *optic chiasma*. Superior extension of the anterior lobe as a result of growth of an adenoma can compress decussating (crossing) optic nerve fibers in the chiasma, leading to visual field defects such as *bitemporal hemianopsia* (ie, loss of peripheral vision resulting from bilateral loss of afferent input from the nasal hemiretinas) and can even lead to hypothalamic dysfunction.

Hypophyseal Portal Circulation

An important vascular connection links the fenestrated capillary plexus of the median eminence and infundibular stalk with that of the anterior pituitary. Termed the *hypophyseal portal system,* this essential link between the hypothalamus and the anterior lobe of the pituitary consists primarily of long portal venules and veins (Fig. 9-25). It is a direct route that readily permits hypothalamic releasing and inhibiting hormones to reach target cells in this lobe. Most of the blood reaching the anterior pituitary is supplied by the hypophyseal portal vessels. The necessary oxygenated blood comes from capsular branches of the inferior hypophyseal arteries. The posterior lobe is supplied almost entirely by the inferior hypophyseal arteries.

The various releasing and inhibiting hormones that continuously regulate the output of anterior pituitary hormones are listed in Table 9-1. The neuronal cell bodies in which these hormones are synthesized lie in a number of separate or overlapping locations in the hypothalamus. Their axons extend in the *tuberoinfundibular tract* to the median eminence and infundibular region, where

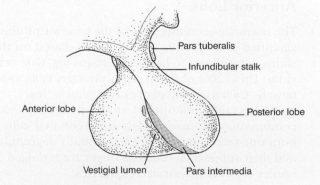

FIGURE 9-24 Main regions of the pituitary.

Pars tuberalis

Infundibular stalk

Anterior lobe

Posterior lobe

Vestigial lumen

Pars intermedia

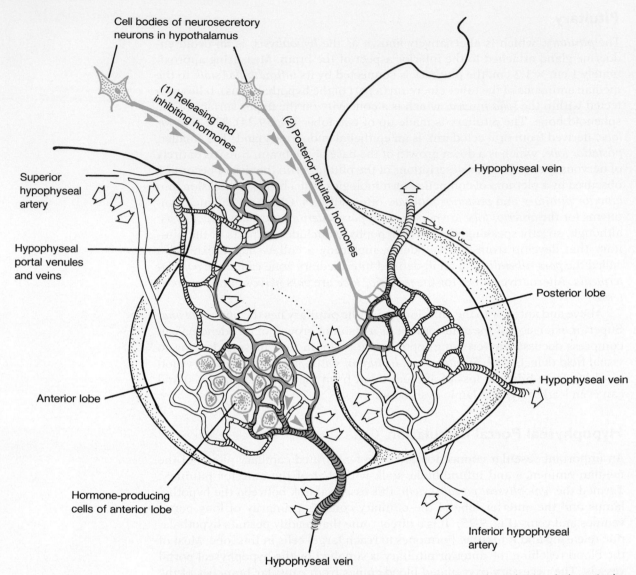

FIGURE 9-25 Blood supply of the pituitary. The hypophyseal portal circulation, which carries hypothalamic releasing and inhibiting hormones, is shown on the left. Blood flow is indicated by open arrows. Hormone transport is indicated by solid arrowheads.

their terminals lie in intimate contact with the fenestrated capillary plexuses that drain into the hypophyseal portal vessels (see Fig. 9-25).

Anterior Lobe

The hormone-secreting cells of the anterior pituitary *(chromophils)* are broadly classified as *acidophils* and *basophils,* based on their affinity for acid or basic stains, which have to be special stains (eg, Gomori) for the difference to be obvious. Up to 20% of the anterior pituitary cells appear smaller and stain less intensely. Called *chromophobes* (Gr. *phobia,* fear), these smaller cells do not contain detectable amounts of stored hormone and are believed to represent a combination of incompletely differentiated cells and functionally exhausted hormone-secreting cells in an essentially degranulated state. The secretory cells and their supporting reticular fibers are arranged as thick branching cords that border on wide fenestrated capillaries.

TABLE 9-1

REGULATION OF RELEASE OF ANTERIOR PITUITARY HORMONES BY HYPOTHALAMIC REGULATORY HORMONES

GROWTH HORMONE (GH)
Releasing hormone (GRH)

Inhibiting hormone (GIH; somatostatin)

PROLACTIN (PRL)
Releasing hormone (PRH)*

Inhibiting hormone (PIH; dopamine)

ADRENOCORTICOTROPHIC HORMONE (ACTH)
Corticotropin-releasing hormone (CRH)

THYROID-STIMULATING HORMONE (TSH)
Thyrotropin-releasing hormone (TRH)*

FOLLICLE-STIMULATING HORMONE (FSH) AND LEUTEINIZING HORMONE (LH)
Gonadotropin-releasing hormone (GnRH)

* Prolactin is also released in response to TRH

TABLE 9-2

HORMONES SECRETED BY ANTERIOR PITUITARY CELLS

ACIDOPHILS
Somatotrophs

    Growth hormone (GH, somatotropin)

Mammotrophs

    Prolactin (PRL)

Mammosomatotrophs

    Prolactin (PRL)

    Growth hormone (GH)

BASOPHILS
Corticotrophs

    Adrenocorticotrophic hormone (ACTH*, corticotropin)

Thyrotrophs

    Thyroid-stimulating hormone (TSH, thyrotropin)

Gonadotrophs

    Follicle-stimulating hormone (FSH)

    Luteinizing hormone (LH)

Corticothyrotrophs

    Adrenocorticotrophic hormone (ACTH)

    Thyroid-stimulating hormone (TSH)

Corticogonadotrophs

    Adrenocorticotrophic hormone (ACTH)

    Follicle-stimulating hormone (FSH)

    Luteinizing hormone (LH)

* α-MSH activity in ACTH; γ-MSH is also produced from pro-opiomelanocortin

Table 9-2 lists the various types of pituitary acidophils and basophils. They include "hybrid" chromophils capable of producing more than one hormone.

The general distribution of the different types of acidophils and basophils, the hormones they produce, and the relative proportions of each type, are shown in Fig. 9-26. Roughly 50% of the chromophils present in the lateral wings of a horizontal section are somatotrophs; the remainder are mostly mammotrophs. Thyrotrophs lie nearer to the anterior border. Gonadotrophs are widely dispersed throughout the lobe. Corticotrophs lie in the anteromedial region between the lateral wings. They also tend to invade the pars intermedia and anterior border of the posterior lobe.

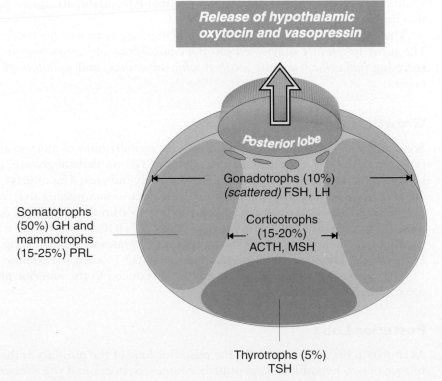

Release of hypothalamic oxytocin and vasopressin

Posterior lobe

Gonadotrophs (10%)
(scattered) FSH, LH

Somatotrophs
(50%) GH and
mammotrophs
(15-25%) PRL

Corticotrophs
(15-20%)
ACTH, MSH

Thyrotrophs (5%)
TSH

FIGURE 9-26 Overall distribution of chromophils in the anterior pituitary. (See text for details.)

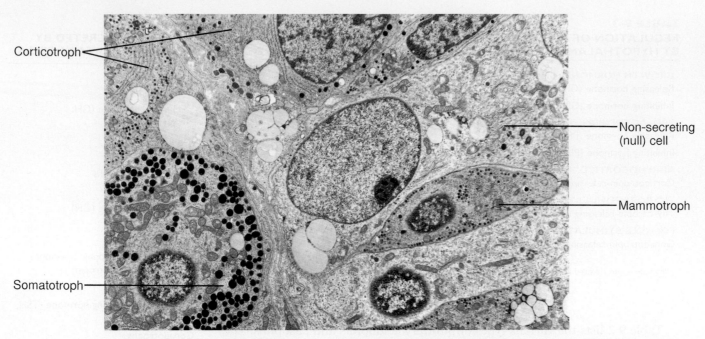

Corticotroph

Non-secreting (null) cell

Mammotroph

Somatotroph

FIGURE 9-27 Somatotroph, corticotrophs, mammotrophs, and null cells of the human anterior pituitary (electron micrograph).

The EM appearance of somatotrophs, corticotrophs, mammotrophs, and non-secreting (null) cells is illustrated in Fig. 9-27.

Corticotrophs produce the polypeptide hormone *ACTH,* along with three additional peptide hormones, by first synthesizing a large precursor molecule called *pro-opiomelanocortin* and then progressively hydrolyzing this as shown in Fig. 9-28. Both γ-MSH and the α-MSH activity of ACTH in patients with elevated levels of ACTH (eg, in primary adrenocortical insufficiency; see Table 2-7) can cause hyperpigmentation (*hypermelanosis*) of the skin by stimulating melanin synthesis in melanocytes. β-Endorphin and met-enkephalin are opioid peptides that have analgesic activity.

The majority of *pituitary tumors* are benign *adenomas* or *microadenomas.* The most frequently diagnosed pituitary adenomas are *prolactinomas,* non-secreting *null cell adenomas, corticotrophic adenomas,* and *somatotrophic adenomas.*

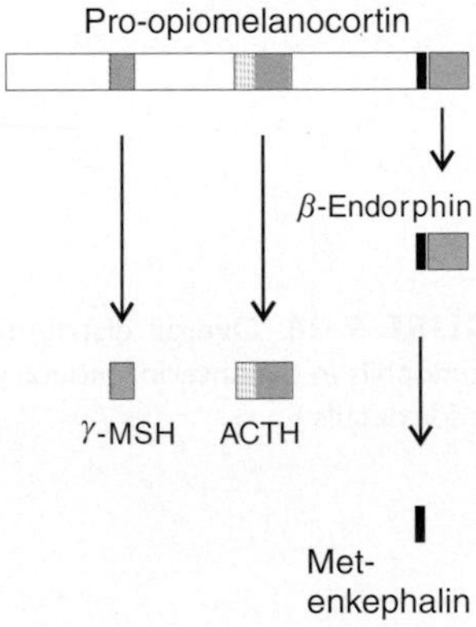

Growth Hormone

Some metabolic actions of GH are direct, eg, mobilization of glucose and free fatty acids. However, the stimulatory effects of GH on skeletal growth, protein synthesis, and cellular proliferation are primarily indirect. The indirect effects are mediated by *insulin-like growth factors* called *somatomedins* that are produced in the liver and other tissues in response to stimulation by GH. *Somatomedin C,* known also as *insulin-like growth factor I* (IGF-I), is the chief stimulus for augmented chondrogenesis in the epiphyseal plates of growing long bones. Furthermore, chondrocytes are able to produce IGF-I locally in response to GH.

The various actions of all the hormones produced in the anterior pituitary are summarized in Table 9-3.

Pro-opiomelanocortin

β-Endorphin

γ-MSH   ACTH

Met-enkephalin

FIGURE 9-28 Pituitary corticotrophs can produce ACTH, γ-MSH, β-endorphin, and met-enkephalin as a result of post-translational processing, through progressive proteolytic cleavage of the pro-opiomelanocortin molecule. A part of the ACTH molecule also has α-MSH activity (pale, striped region).

Posterior Lobe

As shown in Figs. 9-25 and 9-26, the posterior lobe of the pituitary is the site of release of two hypothalamic peptide hormones, *oxytocin* and *vasopressin* (anti-

TABLE 9-3

ACTIONS OF HORMONES SECRETED BY CELLS OF THE ANTERIOR PITUITARY

Hormone	Primary Target Cells	Main Effects
Growth hormone (protein)	Chondrocytes of epiphyseal growth plates; other cells	With some actions mediated by somatomedins (insulin-like growth factors), promotes protein synthesis, body growth, and utilization of carbohydrates and lipids
Prolactin (protein)	Mammary alveolar epithelial cells	Elicits further development of breast tissue in pregnancy; stimulates secretion of milk
Adrenocorticotrophic hormone (polypeptide)	Cells in adrenal cortex	Enlarges adrenal cortex and increases output of adrenal corticosteroids
Thyroid-stimulating hormone (glycoprotein)	Follicular epithelial cells of thyroid	Augments secretory activity of follicular epithelial cells and elicits their hypertrophy and hyperplasia
Follicle-stimulating hormone (glycoprotein)	Follicular (granulosa) cells of ovarian follicles	Promotes growth and maturation of ovarian follicles
	Sertoli cells of testis	Promotes binding of testosterone by augmenting secretion of androgen-binding protein
Luteinizing hormone (glycoprotein)	Ovarian thecal, granulosa, and luteal cells	Elicits ovulation and induces luteinization in ovarian follicles
	Interstitial (Leydig) cells of testis	Augments secretion of testosterone
Melanocyte-stimulating hormone (peptide)*	Melanocytes of skin	Promotes synthesis of melanin

*Activity mostly due to ACTH.

diuretic hormone, ADH). Each of these hormones is produced by a separate group of hypothalamic neurons. The cell bodies of the neurons that produce *oxytocin* are located chiefly in the *paraventricular nucleus*, whereas those that produce *vasopressin* are located chiefly in the *supraoptic nucleus*. In each case, the peptide hormone is transported down the axon in association with a protein known as a *neurophysin*, which is a part of the hormone precursor. By the time the secretory granules reach the axon terminals, the hormone has become fully cleaved from its precursor. The hormone-containing secretory granules are stored in axon terminals that are intimately associated with fenestrated capillaries. In pituitary sections, intracellular accumulations of these secretory granules sometimes appear as irregular basophilic masses known as *Herring bodies*. Inconspicuous glial cells called *pituicytes* also are present; they are believed to serve some supporting function.

Oxytocin (Gk. *oxys*, swift; *tokos*, birth) is used clinically to induce labor and to control postpartum bleeding. It elicits peristaltic contractions of the myometrium and, thereby, expedites parturition. Another important action of oxytocin is that during breast feeding, it elicits contraction of the myoepithelial cells in the breast, causing ejection of milk from the secretory alveoli.

Vasopressin (arginine vasopressin, ADH) promotes water resorption in the kidneys (as outlined under Collecting Ducts in Chap. 7). It also stimulates secretion of ACTH. Relatively high concentrations of vasopressin have marked vasoconstrictor activity.

Between the posterior lobe and the anterior lobe of the pituitary lies the *pars intermedia,* which is rudimentary and ill-defined. It is generally only distinguishable by the presence of a few vestigial colloid-filled cysts. The fibrous *capsule* that encloses the pituitary and the shelf-like *diaphragma sellae* that covers it superiorly are both derived from the dura mater.

Pancreatic Islets

The *pancreatic islets (islets of Langerhans)* are separate, irregularly shaped groups of up to several hundred endocrine secretory epithelial cells (Fig. 9-29). Islets are scattered throughout the pancreas, particularly its tail. Their total number is estimated to be one to two million. The secretory epithelial cells of the islet are closely associated with fenestrated capillaries and are arranged as anastomosing cords. Surrounding the islet is a thin sheath of loose connective tissue with reticular fibers that support the secretory cells. Autonomic efferent nerve endings are present on some of the secretory cells. Four different types of secretory cells have been identified in the islets. *A (α) cells,* which are large and stain pink with Gomori stain (a special staining technique), secrete *glucagon. B (β) cells,* which are smaller and stain blue with this stain, secrete *insulin.* B cells are more numerous than the other cell types. In addition, there are some *D (δ) cells,* which secrete *somatostatin,* and small numbers of *F cells,* which secrete *pancreatic polypeptide.* Neither the D nor the F cells are specifically recognizable in routine histological sections, even with Gomori staining. Immunocytochemical staining is required to identify the four different cell types unequivocally, but their secretory granules do show some consistent differences at the EM level (Fig. 9-30).

Because the hormones made by the islet cells have a variety of stimulatory and inhibitory effects on the secretory activities of the other islet cells (Fig. 9-31), juxtaposition of the different cells within the islet is believed to facilitate mutual paracrine signaling. A cells respond to a drop in plasma glucose (ie, *hypoglycemia*) by secreting glucagon. B cells respond to a rise in the concentration of plasma glucose (ie, *hyperglycemia*) by secreting insulin. Cholinergic impulses

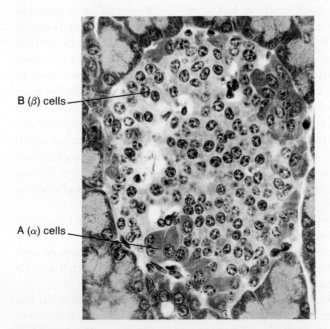

B (*β*) cells

A (*α*) cells

FIGURE 9-29 A and B cells in a pancreatic islet (Gomori stain, guinea pig pancreas).

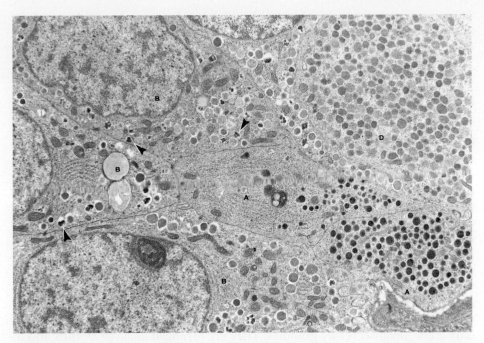

FIGURE 9-30 A, B, and D cells in a pancreatic islet (electron micrograph, human pancreas). Cell types are labeled. Arrowheads indicate insulin-containing B cell granules that have irregularly shaped crystalline contents.

from the right vagus (parasympathetic), and also β-adrenergic receptor (sympathetic) stimulation, increase the secretion of both insulin and glucagon. α-Adrenergic receptor (sympathetic) stimulation inhibits the secretion of both hormones. The role of autonomic regulation seems to be to maintain normal responsiveness of these cells to plasma glucose levels, and paracrine signaling from one cell type to another is presumed to fine-tune the hormonal output of each islet.

Pancreatic polypeptide reduces exocrine secretory activity in the pancreas, delays contraction of the gallbladder, and decreases motility of the intestine. Its overall role appears to be that of slowing down nutrient absorption. *Glucagon* promotes the conversion of glycogen to glucose in hepatocytes and increases glucose production from pyruvate. A rapid and important action of *insulin* is to promote the facilitated diffusion of glucose across the cell membrane, especially in skeletal muscle fibers and adipocytes. This is accomplished by insertion of additional glucose transporters (GLUT 4 molecules) into the cell membrane. Other important effects of insulin are that it promotes the synthesis of (1) glycogen in hepatocytes and muscle fibers, and (2) triglycerides in adipose tissue. Also, it stimulates cell growth by increasing the rate of protein synthesis.

Diabetes Mellitus

The disease *diabetes mellitus* (Gk. *diabētēs*, siphon; L. *mellitus*, sweetened with honey) is characterized by an osmotic diuresis due to the presence of glucose in the urine (*glycosuria*). The glycosuria is a manifestation of *hyperglycemia* resulting from insufficient lowering of the blood glucose level by insulin. The amount of glucose in the urinary filtrate exceeds the amount that can be resorbed by the renal tubules, and the excess is lost in the urine. *Type I*, insulin-dependent diabetes mellitus is due to an insulin deficiency. Autoimmunity is implicated as a potential etiological factor. *Type II*, late onset, non-insulin-dependent diabetes is characterized by a decreased response of the target cells to insulin, ie, insulin refractoriness. Circulating insulin levels may be decreased, normal, or increased.

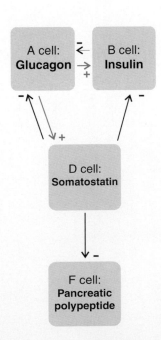

FIGURE 9-31 Local regulation of pancreatic islet cell hormone secretion.

This type of diabetes is associated with a high incidence of obesity. An excessive mass of target cells can potentially raise the demand for insulin to a point where it exceeds the supply. Tissue responsiveness to insulin is decreased in roughly 50% of the cases.

Parathyroids and C Cells

The indistinctly lobulated *parathyroids,* derived from endoderm, are small, ovoid glands that lie along the posterior borders of the lobes of the thyroid, internal to its fascial sheath. Generally, there are four parathyroid glands, but in certain cases, there are two or six of them. Their largest diameter is approximately 5 mm. Although every precaution is taken to preserve integrity of the parathyroids, total thyroidectomy and the resection of laryngeal or esophageal carcinomas are associated with a considerable risk of damage or unintentional removal of parathyroids. In subtotal thyroidectomy, small regions of the thyroid gland are purposely retained on both sides of the trachea to protect the parathyroids, their local blood supply, and the recurrent laryngeal nerves.

Until a few years before puberty, the endocrine cells present in the parathyroids are exclusively *chief (principal) cells,* which secrete *parathyroid hormone* (PTH). These small cells are characterized by a central, spherical nucleus and only a few small secretory granules. They are arranged as large clumps and irregular wide cords supported by reticular fibers. Fenestrated capillaries are also present. A few years before puberty, groups of acidophilic *oxyphil cells* (Gk. *oxys,* acid) begin to appear among the chief cells (Fig. 9-32). Oxyphil cells, which have more cytoplasm and are, therefore, somewhat larger, contain abundant mitochondria. They are widely regarded as chief cells in a non-secretory state, but their functional significance is uncertain.

PTH is an essential hormone because it maintains the required blood Ca^{2+} level. The chief cells possess a Ca^{2+} receptor and secrete PTH when the plasma Ca^{2+} is low. When the plasma Ca^{2+} is high, their secretory activity is inhibited, and a greater proportion of their stored hormone becomes degraded. Hydroxylated metabolites of vitamin D also inhibit PTH secretion. Release of Ca^{2+} from bone mineral by PTH is mediated chiefly by *osteoclasts.* PTH increases (1) the number of osteoclasts present on bone surfaces, and (2) the size and resorptive

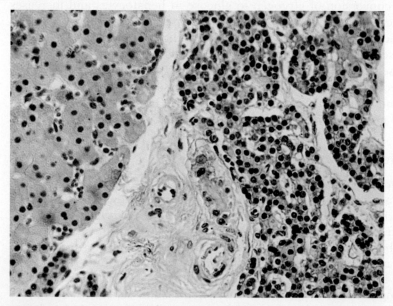

FIGURE 9-32 Parathyroid gland, showing its chief cells on the right and its oxyphil cells on the left.

activity of the ruffled borders on osteoclasts. In addition, PTH increases resorption of Ca^{2+}, and decreases resorption of phosphate, from the renal tubules. It also enhances the synthesis of a hydroxylated derivative of vitamin D_3 (1,25-di-hydroxycholecalciferol) that promotes the absorption of dietary Ca^{2+}.

Hypocalcemia due to PTH deficiency results in *tetany* (involuntary muscle spasms such as laryngeal and carpopedal spasms). Spasms of the laryngeal muscles close the glottis and obstruct the airway. If prolonged, they can cause fatal asphyxia. Spasms affecting the upper extremity cause the elbow and wrist to flex, the metacarpophalangeal joints to flex, the fingers to extend, and the thumb to adduct. Recurring painful cramps of the foot result in plantar flexion of the toes. Under hypocalcemic conditions, motor nerve fibers and the other parts of the nervous system become hyperexcitable. Heightened neural excitability and excessive stimulation at motor end plates results in prolonged involuntary contractions of skeletal muscle fibers.

Overproduction of PTH, eg, due to a parathyroid adenoma or the continuous secretion of a PTH-mimicking product by a non-parathyroid malignancy, produces *hypercalcemia*, ectopic calcification of soft tissues, kidney stones, and excessive bone resorption, leading to multiple bone cysts and spontaneous fractures. It may also result in neuromuscular and behavioral symptoms.

Calcitonin, the secretory product of *C cells* of the thyroid, counterbalances the action of PTH by lowering the plasma Ca^{2+} level. It reduces the rate at which osteoclasts, or their precursors, are recruited for bone resorption. It also reduces bone resorption by decreasing the size and resorptive activity of ruffled borders on osteoclasts, and promotes Ca^{2+} excretion by the kidney tubules. No serious clinical consequences result from a calcitonin excess or deficiency. Since calcitonin inhibits bone resorption, it has found limited application in the treatment of osteoporosis.

ESSENTIAL FEATURES OF THE FEMALE REPRODUCTIVE SYSTEM

An understanding of reproduction in the female requires a certain level of familiarity with (1) the interactions that occur between the hypothalamus, anterior pituitary, ovarian follicles, and endometrium, (2) the cyclic histological and functional changes that ensue in the ovarian follicles and endometrium, and (3) the hormonal and paracrine signaling that takes place between many of the cells involved. Much of this information is an outcome of investigations into modes of action of (1) administered hormonal contraceptives and (2) techniques that result in successful in vitro fertilization. Its diverse clinical applications include management of anovulation, other menstrual disorders, subnormal fertility, and breast cancer.

Ovaries and Ovarian Follicles

The paired *ovaries* are situated on each side of the uterus, in the pelvic cavity. Each ovary has a covering of simple cuboidal epithelium, a thick cortex containing *ovarian follicles,* and an indistinct central medulla provided with many blood vessels (Fig. 9-33). The various types of maturing follicle shown in Figs. 9-33 and 9-34 include (1) superficial *primordial follicles* with flat *follicular epithelial (granulosa) cells* surrounding a central *primary oocyte*, (2 and 3) *primary follicles* (known also as *preantral follicles*) with two or more layers of cuboidal follicular cells, but no antrum, surrounding the oocyte, (4) *secondary follicles* with a forming antrum, (5 and 6) *atretic follicles* (meaning ones that are no longer a hole, in other words, follicles that are gradually becoming filled with

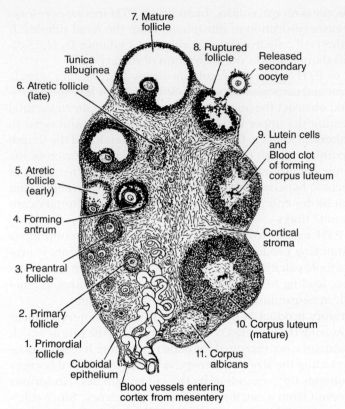

FIGURE 9-33 Stages of ovarian follicular maturation, luteinization, and residual scarring.

other kinds of cells), and (7) *mature (tertiary, Graafian) follicles,* one of which is generally dominant and ruptures at ovulation. The germ cell in the maturing follicles is the primary oocyte. It divides to form the secondary oocyte just before ovulation (see below).

Maturation of ovarian follicles and secretion of estrogen by the follicular cells are stimulated by FSH. Primordial follicles are still unresponsive to FSH. Every 28 days or so, the follicular cells of 20 to 50 such follicles acquire more FSH receptors and begin to respond to FSH. Follicular enlargement is due to their hypertrophic and hyperplastic response to this hormone. The process of follicular maturation takes 3 months to reach completion. It can fail at any stage, resulting in follicular atresia. *Atretic follicles* show histological evidence of degeneration, eg, pyknosis of follicular cell nuclei, disappearance of follicular cells (Fig. 9-35), loss of the zona pellucida (the extracellular glycoprotein layer surrounding the oocyte), shrinkage of the oocyte or karyolysis of its nucleus, or invasion of the follicle by neutrophils.

The region of stroma that lies immediately external to the basement membrane of the follicular epithelium is known as the *theca* (see Fig. 9-34C). Its inner part, the *theca interna,* is richly vascularized; the outer part, the *theca externa,* is fibrous. At the secondary follicle stage, exudate formed from the theca interna vessels begins to collect in the follicle as coalescing pools. The nutritive *follicular fluid* that accumulates in this manner eventually occupies the entire antrum.

Oogenesis

Table 9-4 outlines some key stages of *oogenesis,* starting with the *primordial female germ cells* that migrate to the ovaries from the embryonic yolk sac. The

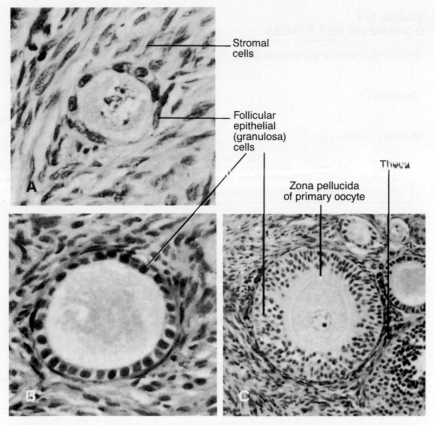

FIGURE 9-34 Early stages of ovarian follicular maturation. (**A**) Primordial follicle. (**B**) Early primary follicle. (**C**) Maturing primary follicle (preantral stage).

postnatal *primary oocytes* are fully differentiated diploid oogonia that have commenced their *first meiotic division (meiosis I)*. At the end of *prophase I* (which is a prenatal stage), they pass into a prolonged resting state called *dictyotene,* and they remain in this state until puberty has occurred. The process of meiosis is resumed only in dominant follicles, which just before the time of ovulation, are mature enough to rupture at the ovarian surface. The delay incurred before the completion of meiosis I can be as long as 55 years.

REVIEW ITEM 9-2

What well-known syndrome is associated with late middle-age pregnancies?

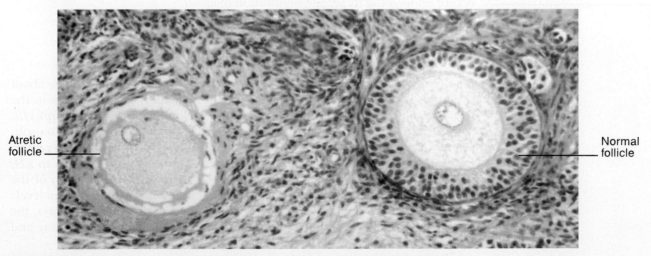

FIGURE 9-35 Normal ovarian primary follicle compared with an ovarian follicle that shows histological signs of atresia (degenerated follicular cells).

TABLE 9-4
OOGENESIS: KEY STAGES

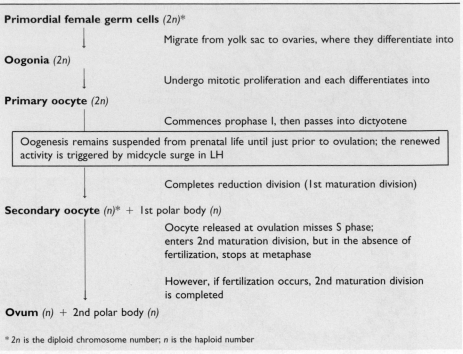

Primordial female germ cells *(2n)**

↓   Migrate from yolk sac to ovaries, where they differentiate into

Oogonia *(2n)*

↓   Undergo mitotic proliferation and each differentiates into

Primary oocyte *(2n)*

        Commences prophase I, then passes into dictyotene

> Oogenesis remains suspended from prenatal life until just prior to ovulation; the renewed activity is triggered by midcycle surge in LH

↓   Completes reduction division (1st maturation division)

Secondary oocyte *(n)** + 1st polar body *(n)*

        Oocyte released at ovulation misses S phase;
        enters 2nd maturation division, but in the absence of
        fertilization, stops at metaphase

        However, if fertilization occurs, 2nd maturation division
↓   is completed

Ovum *(n)* + 2nd polar body *(n)*

* *2n* is the diploid chromosome number; *n* is the haploid number

> **KEY CONCEPT**
>
> Meiosis produces haploid germ cells

> **KEY CONCEPT**
>
> The complement of primary oocytes decreases with time; 99.9% of ovarian follicles undergo atresia.

Resumption of meiosis and rupture of the dominant follicle are responses to the surge in LH that occurs in the middle of the ovarian cycle, which is also known as the *menstrual* (L. *mensis,* month) or *uterine* cycle (see Fig. 9-40). The primary oocyte divides unequally, producing a *secondary oocyte* and the *first polar body,* both of which are *haploid.* The secondary oocyte is released at ovulation, which is conventionally accepted as occurring on day 14 of the cycle. The secondary oocyte begins meiosis II, but becomes arrested at the metaphase stage of the second maturation division. If fertilization occurs, the cell completes this division and goes on to form the *ovum* and *second polar body.* The *reduction division,* which results in progression from the diploid to the haploid chromosome number, occurs between the *primary* and the *secondary oocyte* stages. The secondary oocyte does *not* go through an S phase (DNA synthesis) before undergoing its second maturation division.

Corpus Luteum

A second important consequence of the midcycle rise in LH that brings about ovulation is that it causes *luteinization* of the follicular granulosa cells in the ovulated follicle. This effect is manifested as development of a yellow *corpus luteum* (L. *luteus,* yellow). As indicated in Fig. 9-38, luteinization depends on subsequent acquisition of the LH receptor as a supplement to the FSH receptor. Luteinizing granulosa cells start producing *progesterone* in response to *LH,* while continuing to produce *estrogen* in response to *FSH.* Stimulation of the lutein cells by LH and FSH causes circulating progesterone and estrogen levels to rise in the third week (Fig. 9-36). However, after approximately 12 days, the corpus luteum involutes, unless fertilization ensues, and the progesterone and estrogen levels show a subsequent rapid decline (Fig. 9-36).

Distinctive histological features of the corpus luteum that may aid in its recognition are (1) the presence of large, pale-staining *follicular lutein cells,* de-

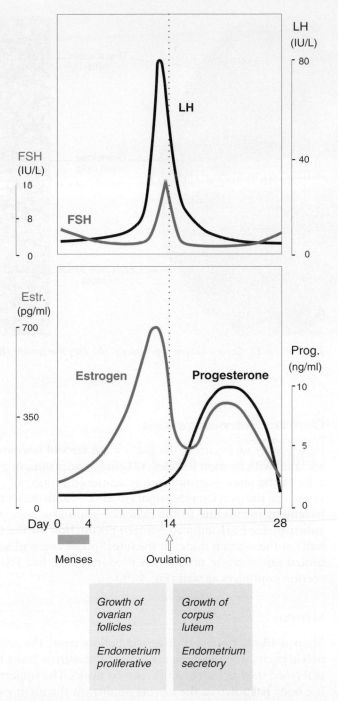

FIGURE 9-36 LH, FSH, estrogen, and progesterone levels in the two main phases of the menstrual cycle.

rived from the follicular granulosa cells, and smaller peripheral *theca lutein* cells (Fig. 9-37), and (2) the presence of central remnants of the *blood clot* formed following ovulation.

When the corpus luteum involutes, it becomes replaced by a rounded or ovoid scar known as a *corpus albicans* (see Fig. 9-33). This process of scarring starts with fibroblast invasion and generally progresses to hyalinization, meaning that much collagen is laid down, becomes pale-staining, and acquires a homogeneous appearance due to tight packing.

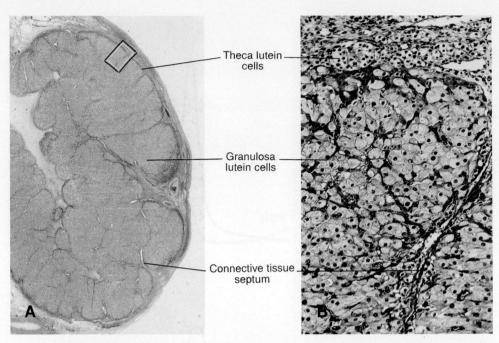

FIGURE 9-37 Corpus luteum of pregnancy. (**A**) Very low power. (**B**) Details of boxed-in area in A.

Ovarian Steroidogenesis

Figure 9-38 summarizes the patterns of steroid hormone synthesis that are associated with ovarian follicles. LH elicits the production of *androgens* by stromal cells of the *theca interna*, also by scattered groups of stromal cells collectively known as the ovarian *interstitial gland*. The androgens pass across the follicular basement membrane to the *follicular granulosa cells*, which utilize them as a substrate for FSH-induced *estrogen* production during the follicular phase (first half) of the ovarian cycle. In the luteal phase (second half) of the cycle, LH-promoted *progesterone* production predominates, but FSH-promoted *estrogen* secretion continues as well (Fig. 9-38).

Uterus

Shaped like a flattened, inverted hollow pear, the *uterus* lies centrally in the pelvic cavity. Its upper part is termed the *uterine body;* the narrower, lower part is termed the *uterine cervix* (L. *cervix*, neck). The uppermost portion of the uterine body is known as the *uterine fundus*. At the *uterine ostium* (ie, *external os* of the cervix), the distal end of the cervical canal opens into the vagina.

The substantial muscular part of the uterine wall is called the *myometrium* (Gk. *metra*, womb). It is made up of three indistinct layers of smooth muscle, the middle layer of which is circular and contains relatively large blood vessels. Uterine smooth muscle cells respond to the high estrogen levels attained in pregnancy by undergoing both hypertrophy and hyperplasia. Oxytocin promotes myometrial contractions and, therefore, is used for the induction of labor.

The muscular walls of the bilateral *uterine tubes (Fallopian tubes* or *oviducts)* undergo peristaltic contractions capable of propelling liberated oocytes to the uterus. Fertilization generally occurs in the *ampulla*, which is a fairly wide segment that borders on the fimbriated, funnel-shaped proximal end of the tube associated with the ovulating ovary. The ampulla is characterized by an elaborate pattern of folding of its ciliated epithelium (Fig. 9-39A). The simple columnar

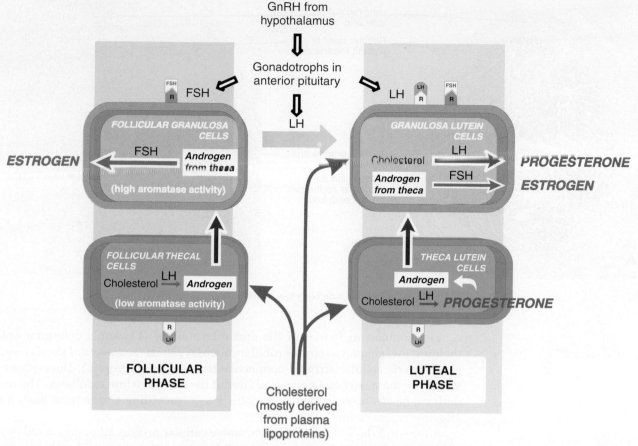

FIGURE 9-38 Production of ovarian steroid hormones involves metabolic cooperation between (1) theca interna stromal cells and (2) granulosa follicular epithelial cells. During the follicular phase of the ovarian cycle, theca interna cells (and other interstitial cells) respond to LH by producing the androgenic steroids dehydroepiandrosterone (DHA), androstenedione, and testosterone from cholesterol. Liberated thecal androgens traverse the follicular basement membrane and enter the follicular granulosa cells, where FSH promotes their aromatization to the estrogens estradiol and estrone. In the luteal phase of the cycle, the chief steroid produced by both types of lutein cells in response to LH is progesterone.

epithelial lining of the tube incorporates secretory cells as well as ciliated cells. It is widely assumed that their secretory product is nutritive and that ciliary activity of the epithelium contributes to transport and nourishment of the oocyte or zygote.

Endometrium

The *endometrium* is the functionally important *mucosal lining* of the uterus. It is the normal site of implantation of the blastocyst. As summarized in Fig. 9-40, cyclic changes in structure and function of this layer reflect variation in circulating levels of ovarian steroid hormones. In response to *estrogen* secreted in the first half of the ovarian cycle, the endometrium undergoes *proliferative* changes that restore it after its partial destruction through menstruation; accordingly, this portion of the cycle is often referred to as the *proliferative, estrogenic,* or *follicular phase* of the *menstrual cycle.* In response to *progesterone* secreted with estrogen in the second half of the cycle, the endometrium undergoes *secretory* changes that prepare it for implantation of the blastocyst. The second half is widely known as the *secretory* or *progestational phase* of the menstrual cycle.

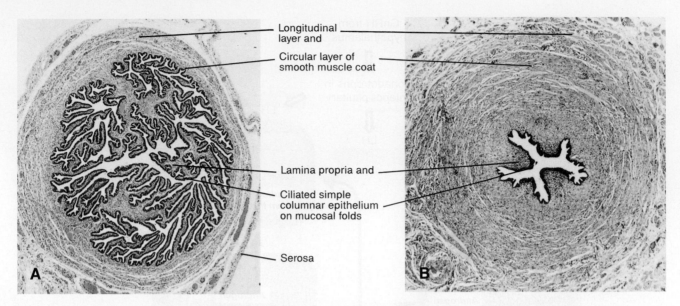

Longitudinal layer and

Circular layer of smooth muscle coat

Lamina propria and

Ciliated simple columnar epithelium on mucosal folds

Serosa

FIGURE 9-39 Uterine tube (very low power). (**A**) Ampulla. (**B**) Isthmus.

The component tissues of the endometrium are (1) simple columnar epithelium, invaginated as simple tubular mucosal glands (*endometrial glands*), and (2) relatively cellular stromal connective tissue (*lamina propria*). During menstruation, the superficial *functional layer* of the endometrium exfoliates. The underlying *basilar layer,* however, remains intact, providing a structural basis for effective regeneration.

After 4 to 5 days of menstruation, active cellular proliferation promoted by a rising estrogen level leads to substantial endometrial thickening. Hence, endometrium obtained during the *proliferative phase* is characterized by the presence of lengthening straight endometrial glands (Fig. 9-41A) and an increased proportion of mitotic figures. In the *secretory phase*, the glands hypertrophy and take on a sacculated appearance that results from accumulation of *glycogen*, their secretory product (Fig. 9-41B). This change is a response to *progesterone,* which the ovaries secrete only in the second half of the cycle (see Fig. 9-36). The hypertrophied secretory cells appear pale and ragged, and there is stromal edema. In the *ischemic (premenstrual) phase,* falling levels of progesterone and estrogen (especially progesterone) fail to maintain suitable conditions for implantation. *Spiral (coiled) arteries* supplying the functional layer of endometrium become elongated during the secretory phase. During the ischemic phase, they undergo intermittent vasoconstriction that becomes increasingly prolonged, and small pools of extravasated blood begin to appear in the stroma. In the *menstrual phase,* resulting ischemic necrosis of the functional layer leads to its exfoliation (Fig. 9-41C). Bleeding occurs from the raw endometrial surface because blood clots do not form in the bleeding vessels. The basilar layer has an uninterrupted, independent blood supply from straight branches of the uterine artery, and therefore it survives. Endometrial bleeding can also occur (1) as a delayed response to a substantial drop in the estrogen level, eg, when a dominant follicle ruptures without releasing its oocyte (ie, in an *anovulatory cycle*), and (2) dysfunctionally when high estrogen levels are maintained in the absence of a cyclic rise and fall of the progesterone level.

Uterine Cervix

The *uterine cervix* has strong, fibrous walls made up of dense ordinary connective tissue with only a small proportion of smooth muscle. Its mucosa does not

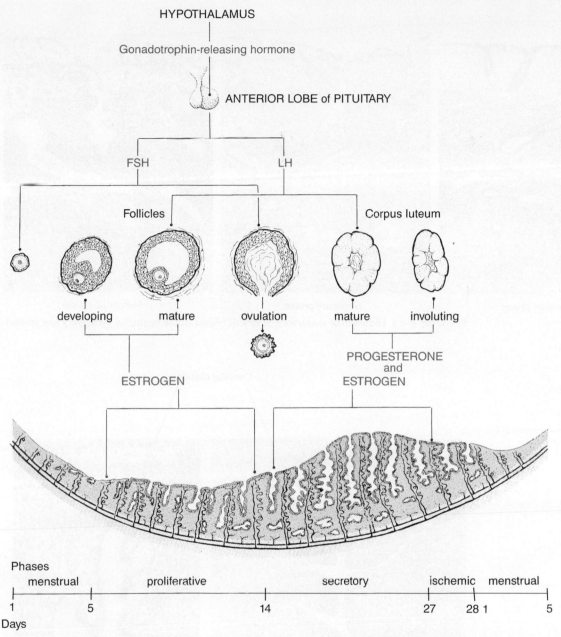

HYPOTHALAMUS

Gonadotrophin-releasing hormone

ANTERIOR LOBE of PITUITARY

FSH   LH

Follicles   Corpus luteum

developing   mature   ovulation   mature   involuting

ESTROGEN   PROGESTERONE
and
ESTROGEN

Phases
menstrual   proliferative   secretory   ischemic menstrual

1   5   14   27   28 1   5
Days

FIGURE 9-40 Effect of stimulation of ovarian steroid secretion on endometrial appearance over the course of the menstrual cycle.

exfoliate during menstruation. Although this part of the uterus undergoes little or no expansion during pregnancy, it is necessary for the cervix to dilate in preparation for parturition. In the later stages of pregnancy, the fibrous tissue in the cervical wall becomes more pliable as a result of the action of the polypeptide hormone *relaxin,* secreted by the corpus luteum of pregnancy and endometrial decidual cells under the implantation site. Relaxin generally also brings about a slight relaxation of the pubic symphysis by eliciting partial replacement of the fibrocartilage with connective tissue that has more flexibility. Osteoclasts as well as fibroblasts seem to be involved, and the induced changes include an altered state of aggregation of the collagen fibrils.

The *cervical canal* is lined by a simple columnar *mucus-secreting epithelium* that is invaginated as numerous folds and associated branching tubular mucosal

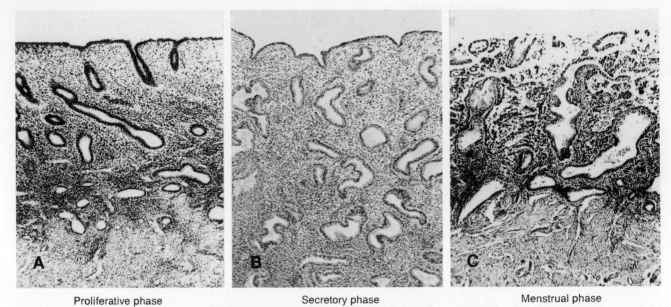

Proliferative phase   Secretory phase   Menstrual phase

FIGURE 9-41 Endometrial appearance at various phases of the menstrual cycle (very low power).

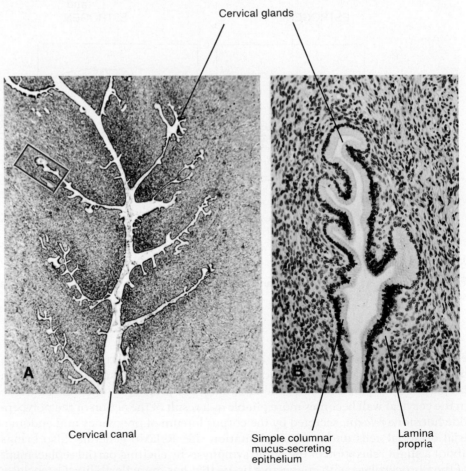

Cervical glands

Cervical canal

Simple columnar mucus-secreting epithelium

Lamina propria

FIGURE 9-42 (**A**) Cervical canal (very low power). (**B**) Cervical mucous gland (medium power).

glands called *cervical (endocervical) glands* (Fig. 9-42). Some of the columnar cells are ciliated. The *cervical mucus* produced by the epithelium shows cyclic steroid hormone-dependent variation in quantity and viscosity. When the estrogen level rises in the proliferative phase, the mucus becomes alkaline and increasingly copious and thin in consistency. When the progesterone level also rises in the secretory phase, less mucus is produced, and it becomes less alkaline and more viscid, and accordingly presents more of a barrier to migrating spermatozoa.

Exocervix and Vagina

In the vicinity of the external os of the exocervix (uterine ostium), the simple columnar epithelial lining of the cervical canal borders on the stratified squamous non-keratinizing epithelium of the vagina. This borderline, described as the *squamocolumnar junction,* is abrupt and variable in position, as discussed in part D9-8 of the Discussion section of this chapter.

In contrast to the cervix, the *vagina,* a flattened sheath-like tube with strong fibromuscular walls, lacks mucosal glands (Fig. 9-43). Its stratified squamous non-keratinizing epithelial lining, accordingly, requires cervical mucus for it to stay moist. During a woman's reproductive years, the epithelial lining of this part of the reproductive tract becomes fairly substantial as a result of basal and parabasal cellular proliferation in response to repeated estrogenic stimulation. However, with the considerably lower estrogen levels found before puberty and after menopause, this epithelium can be quite thin, and during childhood vaginal infections are not uncommon. Estrogen is often effective in treating such infections because it thickens the vaginal epithelium.

Estrogenic stimulation also promotes the storage of glycogen and lipids in vaginal epithelial cells, which gives these cells a pale, empty appearance in H&E sections. The glycogen content becomes maximal at the time of ovulation. Its usual role is to give rise to lactic acid as a consequence of bacterial action. The acidic conditions inhibit growth of microorganisms and promote an appropriate microflora (eg, lactobacilli) in the cervical mucus within the vaginal lumen. A cytological sign of estrogenic stimulation, detectable in exfoliated cells obtained from the vaginal surface, is an increasing tendency toward acidophilic staining when special stains, eg, *Papanicolaou stain,* are used. This stain also has useful application in screening for the early stages of cervical carcinoma (see part D9-8 of the Discussion section of this chapter).

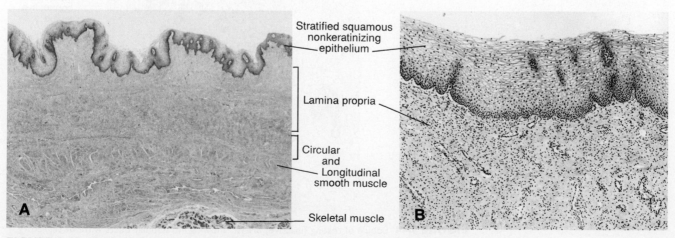

FIGURE 9-43 (**A**) Vagina (very low power). (**B**) Vaginal mucosa (very low power).

Breast

The paired *mammary glands* (*breasts*) are each made up of 15 to 25 lobes. Each lobe represents a compound alveolar gland with a *lactiferous duct* that dilates as a *lactiferous sinus* near its surface opening, an orifice on a nipple. The stromal fibrous tissue that connects the lobes contains abundant *adipose tissue* when the breast is in the non-lactating condition.

The prepubertal breast is represented by a rudimentary epithelial duct system. Increased levels of estrogen at puberty (1) stimulate further growth of the duct system, and (2) promote adipocyte differentiation from stromal cells. Breast enlargement at puberty is chiefly a consequence of lipid deposition in the recently supplemented population of adipocytes. Breast development remains arrested at this stage until pregnancy, when further proliferative and secretory changes occur in response to the high estrogen, progesterone, prolactin, and chorionic somatomammotropin levels that are attained. These changes prepare the breast for lactation.

Resting Breast

Mature breast tissue that has not yet undergone the secretory response is described as the *resting* (*inactive*) breast. Each lobe is represented by a number of small lobules that essentially contain only *ducts* (Fig. 9-44). The walls of the larger ducts appear as a double layer of low columnar or cuboidal epithelial cells, the outermost layer of which represent contractile myoepithelial cells. The smaller ducts are lined by a single layer of cuboidal cells. The intralobular con-

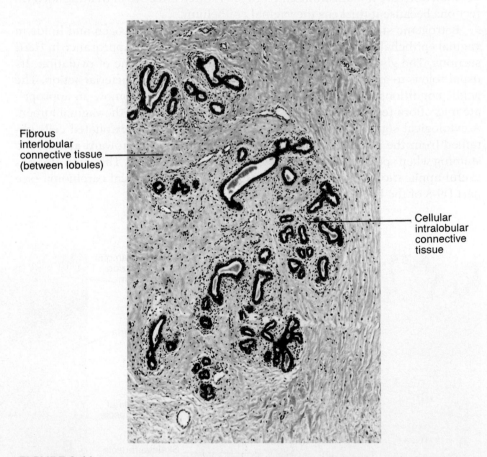

Fibrous interlobular connective tissue (between lobules)

Cellular intralobular connective tissue

FIGURE 9-44 Lobule of resting (inactive) breast, showing intralobular ducts without secretory alveoli.

nective tissue that supports the ducts, derived through down-growth of the papillary layer of dermis, is relatively cellular. The interlobular connective tissue in which the lobules lie scattered, representing the reticular layer of dermis, is dense ordinary connective tissue. Regions of interlobular adipose tissue also are present. Recognition of (1) a diffuse lobular pattern and (2) a virtual absence of secretory units is the key to distinguishing resting breast from other types of glands.

Breast discomfort or tenderness occurring in the second half of the menstrual cycle may result from progesterone-promoted edema of the breast connective tissue.

Lactating Breast

The additional epithelial proliferation necessary to complete full growth of the breast's branched duct system is elicited by high estrogen levels during the first half of pregnancy. The terminal branches of the duct system then undergo further differentiation, becoming *secretory alveoli*. A network of contractile myoepithelial cells forms around each alveolus. The proliferative changes prepare the breast for the predominantly progesterone-induced secretory changes that ensue in the second half. In addition to estrogen and progesterone, PRL, GH, thyroid hormone, chorionic somatomammotropin, adrenal glucocorticoids, and insulin contribute to full lobuloalveolar differentiation and growth, and promote secretory activity of the alveoli. As may be seen in Fig. 9-45, many of the alveoli become filled with their secretion (*colostrum*), and the lobules become easier to discern. The interlobular connective tissue between them becomes reduced to fairly vascular fibrous septa. Different amounts of stored secretion characterize the individual lobules, and different degrees of distention characterize the individual alveoli of each lobule. This highly lobular, secretory appearance becomes even more accentuated during postpartum breast feeding.

For the first 5 days after parturition, colostrum is secreted. This is followed by transitional milk. Mature milk is secreted at 10 days. The compositions of colostrum and mature breast milk are compared in Table 9-5.

The action of PRL in bringing about milk secretion is antagonized by high estrogen levels. Secretion of colostrum and milk, therefore, remains inhibited

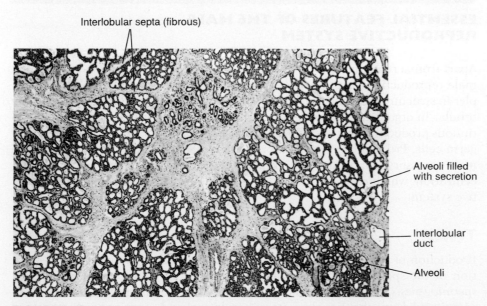

Interlobular septa (fibrous)

Alveoli filled with secretion

Interlobular duct

Alveoli

FIGURE 9-45 Breast tissue, showing secretory changes in preparation for lactation (5th month of pregnancy).

TABLE 9-5
COLOSTRUM AND BREAST MILK (HUMAN): KEY CONSTITUENTS

Constituent	Colostrum	Mature Milk
Triglycerides	+	+ +
Lactose	+	+ +
Immunoglobulins, eg, IgA	+ +	+
Lactoferrin	+ +	+
Casein	+	+
α-Lactalbumin	+	+
Sodium	+ + +	+
Chloride	+ + +	+
Calcium	+	+
Phosphate	+	+
Vitamins	+	+

throughout pregnancy. Expulsion of the placenta at parturition results in a rapid decline in estrogen (and progesterone) levels that initiates lactation. Breast feeding generally results in postpartum amenorrhea of variable duration. Sustained lactation is dependent on continuing PRL secretion.

Breast feeding also depends on *oxytocin* release from the posterior pituitary. This hormone acts on myoepithelial cells of the breast, causing their contraction and resulting in *milk ejection*. Afferent impulses from a suckled nipple pass via the spinal cord to the hypothalamus and trigger release of oxytocin from axon terminals of hypothalamic neurons that produce it. This response, called the *milk ejection reflex*, is subject to inhibition by psychological factors such as stress. PRL release is regulated by a similar neuroendocrine reflex, since the same afferent impulses suppress release of hypothalamic PIH (dopamine) and, hence, ensure continuing PRL secretion by anterior pituitary mammotrophs.

ESSENTIAL FEATURES OF THE MALE REPRODUCTIVE SYSTEM

Apart from a remarkable diversity of lining epithelia in the various parts of the male reproductive tract, the *male reproductive system* seems substantially simpler in structure and function when compared with the female system. Basically tubular in organization, it is a somewhat convoluted linear system for the continuous production, storage, and intermittent emission of *spermatozoa*, the male germ cells. Production of spermatozoa, and adequate secretory activity of the male accessory glands, depend on maintenance of a local high androgen concentration, which represents a further essential function of the male reproductive system.

Testes

Production of spermatozoa (*spermatogenesis*), including complex transformation of the spermatozoon's precursor (the spermatid) into spermatozoa, ie, *spermiogenesis*, takes place in the *testes*. Each of these paired organs has an associated *epididymis* that lies along its posterolateral and superior borders.

The structural and functional unit of a testis is the looped *seminiferous tubule,* of which there are up to 1,000 in each testis. Both ends of each tubule connect with the *rete testis,* a system of anastomosing small tubules that, in turn, opens into the *ductuli efferentes, ductus epididymis,* and *ductus deferens* (Fig. 9-46). Incomplete *lobules,* each tightly packed with one to four convoluted seminiferous tubules, are demarcated by fibrous *septa* that extend inward from the *tunica albuginea* (the thick, mesothelium-covered capsule of the testis).

Spermatogenesis

Table 9-6 outlines the chief stages of spermatogenesis, starting with the *primordial male germ cells* that migrate to the testes from the embryonic yolk sac. *Spermatogonia* are present in the prepubertal testes. They undergo mitosis in late adolescence, producing *primary spermatocytes*. The cells of this series, as far as and including primary spermatocytes, are diploid. After puberty, primary spermatocytes enter the reduction division of meiosis I, producing secondary spermatocytes, which are haploid. Without first passing through an S phase, secondary spermatocytes undergo the second maturation division, producing haploid *spermatids* that undergo morphological transformation into *spermatozoa*.

A fundamental difference between meiosis in males and the equivalent process in females is that the supply of primary oocytes becomes progressively depleted over a woman's lifetime, whereas the supply of primary spermatocytes is sustained, even in old men. This is because the spermatogenic cell population is essentially a *continuously renewing* system that depends on spermatocyte replacement from *stem cells*.

The potential for such renewal lies at two consecutive levels. The spermatogenic stem cells are called *type A spermatogonia*. Under normal circumstances, a subtype of the type A spermatogonium that is known as the *pale type A spermatogonium* because its nucleus stains rather lightly, serves as a renewing stem cell. In other words, its progeny have an equal chance of remaining as pale type A cells (self-renewal) or differentiating further, becoming type B spermatogonia (differentiation). *Type B spermatogonia* are differentiating progenitors that give rise to primary spermatocytes but lack the capacity to self-renew. A third class of spermatogonium has also been identified. Known as the *dark type A spermatogonium* because its nucleus stains a little more intensely, it remains out of cycle until the supply of pale type A spermatogonia becomes critically depleted. Hence, it is regarded as a higher-level, "reserve" stem cell that can supplement

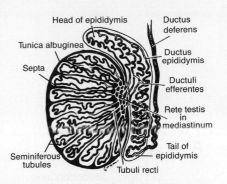

FIGURE 9-46 Testis and epididymis: constituent tubules and associated ducts.

> **KEY CONCEPT**
>
> The spermatogenic cell population is self-renewing.

TABLE 9-6
SPERMATOGENESIS: KEY STAGES

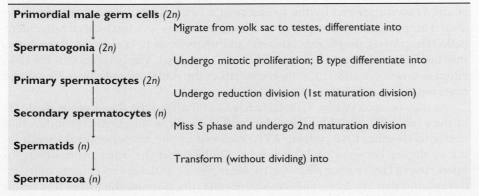

Primordial male germ cells *(2n)*	
↓	Migrate from yolk sac to testes, differentiate into
Spermatogonia *(2n)*	
↓	Undergo mitotic proliferation; B type differentiate into
Primary spermatocytes *(2n)*	
↓	Undergo reduction division (1st maturation division)
Secondary spermatocytes *(n)*	
↓	Miss S phase and undergo 2nd maturation division
Spermatids *(n)*	
↓	Transform (without dividing) into
Spermatozoa *(n)*	

cell renewal if proliferation of the renewing stem cells is impaired. The hierarchy of the three types of spermatogonia is therefore:

Dark type A (reserve) → Pale type A (renewing) → Type B (differentiating)

The differentiating progeny cells of dividing spermatogonia gradually approach the seminiferous tubular lumen. Each time they divide, they remain interconnected by fine *intercellular bridges* that become severed only in the final stages of spermiogenesis. Because of these bridges, cytoplasmic continuity exists between each cohort of synchronously developing clonal progeny cells of single spermatogonia.

Production of spermatozoa from spermatogonia (ie, spermatogenesis) is completed in 64±4 or 5 days. During the next 10 days or so, the newly produced spermatozoa passing along the ductus epididymis undergo a maturation process, after which they acquire the capacity for fertilization.

Spermiogenesis

Four key stages of spermatid transformation into spermatozoa are shown in Fig. 9-47A through 9-47D. The newly formed *spermatid* is a haploid spherical cell with the usual complement of cytoplasmic organelles. One of the first changes is that the Golgi region becomes closely approximated to the nucleus, giving polarity to the cell. The paired centrioles migrate to the caudal pole of the nucleus (Fig. 9-47A). A large Golgi saccule known as the *acrosome vesicle* (Gk. *akron,* extremity) spreads out over the anterior pole of the nucleus, forming a flattened, cup-shaped structure called the *head cap*. The acrosome plays an important role in penetration of the investments surrounding the secondary oocyte after ovulation. It contains a trypsin-like protease, lysosomal hydrolases, and hyaluronidase. On the opposite (caudal) side of the cell, the axoneme (shaft) of the *flagellum* (tail) grows out from the distal centriole (Fig. 9-47B). This centriole, initially aligned with the axoneme, then disappears, along with a ring-shaped *annulus,* which forms around it. A second annulus forms externally to the first and then migrates caudally. Also, another temporary structure called a *spindle-shaped body* develops and then disappears. The nucleus becomes ovoid and gradually lengthens; its chromatin becomes increasingly condensed and electron dense. Some reduction in cell volume is achieved through the elimination of residual cytoplasm (Fig. 9-47B). Finally, the *middle piece (midpiece)* becomes increasingly distinct from the *principal piece* (see Fig. 9-49). This is mainly because the *mitochondria* migrate to the proximal end of the axoneme, where they become arranged helically as the *mitochondrial sheath* that characterizes the middle piece of the spermatozoon (see Fig. 9-47D).

Each *spermatozoon* is made up of a head, midpiece, principal piece, and end piece (Figs. 9-48, 9-49). The ellipsoidal head contains the elongated *nucleus* with its acrosomal *head cap*. The midpiece, representing the proximal part of the flagellum, is characterized by the presence of a helical arrangement of *mitochondria*. The principal piece contains a supplementary cytoskeletal arrangement called the *fibrous sheath* that converts sliding movement between microtubules into lashing movement of the flagellum (L. for whip). The end piece of the flagellum is simpler in construction. It consists of the remainder of the axoneme and covering cell membrane.

As may be seen in Fig. 9-48, the *axoneme* (shaft) of the flagellum is made up of the usual nine peripheral doublets and two central single microtubules that characterize cilia. Energy from ATP produced by the mitochondrial sheath induces sliding between each peripheral doublet and the adjacent doublet. An outer ring of large *coarse fibers* (*outer dense fibers*), and a *dorsal column* and *ventral column* that are interconnected by *fibrous ribs,* harness the forces that result from this sliding movement and apply them to propulsive lashing of the flagel-

A Golgi region

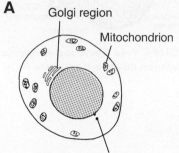

Mitochondrion

Centrioles

B Acrosome and head cap

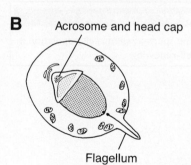

Flagellum

C Residual cytoplasm

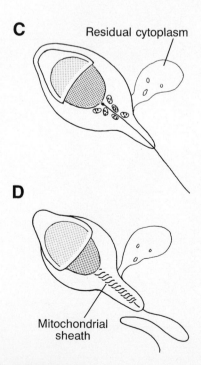

D

Mitochondrial sheath

FIGURE 9-47 Key stages of spermiogenesis. (See text for details.)

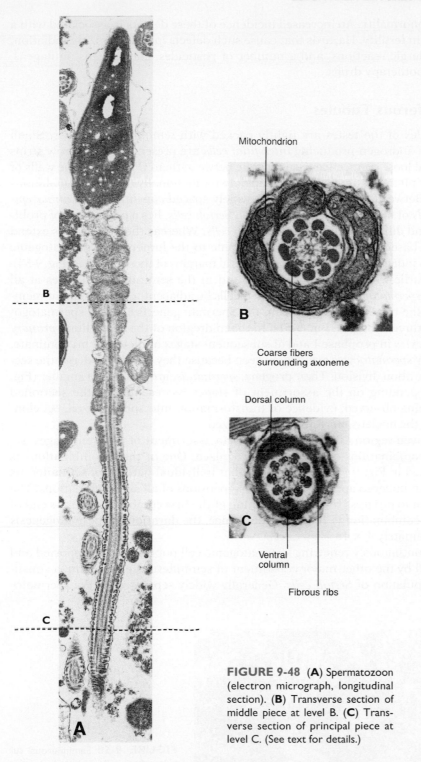

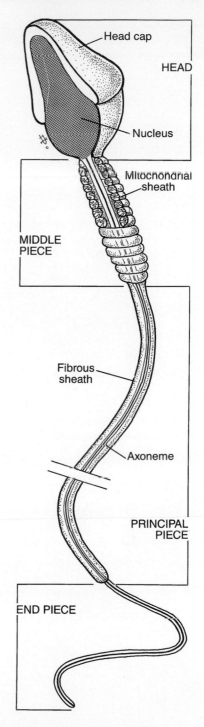

FIGURE 9-48 (**A**) Spermatozoon (electron micrograph, longitudinal section). (**B**) Transverse section of middle piece at level B. (**C**) Transverse section of principal piece at level C. (See text for details.)

FIGURE 9-49 Main parts of a spermatozoon.

lum. Men with *Kartagener syndrome* and other *immotile cilia* (*ciliary dyskinesia*) *syndromes* are usually sterile because a structural defect, lack, or transposition of any of the axonemal microtubules, or defective action of their dynein arms (an ATPase), is manifested as a lack of propulsion.

Sperm counts are normally more than 100 million spermatozoa per milliliter of semen. Counts below 20 million/mL generally indicate sterility. The average ejaculate volume is 3 mL, 80% of which represents prostatic fluid and the secretion of seminal vesicles. Up to 20% of spermatozoa show some kind of morphological abnormality. An increased incidence of these defects is associated with a decrease in fertility. Hazards that cause such defects include ionizing radiation, severe allergic reactions, and a number of pesticides, carcinogens, mutagens, and chemotherapy drugs.

Seminiferous Tubules

The lobules of the testes are tightly packed with *seminiferous tubules*. Small groups of androgen-producing *interstitial cells* are present in the narrow strips of stromal loose connective tissue that lie between them (Fig. 9-50). The walls of each seminiferous tubule are made up of two functionally different populations of cells. Between the interconnected, widely spaced *constitutive columnar epithelial cells* of the tubule, which are called *Sertoli cells,* lies a population of proliferating and differentiating *spermatogenic cells*. Whereas the Sertoli cells extend from the basement membrane of the tubule to the lumen, the spermatogenic cells lie in individual pockets along the lateral margins of these cells (see Fig. 9-54).

The earliest spermatogenic cells, found in the seminiferous tubules at all ages, are *spermatogonia*. These rounded cells lie adjacent to the basement membrane of the tubule. As explained in the Spermatogenesis section, spermatogonia have three subtypes (Fig. 9-51). In the midregion of the epithelium, *primary spermatocytes* in prophase I and at subsequent stages of meiosis I predominate. *Secondary spermatocytes* are seldom seen because they rapidly undergo the second maturation division. Their progeny, *spermatids,* are somewhat smaller (Fig. 9-51). Depending on the assortment of stages represented in the sectioned tubule being observed, evidence of transformation into spermatozoa, eg, elongation of the nucleus, may also be recognized.

Any given region of the tubule shows an assortment of different stages, six specific combinations of which are recognized. One of these combinations is represented in Fig. 9-51. It so happens that individual patches of seminiferous epithelium undergo approximately four repetitions of all six combinations. The time taken to progress from the beginning of the first combination to the end of the sixth combination is 16 days or so; hence, the duration of spermatogenesis is approximately 4 × 16 = 64 days.

The continuously renewing spermatogenic cell population is supported and nourished by the other major constituent of seminiferous epithelium, a constitutive population of *Sertoli cells*. Generally widely separated by the spermato-

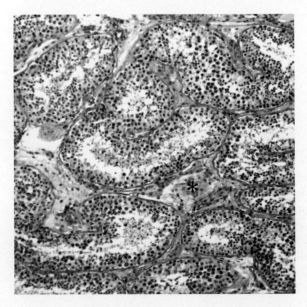

FIGURE 9-50 Seminiferous tubules of testis (low power), showing a group of interstitial cells (indicated by asterisk).

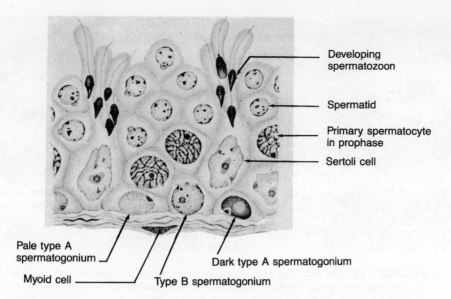

Developing
spermatozoon

Spermatid

Primary spermatocyte
in prophase

Sertoli cell

Pale type A
spermatogonium

Myoid cell

Dark type A spermatogonium

Type B spermatogonium

FIGURE 9-51 Cellular composition of a representative region of seminiferous epithelium. This is a specific cellular association known as Stage I. Five other specific associations between spermatogenic and Sertoli cells also exist.

genic cells that they are nurturing, these non-dividing tall columnar secretory cells may be recognized by their distinctive, irregularly shaped elongated nucleus (see Fig. 9-51). Because spermatogenic cells lie in pockets in the peripheral cytoplasm of Sertoli cells, lateral Sertoli cell borders are difficult to distinguish. The fluid secretion produced by Sertoli cells, termed *testicular fluid*, contains an *androgen-binding protein* (ABP). This protein passes with the testicular fluid into the lumen of the seminiferous tubule, where it maintains a local high concentration of testosterone. *Secretion of ABP* by Sertoli cells is promoted by *FSH*. Testosterone may synergize in this action. Rising levels of *inhibin*, a polypeptide produced by Sertoli cells when they are acted upon by FSH, suppress further release of FSH. Additional functions of Sertoli cells include maintenance of an indirect nutrient supply to the spermatogenic cells, maintenance of the blood–testis barrier (see below), and phagocytosis of degenerating germ cells and residual cytoplasm from spermatids.

Surrounding the seminiferous tubules, external to their basement membrane, are a few layers of flattened cells called *myoid cells* (see Fig. 9-51). These resemble smooth muscle cells, except that they are squamous. Myoid cell contraction may produce slight peristalsis of the tubular wall.

The *interstitial (Leydig) cells* that lie between the seminiferous tubules are fairly large cells with a central round to ovoid nucleus (Fig. 9-52). These cells produce *testosterone*. They are typical steroid-secreting cells with droplets of stored lipid and an extensive sER. They also contain crystalloid inclusions of distinctive internal structure but of unknown function (*crystals of Reinke*, Fig. 9-53). The stroma in which the interstitial cells lie contains unfenestrated blood capillaries (see Fig. 9-52) and lymphatic capillaries.

Secretion of testosterone by interstitial cells is promoted by *LH*. Rising levels of testosterone suppress the further release of LH. Relatively high local concentrations of testosterone (the active form of which, in certain target cells, is *dihydrotestosterone*, DHT) are a critical requirement for late stages of spermatogenesis, notably, late maturation of spermatids. This requirement probably reflects a testosterone-dependent effect mediated by Sertoli cells. Furthermore, FSH stimulation of Sertoli cells is necessary for the completion of spermatid maturation. Another effect of FSH is to increase LH receptor expression on intersti-

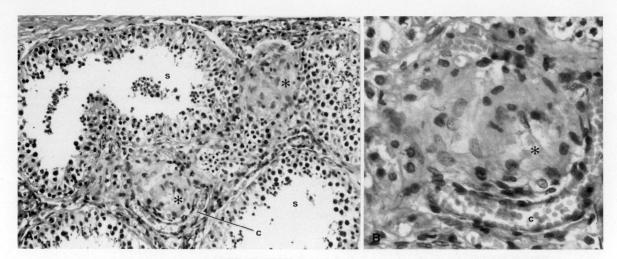

FIGURE 9-52 Interstitial cells of the testis. (**A**) Two groups of interstitial cells, indicated by asterisks. (**B**) The lower group of cells in more detail. A wide capillary (**C**) borders on these cells.

tial cells. Adequate secretion of both FSH and LH is, therefore, essential for a normal level of male fertility.

Blood–Testis Barrier

The interior of the seminiferous tubules constitutes a separate compartment with its own distinctive molecular and ionic composition. It contains relatively high testosterone, ABP, and K$^+$ concentrations, but low Na$^+$ and total protein concentrations. As in certain other columnar epithelia, the lateral borders of the constituent columnar (ie, Sertoli) cells of seminiferous tubules are joined by *continuous tight junctions*. These junctions seal off an *adluminal compartment* from a *basal compartment* lying at the periphery of the tubule (Fig. 9-54). Even though a diffusion barrier exists between the intercellular space and the lumen, successive generations of proliferating and differentiating spermatogenic cells pass toward the lumen by moving radially between the lateral borders of neighboring Sertoli cells. This means that the spermatogenic cells are required to pass through the tight junctions to enter the adluminal compartment. The tight junctions collectively produce a permeability barrier termed the *blood–testis barrier*. This barrier greatly limits the diffusion of macromolecules without restricting passage of water, ions, or steroid hormones. Essential nutrients and cytokines can reach the differentiating and maturing spermatogenic cell population indirectly from Sertoli cells. When spermatocytes pass through the tight junctions, new junctions form behind them, maintaining integrity of the permeability barrier. Spermatogonia lie in the basal compartment. Spermatocytes in prophase I and all subsequent stages of spermatogenesis lie in the adluminal compartment.

A widely accepted working hypothesis about the functional significance of the blood–testis barrier is that it is essentially protective. By maintaining a comparatively high intraluminal concentration of ABP, and therefore testosterone, it maintains a protected, favorable microenvironment for spermatogenic differentiation. To a certain extent, it may also protect the spermatogenic cells from circulating exogenous toxic chemicals and mutagens. Another putative role of the barrier is to reduce the risk that newly expressed antigens on the meiotic progeny cells (ie, antigens that do not begin to appear until the second decade of life) will trigger destructive immune responses. Even when immune responses do occur, the differentiating germ cells within the seminiferous tubules

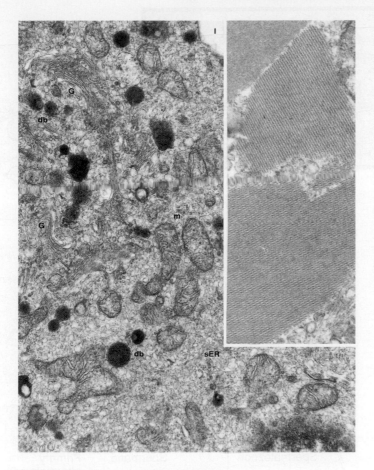

FIGURE 9-53 Interstitial cells of the testis (electron micrograph). Part of the nucleus (N) is discernible at bottom right. Dense bodies (db) representing lipochrome pigment, smooth-surfaced endoplasmic reticulum (sER), Golgi stacks (G), and mitochondria (m) are recognizable in the cytoplasm. Crystals of Reinke are shown in the inset. Tubules of sER are discernible between them.

are fairly well protected from contact with macromolecular antibodies by the permeability barrier maintained by the Sertoli cells.

Prostate

The prostate is a clinically important part of the male reproductive tract because (1) it is extremely likely to undergo benign hyperplasia, and (2) approximately 10% of men in the United States develop clinical manifestations of prostatic carcinoma. Prostatic cancer is currently the malignancy that is most commonly diagnosed in men.

The *prostate* surrounds the urethra at the base of the bladder. Roughly the shape and size of a horse chestnut, it is a conglomeration of 30 to 50 compound tubuloalveolar glands. Positioned between the anteromedial, predominantly stromal part of the gland and the posterior, predominantly glandular part, lies the *prostatic urethra*. The glandular part consists of an anterior and anterolateral *peripheral zone*, paired *central zones*, small paired *transitional zones*, and a *periurethral glandular zone*. *Prostatic carcinomas* arise chiefly, but not exclusively, from the *main glands* (Fig. 9-55) in the peripheral zone. The *mucosal glands* present in the transitional zones and periurethral zone are the most likely sites to undergo *benign prostatic hyperplasia* (BPH).

Sections of prostate are characterized by the presence of numerous irregularly shaped secretory units that have an elaborate folded appearance (Fig. 9-56). With adequate testosterone levels, the secretory cells are tall columnar. Small non-secreting basal cells are also usually present, irregularly distributed between tall secretory cells, so that even though the epithelium may have a simple columnar appearance, it is generally pseudostratified. Intraluminal calcified

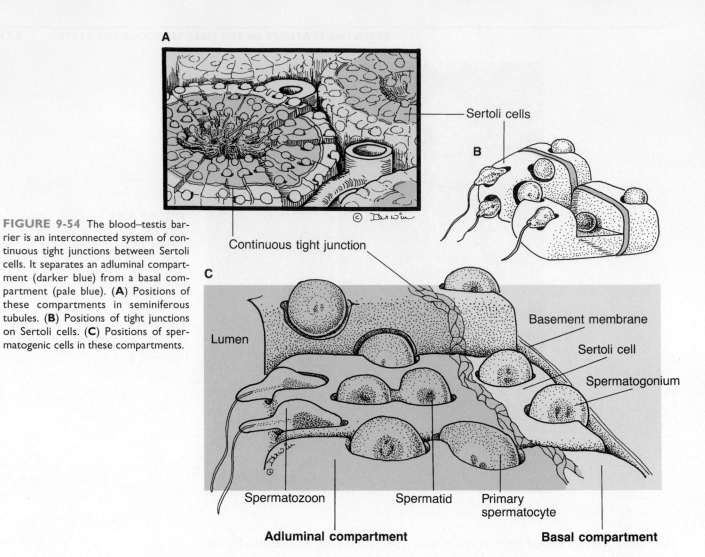

- Sertoli cells

B

Continuous tight junction

A

© Derwin

C

Lumen

Basement membrane

Sertoli cell

Spermatogonium

Spermatozoon

Spermatid

Primary spermatocyte

Adluminal compartment

Basal compartment

FIGURE 9-54 The blood–testis barrier is an interconnected system of continuous tight junctions between Sertoli cells. It separates an adluminal compartment (darker blue) from a basal compartment (pale blue). (**A**) Positions of these compartments in seminiferous tubules. (**B**) Positions of tight junctions on Sertoli cells. (**C**) Positions of spermatogenic cells in these compartments.

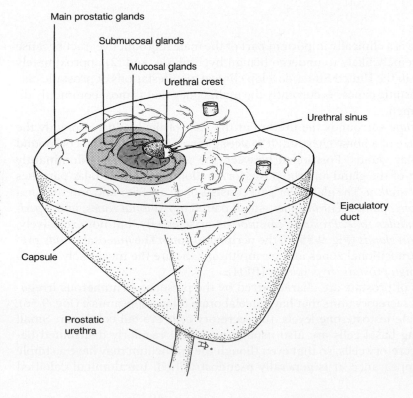

Main prostatic glands

Submucosal glands

Mucosal glands

Urethral crest

Urethral sinus

Ejaculatory duct

Capsule

Prostatic urethra

FIGURE 9-55 Prostate (inferior region), indicating the positions of the mucosal, submucosal, and main prostatic glands, and their relation to the prostatic urethra.

Fibromuscular stroma | Secretory units with folded epithelium | Secretory epithelium (tall columnar) | Calcified concretion

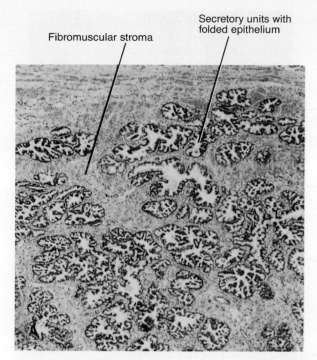
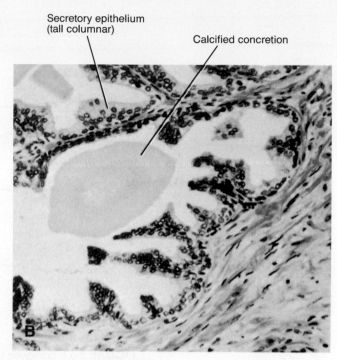

FIGURE 9-56 (**A**) Prostate (very low power). (**B**) Prostatic secretory unit containing a calcified concretion (medium power). Some smooth muscle fibers (*dark gray*) may be discerned in the fibromuscular stroma at lower right in **B**.

prostatic *concretions* may be present, eg, in older men (Fig. 9-56B). The prostatic *stroma* and *capsule* are both *fibromuscular,* ie, made up of smooth muscle intermixed with dense ordinary connective tissue, a distinctive combination that is unique to the prostate.

Prostatic fluid is thin, milky, and slightly acidic. Its contents include citrate, spermine, polyamines, fibrinolytic enzymes, and binding proteins. In addition, it contains *prostate-specific antigen* (PSA) and *prostatic acid phosphatase* (PAP). PSA, which is produced by normal as well as malignant prostatic secretory epithelial cells, is a serine protease that resembles kallikrein. It brings about the liquefaction of semen. Both PSA and PAP can be used as markers for following the progression of prostatic cancer.

Other Ducts and Accessory Glands

The spermatozoa produced in each testis pass through approximately 12 ciliated *ductuli efferentes* to the associated *ductus epididymis* (Fig. 9-57). This highly convoluted duct is lined with a pseudostratified columnar epithelium. *Stereocilia* (Gk. *stereos,* solid), which are bundles of long, immotile microvilli, are present on the luminal border of the lining cells. This epithelium resorbs substantial amounts of testicular fluid and secretes maturation factors. During emission, peristalsis of the thick muscular walls of the *ductus deferens* moves spermatozoa from the ductus epididymis, in which they are stored, to the *urethra*. The ductus deferens has a pseudostratified columnar epithelium with stereocilia (Fig. 9-58). In the spermatic cord, it is associated with accompanying arteries, nerves, lymphatics, and cremaster muscle. The pampiniform plexus of anastomosing veins, which wind around the duct like tendrils (L. *pampinus,* tendril), is a site where the veins commonly become varicose.

Vasectomy (bilateral ligation of the ducti deferentes, which are also known as the vasa deferentia) prevents transfer of spermatozoa from the ducti epidi-

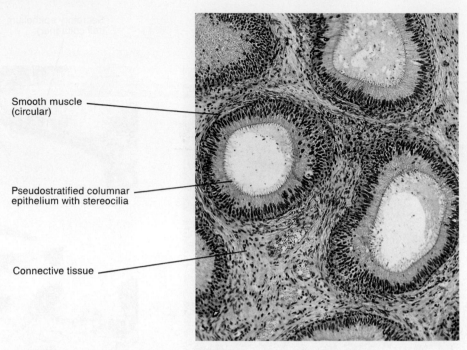

Smooth muscle
(circular)

Pseudostratified columnar
epithelium with stereocilia

Connective tissue

FIGURE 9-57 Epididymis (medium power), showing the ductus epididymis.

dymides and is, therefore, an effective means of birth control. Although this procedure is potentially reversible, it is accompanied by an increased risk of development of autoimmunity to spermatozoal antigens. Production of immobilizing or agglutinating antibody can lead to permanent decrease in fertility.

The *seminal vesicles* are elongated structures that open into the distal end of the ducti deferentes. Each seminal vesicle represents an unbranched, convoluted tubular diverticulum of the duct. Histological sections of seminal vesicle,

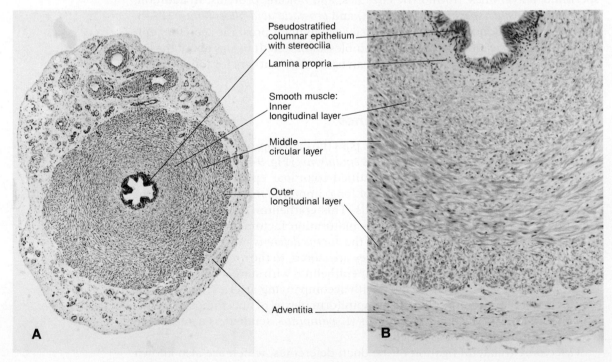

Pseudostratified
columnar epithelium
with stereocilia

Lamina propria

Smooth muscle:
Inner
longitudinal layer

Middle
circular layer

Outer
longitudinal layer

Adventitia

A

B

FIGURE 9-58 (**A**) Ductus deferens (very low power). (**B**) Details of the wall structure of this duct.

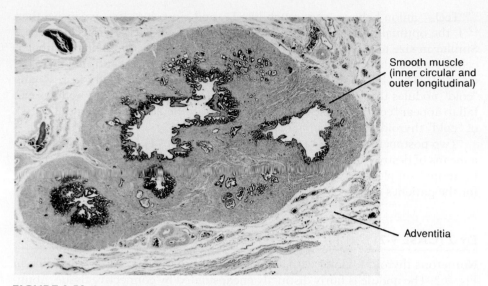

Smooth muscle (inner circular and outer longitudinal)

Adventitia

FIGURE 9-59 Seminal vesicle (very low power).

therefore, usually show several sections of the single tortuous, muscular-walled tube (Fig. 9-59). Its many convolutions are bound together by their fibroelastic adventitia. The epithelial lining, which is elaborately folded and is made up of tall columnar secretory cells, can be either simple columnar or pseudostratified. Secretory activity of these cells is testosterone-dependent. The thick secretion of the seminal vesicles, delivered by way of the *ejaculatory ducts,* is rich in fructose, prostaglandins, and ascorbic acid. Contributing more than half the fluid volume of semen, it is regarded as nutritive to spermatozoa.

The lining epithelium of the *prostatic urethra* is transitional proximally and pseudostratified or stratified columnar distally. The *membranous urethra* (which traverses the urogenital diaphragm) has a stratified columnar lining. The *spongy part* of the urethra (*penile urethra*) is lined with the same epithelium, except distally in the navicular fossa, where epidermis is present. A characteristic feature of the male urethra is that it has numerous small diverticula.

CASE DISCUSSIONS

D9-I (CASE 9-1)

In the thyroid nodule illustrated in Fig. 9-1, tree-like branching of the fibrovascular stroma raises the covering layer of cuboidal epithelial cells into papillae. Follicular organization is absent from this part of the nodule. Some of the large nuclei seen in the epithelial cells are unusually pale-staining and, accordingly, are sometimes described as "orphan Annie eye" nuclei (indicated in Fig. 9-1A). In most other respects, the covering epithelial cells resemble large thyroid follicular epithelial cells, except that there is no recognizable follicular arrangement. Tiny lamellar calcifications (indicated in Fig. 9-1B), known as *psammoma bodies* (Gk. *psammos,* sand), may be recognized in the stroma at the tips of some of the papillae. These are some of the features by which this nodule can be recognized as a *thyroid papillary carcinoma.* In addition, metastatic thyroid papillary carcinoma was identified in the resected cervical node.

Although sodium (^{99m}Tc)pertechnetate was employed in this case for the thyroid scan (see Fig. 9-1C), it is not the most informative radionuclide for thyroid scanning, because solitary hypofunctioning nodules do not always show up. The

$^{99m}TcO_4^-$ anion behaves very much like I^-, and since it is less expensive than ^{123}I, the optimal radioisotope for imaging the thyroid, it is often used instead. Similar in size to I^-, the $^{99m}TcO_4^-$ anion enters the thyroid follicular epithelial cells by way of their iodine uptake channels and becomes concentrated there (ie, trapped). The chief drawback associated with its use is difficulty in resolving "cold" nodules that are <1 cm in diameter. Also, hypofunctioning nodules can fail to appear "cold" because of masking by extrafollicular radioisotope. The risk of "cold" thyroid nodules being malignant is 10–20%.

Two postoperative measures for consideration are (1) ^{131}I administration as a means of destroying the remainder of the malignant thyroid cells and (2) daily hormonal supplementation with L-thyroxine (T_4) as a means of compensating for the patient's deficit of thyroid hormone.

D9-2 (CASE 9-2)

Numerous thyroid follicles with a wide range of diameters are recognizable in Fig. 9-2. The nodule is fairly distinctly encapsulated by connective tissue. Abundant, well-stained colloid indicates active thyroglobulin secretion in the nodule. In contrast to the brightly stained nodular follicles, the perinodular follicles (seen at *bottom left*) appear less active, more uniform in diameter, and somewhat more compressed. Also, in the perinodular stroma there is a diffuse infiltration of lymphocytes, together with macrophages and plasma cells. This is evidence of a persisting *chronic thyroiditis*. Under most circumstances, immune responses are not directed against endogenous macromolecules, but in patients with *Hashimoto's thyroiditis,* autoimmunity develops to several of the patient's own thyroid follicular epithelial cell antigens and thyroid colloid antigens. Circulating antibodies directed against such thyroid antigens can be very destructive; hence, autoimmune thyroiditis can result in hypothyroidism. The pathological diagnosis returned for the resected nodule was a benign *thyroid hyperplastic adenomatous nodule* that developed in a background of chronic thyroiditis. This diagnosis was confirmed at operation.

D9-3 (CASE 9-3)

An ultrasound scan of the patient's abdomen in Case 9-3 reveals an unusual abdominal mass. Indicated by dotted cross lines left of *center* in Fig. 9-4, it lies near the right kidney. Figure 9-4 is a sagittal scan of the right upper quadrant of the abdomen (the patient's head lies to the left). From Figs. 9-4 and 9-5, it may be concluded that the abnormal mass lies at the upper (superior) pole of the right kidney, the position normally occupied by the right *adrenal (suprarenal) gland.*

Almost all of Jack's symptoms (but not the osmotic diuresis, which is associated with his glycosuria) are attributable to paroxysmal elevation of blood levels of *epinephrine* and *norepinephrine,* catecholamine hormones produced by the adrenal medulla. Correct diagnosis depends on knowing that the patient's transient episodes of headache, hypertension, heart palpitations (which may be accompanied by tachycardia), and gastrointestinal symptoms could result from paroxysmal episodes of sympathetic overstimulation. The increased output of urinary metanephrine is also an indication of catecholamine overproduction.

The cells seen in Fig. 9-6 resemble chromaffin cells of the adrenal medulla. Furthermore, many of them stain brown with dichromate (or other chromium salts) as a result of oxidation of the catecholamine stored in their secretory granules (the so-called *chromaffin reaction*). From the histological appearance of these hyperplastic cells it is not easy to decide whether they are benign or malignant unless metastases are found as well. However, in this instance, there is much variation in both nuclear morphology and nuclear size. The tumor was diagnosed as a *pheochromocytoma* (Gk. *phaios,* dusky brown). Unlike diabetes mellitus, which is a chronic disease that is quite common, pheochromocytomas are rare, and only 10% of them become malignant. The main benefit of their surgical excision is that it avoids later potentially lethal cardiovascular complications resulting from unregulated catecholamine release.

D9-4 (FIG. 9-3)

Figure 9-3 shows a typical example of a *nontoxic nodular goiter (simple goiter)* taken from a biochemically euthyroid patient. Its large follicles are greatly distended with thyroglobulin-containing colloid, and the follicular epithelial cells look very low and flat. In a normal thyroid, only a few thyroid follicles would be this large and the follicular epithelial cells would be more cuboidal, but there can be substantial variation. Abundance of the follicular epithelial cells in the large follicles in Fig. 9-3 suggests an earlier hyperplastic response to TSH. Large amounts of thyroglobulin have accumulated in these follicles because TSH is no longer stimulating resorptive activity in their flat-looking cells (see Fig. 9-20).

In a *toxic diffuse goiter,* which is a different type of goiter that is clinically associated with hyperthyroidism, the numerous follicular epithelial cells have a columnar shape and the volume of stored thyroglobulin is greatly decreased as a result of rapid resorption (see Fig. 9-20). In toxic diffuse goiters, hypertrophy, hyperplasia, and increased thyroid hormone production are due to the presence of *thyroid-stimulating immunoglobulins* (TSI) that bind to the TSH receptor on these cells and stimulate thyroid growth and thyroid hormone secretion by mimicking prolonged effects of TSH.

D9-5 (CASE 9-4)

The general organization of the tissue seen in Fig. 9-8 is essentially similar to that of the anterior pituitary (adenohypophysis). Adjacent to wide capillaries lie large, irregular clumps of secretory cells each with a substantial spherical nucleus. However, instead of there being the usual mixture of secretory cell types and chromophobes, these cells all have a rather uniform appearance and represent acidophils of a single type. Marked hyperplasia has produced a benign secreting *acidophilic adenoma* known as a *prolactin cell adenoma (prolactinoma).* The resulting *hyperprolactinemia* is causing *galactorrhea,* which is milk production under non-nursing circumstances.

Besides prolactin, there is a requirement for estrogen, progesterone, somatomedins, glucocorticoids, insulin, thyroid hormone, and oxytocin for adequate lactation and breast feeding. In non-pregnant women, prolactin secretion would normally stay inhibited by dopamine from the hypothalamus. Hyperprolactinemia can augment hypothalamic dopamine levels, which in turn may depress GnRH secretion, resulting in low estrogen levels. Failure to menstruate in such a case may indicate inadequate priming of the endometrium by estrogen. However, prolactinoma patients do not invariably have decreased estrogen levels.

An impaired visual field in patients with a pituitary tumor indicates pressure or encroachment on the optic chiasma, which lies immediately anterosuperior to the pituitary stalk.

D9-6 (CASE 9-5)

Whereas the cellular organization seen in Fig. 9-9 is similar to that of Fig. 9-8, the predominant cell type is somewhat smaller, with a relatively small condensed nucleus. Also, fenestrated capillaries are not as conspicuous. Although it is not apparent in H&E sections, the secretory cell in this case is a type of basophil. The patient has a *basophilic adenoma* called a *corticotroph adenoma*. The actively secreting cells in this benign tumor are PAS-positive, since the ACTH that they are overproducing is a glycoprotein.

This patient has *Cushing's disease*. Excessive production of *ACTH* by a pituitary tumor elicits *cortisol* overproduction by the zona fasciculata and zona reticularis of the adrenal cortex. Normally, ACTH secretion would show a diurnal variation, and secretion of this hormone would become inhibited by rising levels of glucocorticoids such as cortisol. In this case, however, the corticotroph adenoma is secreting ACTH autonomously. Excessive unregulated output of ACTH chronically elevates the patient's cortisol level, which in turn leads to fat redistribution and also muscle wasting because of protein catabolism. ACTH causes both the fasciculata and the reticularis of the adrenal cortex to hypertrophy and hypersecrete; hence, androgen levels as well as cortisol levels are elevated in this patient. The response of such patients to CRH is augmented or normal, in contrast to the negligible response shown by patients who have a hypersecreting adrenal tumor. Susceptibility of such patients to infections is chiefly due to the fact that cortisol is anti-inflammatory. At high concentration, cortisol is also immunosuppressive.

D9-7 (CASE 9-6)

The karyotype seen in Fig. 9-10A reveals that this is a male fetus with the expected XY combination. However, the G group contains an extra chromosome 21, indicating *trisomy 21*. The banding pattern (*G bands*) by which the homologues were recognized and matched to each other was produced using the Giemsa stain.

This finding is unwelcome news for Millie because it means that her new baby will have *Down syndrome*. In fact, even if only an additional part of a chromosome 21 (its long arm) were included as a translocation, this would be enough to cause the same syndrome. Thus, the different fetal karyotype shown in Fig. 9-11 contains the usual two chromosome 21s, and in addition the chromosome 14 on the right is somewhat longer than its partner. This extra length is due to translocation of the long arm of a chromosome 21 onto the long arm of a chromosome 14. The chromosome constitution of this other fetus is therefore 46,XX,⁻14,⁺t(14q21q) where t denotes a translocation, q denotes the long arm of the chromosome, − denotes a missing chromosome, and + denotes an added chromosome that is there in its place. Because this female fetus is also virtually trisomic for chromosome 21, it too will have Down syndrome. Either parent can be the translocation carrier for the translocation type of Down syndrome.

An increased risk of Down syndrome is associated with late pregnancies. This syndrome is generally a result of non-disjunction of the mother's paired chromosome 21s in meiosis I. If a secondary oocyte receives two chromosome 21s and then becomes fertilized by a spermatozoon that contributes another, trisomy 21 results. Even though the great majority of conceptuses that are trisomic for chromosome 21 spontaneously abort or are stillborn, Down syndrome ranks highest as the most common chromosomal aberration in newborn babies. It is found in approximately 1 out of every 800 live births. In mothers of Millie's age, the incidence is even higher—approximately 1 out of every 40 live births. Approximately 70% of babies born with Down syndrome exhibit atypical combinations of palmar and plantar ridge patterns and flexion creases. This syndrome is also characterized by the presence of distinctive facial features, a short stature, and a variety of atypical physical characteristics. In addition, mental development is retarded during childhood.

The chromosome constitution of the fetus that Millie is now carrying is correctly recorded as 47,XY,⁺21, the ⁺21 denoting its extra autosome.

D9-8 (CASE 9-7)

In addition to being used for hormonal assessment, the *Pap* (the abbreviated form of *Papanicolaou*) *smear* serves as an easy and rapid means of detecting the presence of atypical cervical epithelial cells that may be associated with an increased risk of cervical cancer. Superficial epithelial cells scraped from the exocervix (portio vaginalis) and posterior fornix are spread out on a slide, fixed in ether-alcohol, and stained with a combination of hematoxylin, orange G, and eosin azure. The majority of cells seen in a normal Pap smear (eg, the smear shown in Fig. 9-12C which was obtained in week 2 of a menstrual cycle) are maturing superficial squamous cells with a characteristic rather small or pyknotic nucleus (see Fig. 9-12C). As the squamous cells mature they become acidophilic (ie, pink-staining). Their maturation and the accompanying accumulation of intracellular glycogen are considered to be an estrogen effect. A few neutrophils also may be present. Teresa's Pap smear, however, contains some *atypical squamous cells* as well as a few pink or blue normal squamous cells and numerous neutrophils. Toward the middle of Fig. 9-12A, lie some smaller blue squamous cells with a relatively large nucleus containing coarse chromatin granules. Termed *dysplastic epithelial cells*, these atypical cells have an increased ratio of nuclear to cytoplasmic volume. In other words, their nucleus appears unusually large compared with that of normal squamous cells of comparable size. Furthermore, some of these atypical cells possess a nucleus that is *hyperchromatic* (dark-staining) or *pleomorphic* (irregular in shape or in some other way variable in appearance). The presence of numerous distinctly atypical squamous cells in a Pap smear is interpreted as being indicative of a *severe dysplasia*.

Pathologists use the term *dysplasia* to denote disorganized (abnormal) tissue growth. As the degree of dysplasia found in the cervical epithelium increases, the risk of cancer arising at the dysplastic site also increases. Foci of severe cervical dysplasia are therefore regarded as having an increased potential for becoming malignant. Dysplasia may be manifested as a change in the appearance of the cells as well as a change in their arrangement. In this case, for example, most of the cells in the epithelium retain a fairly large nucleus. Furthermore, the maturation process remains incomplete and this results in a crowded population of rather small and uniform-looking cells. Significant variation may, nevertheless, occur in nuclear size (see Fig. 9-12D). A severely dysplastic appearance that affects the full thickness of the cervical epithelium is considered indicative of an increased risk of developing cervical cancer. The severe dysplasia indicated by the Pap smear in Fig. 9-12A, and shown on the right in Fig. 9-12C, and also at higher magnification in Fig. 9-12D, is designated *cervical intraepithelial neoplasia*, high grade (CIN III). Below the dysplastic epithelium a local accumulation of small lymphocytes also may be found (see Fig. 9-12C,D). Although such an epithelial dysplasia is often described as cervical intraepithelial neoplasia, there is no microscopic evidence to suggest that any malignant cells have yet invaded the underlying connective tissue. For this reason, such a lesion is often described as *carcinoma in situ* (CIS), meaning that it could be regarded as a potential epithelial malignancy that is still at a preinvasive stage.

If only the basal third of the stratified squamous cervical epithelium has this crowded appearance and the superficial two-thirds appears to mature in the usual manner, the epithelium is described as mildly dysplastic and the lesion is designated CIN I (low grade). If the basal two-thirds of the epithelium looks atypical but the top third shows some maturation, the lesion is described as showing moderate dysplasia and is designated CIN II. There is considered to be an almost 2% risk of progression from CIN to invasive squamous cell carcinoma of the cervix over a period of about 10 years. Cervical screening for dysplasia, early diagnosis, and local ablation of dysplastic epithelium by cryosurgery or other means have markedly reduced the incidence of this formerly prevalent form of cancer in North America. It remains more of a problem elsewhere.

Potential sites of cervical intraepithelial neoplasia turn white following application of 5% acetic acid during colposcopic examination (hence the term *aceto white lesion*). Also, an absence of dark-brown staining following application of an iodine solution indicates patches of epithelium that are not storing normal quantities of glycogen (Schiller's test). In the majority of young women, especially young mothers, part of the exocervix is covered by reddish *endocervical ectropion* (exposed endocervical mucosa). This is because simple columnar epithelium has extended out of the endocervical canal and now covers much of the exocervix. In such cases, the squamocolumnar junction between the endocervical mucosa (mucus-secreting simple columnar epithelium) and the stratified squamous non-keratinizing (more accurately described as *incompletely keratinizing*) epithelial lining of the vagina is situated on the exocervix. Later in life, the endocervical ectropion becomes replaced by new stratified squamous epithelium, with the result that the squamocolumnar junction becomes situated closer to the external os. By menopause, the junction may even recede into the endocervical canal. Consecutive replacement of one type of epithelium by another is believed to involve some re-epithelialization (migration of squamous epithelial cells) as well as a switch in epithelial cell differentiation (*metaplasia*). The area that becomes replaced with a different epithelium in this manner is termed the *transformation zone*. Dysplastic changes and cervical carcinomas occur chiefly in the transformation zone. Human papillomaviruses (HPV 16, 18, and 31) are implicated in the etiology of cervical carcinoma.

Finally, from the histological appearance of the external iliac node shown in Fig. 9-12E, it may be concluded that the cervical lesion in Case 9-7 must also have had a large component of invasive squamous cell carcinoma, and this must have already spread by way of lymphatics to the local regional draining nodes. Most of the node is populated with cells of metastatic *large cell keratinizing carcinoma*, the malignant squamous cells of which have formed some whorls of keratin (*keratin pearls*).

D9-9 (CASE 9-8)

At low magnification, an essentially lobular pattern of duct-like structures (enlarged *terminal ducts*) may be recognized in the section (see Fig. 9-14A,B). This tissue architecture resembles the characteristic organization of its normal counterpart, non-lactating breast tissue. Parts of this section (see Fig. 9-14B) show the second major tissue of the breast, *adipose tissue*, which looks dark yellow in the mastectomy specimen (see Fig. 9-15A). Within the enlarged terminal ducts, and extending from them, groups and islands of morphologically variable (*pleomorphic*) tumor cells are discernible (see Fig. 9-14C). An increased incidence of mitosis (>20 mitotic figures per high power field, with invasion of the adjacent adipose tissue (see Fig. 9-14D) suggests that this tumor is a carcinoma. The pathologist's diagnosis in this case is *moderately to poorly differentiated invasive (infiltrating) ductal carcinoma* and *intraductal carcinoma*. Also noted were a moderate *desmoplastic reaction*, meaning a fibroblastic response to the presence of malignant cells (see Fig. 9-14C), and some tumor cells were found within breast lymphatics. Firmness and immobility of this patient's tumor mass result from the desmoplastic reaction. All the surgical resection margins were found to be free of tumor cells.

Estrogen is a typical steroid hormone that binds to a specific receptor protein present in the cytosol. The hormone-receptor complex then finds its way into the nucleus, where it can affect gene expression and induce cell proliferation. The chief reason for assaying the *estrogen receptor* content of this patient's breast tumor is to determine whether estrogen could be one of the factors stimulating proliferation of its cells. Through a variety of growth-stimulating effects that include involvement of paracrine or autocrine growth factors, estrogen has the potential to promote proliferation of tumor cells that express its receptor.

Breast cancer (*mammary carcinoma*) remains one of the chief causes of death in women. If a breast tumor is still at the hormone-dependent stage of formation, advantage may be taken of its estrogen dependence by administering tamoxifen, an antiestrogen. Tamoxifen binds to the cytosolic estrogen receptor and becomes translocated to the nucleus, where it arrests the transcription of certain genes instead of inducing their transcription.

Some carcinomas that arise from breast epithelium are ER+, ie, positive for the nuclear *estrogen receptor* protein. The cytosolic estrogen receptor protein is not a reliable indicator because it is labile at room temperature. ER+ mammary carcinomas, and also breast tumors that express the *progesterone receptor* protein (PR+ tumors), are more likely to respond to hormonal therapy than the corresponding receptor negative tumors. Patients with breast tumors that are ER+ also have a better chance of survival.

In this patient, no metastatic spread of tumor to the axillary lymph nodes was detected, even though some of the breast lymphatics evidently contained recognizable tumor cells. Because the primary tumor was reported as ER−, the chances of bringing about regression through hormonal or antiestrogen therapy in the event of subsequent recurrence are smaller than in the case of an ER+ tumor. In fact, the proportion of patients with advanced ER− breast cancer showing a favorable response to tamoxifen therapy is only 13%. It should, however, be appreciated that although this patient's tumor was reported as ER−, categorization as "positive" or "negative" is far from absolute because, in this case, a qualitative estimate has been assigned to a measurable quantity. Assessments such as this become meaningful only when the critical levels for supporting nonautonomous growth or achieving clinical responsiveness have been firmly established. Such cutoff points are hard to determine in situations that involve a number of interacting growth factors.

D9-10 (CASE 9-9)

Non-malignant overgrowth of the prostate, termed *benign prostatic hyperplasia* or *nodular prostatic hyperplasia,* is a common condition in elderly men. Its incidence increases from 20% of men in their 50s to 90% of men in their 80s. However, prostatic enlargement is not always detected, and a significant proportion of such men remain essentially asymptomatic.

In view of the fact that either testosterone or its derivative, dihydrotestosterone (DHT), acts as a stimulus for cellular proliferation and secretory activity in the prostate, it remains enigmatic that benign prostatic hyperplasia develops over the years when a man's testosterone levels are declining and his estrogen levels are increasing relative to testosterone. Generally speaking, the periurethral *mucosal glands* undergo benign hyperplasia, whereas the subcapsular *main glands* undergo malignant change (see Fig. 9-55). It is sometimes difficult to recognize any difference between a hyperplastic nodule (see Fig. 9-16A) and the normal prostate (see Fig. 9-16D), but the shape of the nodule itself often can be recognized and the pattern of folding of its secretory epithelium may look slightly different (eg, less elaborate). Nothing in part A of Fig. 9-16 suggests cancer; this part shows only a benign hyperplastic nodule.

The overgrowth of prostatic mucosal glands that occurs in benign prostatic hyperplasia compresses not only the prostatic urethra but also the peripheral main glands of the prostate. Increasing obstruction of the urethra leads to incomplete emptying of the urinary bladder, which predisposes patients to ascending bacterial infections and bladder inflammation, and may even impair renal function. Urinary tract infections are a common complication in benign prostatic hyperplasia.

The most common malignancy affecting the prostate is *prostatic adenocarcinoma* (Gk. *adenos*, gland), which is illustrated in Fig. 9-16B,C. In the upper half of Fig. 9-16B, it may be seen that among a few irregularly distended normal secretory units lie a number of smaller tubular structures that are somewhat different in appearance. Higher magnifications show that all these tubular structures are made up of a single layer of cuboidal epithelial cells that possess a relatively large, spherical nucleus and a prominent nucleolus (see Fig. 9-16C). In contrast, normal prostatic secretory units are made up of tall columnar secretory cells with some small interspersed basal cells (see Fig. 9-16D). The tubular structures can loosely resemble ducts or rudimentary secretory units, and when seen in a malignant tumor, they are a hallmark of a differentiated adenocarcinoma.

Prostatic adenocarcinoma is a leading cause of mortality in high-risk groups of men. This tumor commonly metastasizes to sacral, iliac, and aortic lymph nodes, bones, and the lungs. It may also invade the contiguous pelvic tissues and organs by direct extension, often following a perineurial route. Typically, the metastases in prostatic cancer are sites of increased osteoblastic activity (see explanatory note given for Fig. 4-7). Bone scans are therefore useful for locating these metastases, eg, in vertebral bodies, the pelvis, or ribs (see Fig. 9-17).

BIBLIOGRAPHY

Endocrine

Bonga SEW, Pang PKT. Control of calcium regulating hormones in the vertebrates: Parathyroid hormone, calcitonin, prolactin, and stanniocalcin. Int Rev Cytol 128 : 139, 1991.

Carmichael SW, Winkler H. The adrenal chromaffin cell. Sci Am 253(2):40, 1985.

Deftos LJ, Parthemore JG, Stabile BE. Management of primary hyperparathyroidism. Annu Rev Med 44 : 19, 1993.

Ekholm R. Biosynthesis of thyroid hormones. Int Rev Cytol 120 : 243, 1990.

Farley JR, Tarbaux NM, Hall SL, Linkhart TA, Baylink DJ. The anti-bone-resorptive agent calcitonin also acts in vitro to directly increase bone formation and bone cell proliferation. Endocrinology 123 : 159, 1988.

Fujita H. Functional morphology of the thyroid. Int Rev Cytol 113 : 145, 1988.

Gharib H. A strategy for the solitary thyroid nodule. Hosp Pract 27(9A):53, 1992.

Hedge GA, Colby HD, Goodman RL. Clinical Endocrine Physiology. Philadelphia, W.B. Saunders, 1987.

Horvath E, Kovacs K. Pituitary gland. Pathol Res Pract 183 : 129, 1988.

Jasani B, Schmid KW. Immunocytochemistry in Diagnostic Histopathology. Edinburgh, Churchill Livingstone, 1993.

Jay V, Kovacs K, Horvath E, Lloyd RV, Smyth HS. Idiopathic prolactin cell hyperplasia of the pituitary mimicking prolactin cell adenoma: A morphological study including immunocytochemistry, electron microscopy, and in situ hybridization. Acta Neuropathol (Berl) 82 : 147, 1991.

Kovacs K, Horvath E. Tumors of the Pituitary Gland. Washington, D.C., Armed Forces Institute of Pathology, 1986.

Motta PM, ed. Ultrastructure of Endocrine Cells and Tissues. Boston, Martinus Nijhoff, 1984.

Neville AM, O'Hare MJ. The Human Adrenal Cortex. Berlin, Springer-Verlag, 1982.

Ogren L, Talamantes F. Prolactins of pregnancy and their cellular source. Int Rev Cytol 112 : 1, 1988.

Orci L, Vassalli J-D, Perrelet A. The insulin factory. Sci Am 256(9):85, 1988.

Orth DN. Cushing's syndrome. N Engl J Med 332 : 791, 1995.

Phillips LS, Vassilopoulou-Sellin R. Somatomedins. N Engl J Med 302 : 371, 1980.

Reichlin S. Somatostatin (First of two parts). N Engl J Med 309 : 1495, 1983.

Reichlin S. Somatostatin (Second of two parts). N Engl J Med 309 : 1556, 1983.

Snyder SH. The molecular basis of communication between cells. Sci Am 253(4):132, 1985.

Troncone L, Shapiro B, Satta MA, Monaco F, eds. Thyroid Diseases: Basic Science, Pathology, Clinical and Laboratory Diagnoses. Boca Raton, Fla., CRC Press, 1994.

Tsigos C, Chrousos GP. Differential diagnosis and management of Cushing's syndrome. Annu Rev Med 47 : 443, 1996.

Female Reproductive

Aaltomaa S, Lipponen P, Eskelinen M, Kosma V-M, Marin S, Alhava E, Syrjänen K. Hormone receptors as prognostic factors in female breast cancer. Ann Med 23:643, 1991.

Boon M, Suurmeijer AJH. The Pap Smear, ed 3. Amsterdam, Harwood Academic Publishers, 1996.

Familiari G, Makabe S, Motta PM, eds. Ultrastructure of the Ovary. Boston, Kluwer Academic Publishers, 1991.

Forsling ML. The anatomy of the reproductive tract and the physiology of the menstrual cycle. In: Dooley MM, Brincat MP, eds. Understanding Common Disorders in Reproductive Endocrinology. Chichester, U.K., John Wiley & Sons, 1994.

Guraya SS. The comparative cell biology of accessory somatic (or Sertoli) cells in the animal testis. Int Rev Cytol 160 : 163, 1995.

Howie PW. Natural regulation of fertility. Br Med Bull 49 : 182, 1993.

Johnson MH, Everitt BJ. Essential Reproduction. Oxford, Blackwell Scientific Publications, 1980.

Jordan VC. Resistance to antioestrogen therapy. A challenge for the future. In: Cavalli F, ed. Endocrine Therapy of Breast Cancer III. Berlin, Springer-Verlag, 1989, p 51.

Kemp BE, Niall HD. Relaxin. Vitam Horm 41 : 79, 1984.

Kotsuji F, Tominaga T. The role of granulosa and theca cell interactions in ovarian structure and function. Microsc Res Tech 27 : 97, 1994.

Monaghan P, Perusinghe NP, Cowen P, Gusterson BA. Peripubertal human breast development. Anat Rec 226 : 501, 1990.

Newman-Hirshfield A. Development of follicles in the mammalian ovary. Int Rev Cytol 124 : 43, 1991.

Norman RL, ed. Neuroendocrine Aspects of Reproduction. New York, Academic Press, 1983.

Papanicolaou GN. Atlas of Exfoliative Cytology. Cambridge, MA, Harvard University Press, 1954.

Sidhu KS, Guraya SS. Current concepts in gamete receptors for fertilization in mammals. Int Rev Cytol 127 : 253, 1991.

Male Reproductive

Andriole GL, Catalona WJ. Prostate carcinoma. Annu Rev Med 45 : 351, 1994.

Davidoff MS, Schulze W, Middendorff R, Holstein A-F. The Leydig cell of the human testis: A new member of the diffuse neuroendocrine system. Cell Tissue Res 271 : 429, 1993.

Dufau ML. Endocrine regulation and communicating functions of the Leydig cell. Annu Rev Physiol 50 : 483, 1988.

Forti G, Vannelli GB, Barni T, Balboni GC, Orlando C, Serio M. Sertoli-germ cells interactions in the human testis. J Steroid Biochem Mol Biol 43 : 419, 1992.

Kerr JB. Ultrastructure of the seminiferous epithelium and intertubular tissue of the human testis. J Electron Microsc Tech 19 : 215, 1991.

Lepor H, Lawson RK. Prostate Diseases, Philadelphia, W.B. Saunders, 1993.

Matsumoto AM, Bremner WJ. Endocrine control of human spermatogenesis. J Steroid Biochem 33 : 789, 1989.

Orgebin-Crist MC, Danzo BJ, eds. Cell biology of the testis and epididymis. Ann N Y Acad Sci 513 : 1, 1987.

Paniagua R, Nistal M, Sáez FJ, Fraile B. Ultrastructure of the aging human testis. J Electron Microsc Tech 19 : 241, 1991.

Russell LD, Ettlin RA, Sinha Hikim AP, Clegg ED. Histological and Histopathological Evaluation of the Testis. Clearwater, Fla., Cache River Press, 1990.

Setchell BP. The functional significance of the blood–testis barrier. J Androl 1 : 3, 1980.

Sharpe RM. Follicle-stimulating hormone and spermatogenesis in the adult male. J Endocrinol 121 : 405, 1989.

Trainer TD. Histology of the normal testis. Am J Surg Pathol 11 : 797, 1987.

Tung K. Immunopathology and male infertility. Hosp Pract 23(6):191, 1988.

Yeung CH, Cooper TG, Bergmann M, Schulze H. Organization of tubules in the human caput epididymidis and the ultrastructure of their epithelia. Am J Anat 191 : 261, 1991.

Review Items: Cross References

Information relevant to the Review Items listed in this chapter may be found in the following pages of Cormack, DH. Essential Histology. Philadelphia, J.B. Lippincott, 1993:

REVIEW ITEM	PAGES
9-1	359–360
9-2	359
9-3	363–364 and 369–370

CHAPTER 10

Eyes

CASE 10-1

Marcella Sinclair's eyesight is failing bilaterally in her 48th year. She has great difficulty in reading when the light is poor. Over the last few years, her kidney function has also deteriorated. She was diagnosed as having diabetes mellitus when she was only 6 years old.

Three hours after Marcella gets up one morning, she notices that her vision seems very blurred on the left side. In her left eye, she sees a shower of dark specks that change their position slightly when she shifts her gaze. Within the next 18 months, the visual acuity of her left eye declines to 6/60.

Marcella also has various symptoms of coronary heart disease. At the age of 62, she dies from a massive myocardial infarct.

Figures 10-1A and 10-2A through 10-2C show the degenerative changes that have occurred in Marcella's left eye.

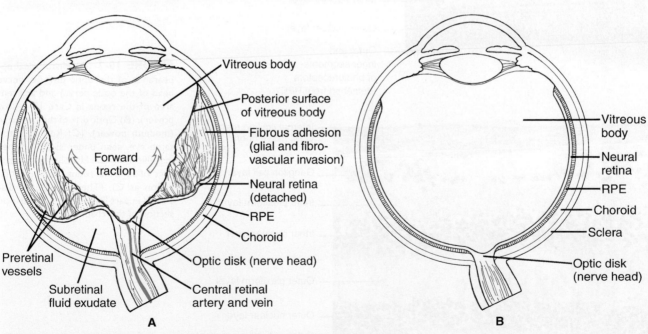

FIGURE 10-1 (**A**) Diagram of the left eye in Case 10-1. (**B**) Diagram of a normal eye.

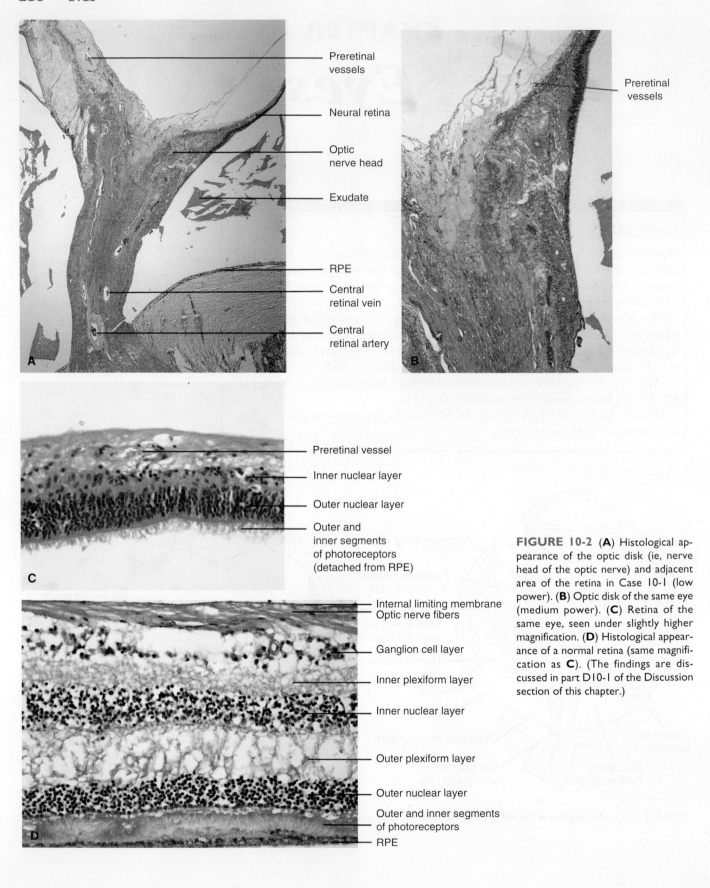

Preretinal vessels

Neural retina

Optic nerve head

Exudate

RPE

Central retinal vein

Central retinal artery

Preretinal vessels

Preretinal vessel

Inner nuclear layer

Outer nuclear layer

Outer and inner segments of photoreceptors (detached from RPE)

Internal limiting membrane
Optic nerve fibers

Ganglion cell layer

Inner plexiform layer

Inner nuclear layer

Outer plexiform layer

Outer nuclear layer

Outer and inner segments of photoreceptors

RPE

FIGURE 10-2 (**A**) Histological appearance of the optic disk (ie, nerve head of the optic nerve) and adjacent area of the retina in Case 10-1 (low power). (**B**) Optic disk of the same eye (medium power). (**C**) Retina of the same eye, seen under slightly higher magnification. (**D**) Histological appearance of a normal retina (same magnification as **C**). (The findings are discussed in part D10-1 of the Discussion section of this chapter.)

ANALYSIS
Case 10-1

What explanation for the patient's visual failure is suggested by the illustrations shown in Fig. 10-1A and Fig. 10-2A?

(The answer is considered in part D10-1 of the Discussion section of this chapter.)

CASE 10-2

Margaret Hanley, aged 47 years, has a 3-year history of dull, poorly localized headaches. The severity of the pain increases if she coughs or bends forward. Analgesics provide little relief, but sitting up generally lessens the intensity of her early morning headaches.

Over the last 4 years, Margaret has developed progressive left-sided weakness. First her left arm was involved, then her left leg. A number of minor seizures occurred that involved her left leg and left hand. She has occasionally experienced facial numbness and tingling.

Physical examination does not indicate any abnormality of her cranial nerves. Her speech sounds normal, and she shows no detectable evidence of mental confusion. However, spastic hemiparesis is noted in both her left arm and left leg. In the left arm, pain, temperature, and discriminative touch sensation are significantly impaired. Only minor use of her left arm is made while walking.

A few hours before Margaret's admission to hospital, she experiences an episode of sudden severe nausea with intermittent momentary dimming of her vision. A CT scan discloses a large abnormal mass in the right frontal lobe of her brain (Fig. 10-3).

The ophthalmoscopic and histological appearances of the patient's optic disks are illustrated in Fig. 10-4A,C,D.

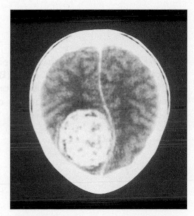

FIGURE 10-3 Axial CT (computed tomography) image of the brain in Case 10-2.

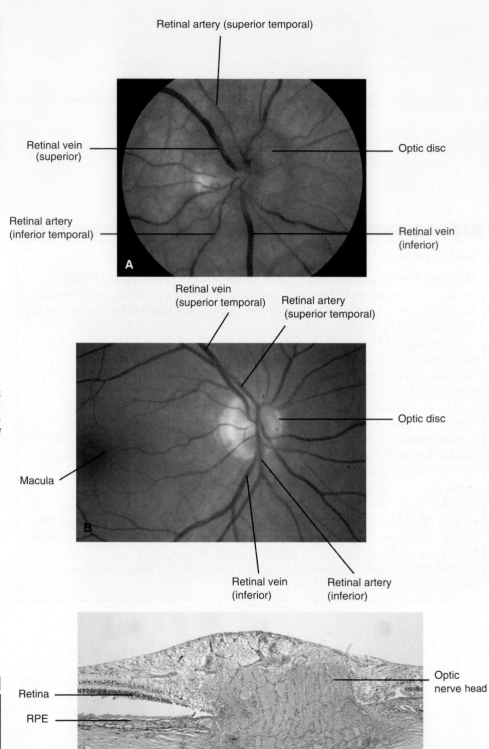

Retinal artery (superior temporal)

Retinal vein (superior)

Optic disc

Retinal artery (inferior temporal)

Retinal vein (inferior)

A

Retinal vein (superior temporal)

Retinal artery (superior temporal)

Optic disc

Macula

B

Retinal vein (inferior)

Retinal artery (inferior)

Retina

RPE

Optic nerve head

C

FIGURE 10-4 (**A**) Ophthalmoscopic view of right fundus in Case 10-2. (**B**) Ophthalmoscopic view of fundus of normal eye. (**C**) Histological appearance of optic disk in Case 10-2 (low power).

ANALYSIS
Case 10-2

What information do parts A, C, and D of Fig. 10-4 disclose about the patient's condition in Case 10-2?

(The answer is considered in part D10-2 of the Discussion section of this chapter.)

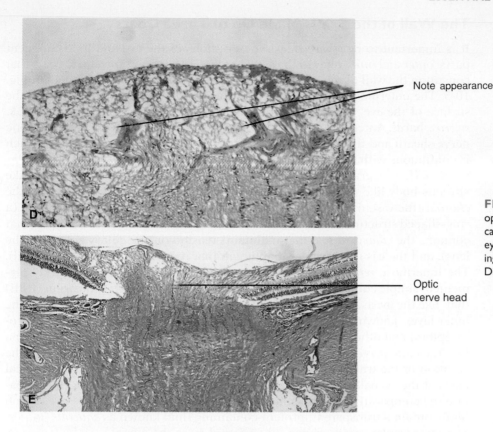

Note appearance

Optic
nerve head

FIGURE 10-4 (Continued) **(D)** Same optic disk (medium power). **(E)** Histological appearance of optic disk in a normal eye (same magnification as **C**). (The findings are considered in part D10-2 of the Discussion section of this chapter.)

ESSENTIAL FEATURES OF THE EYES

The *eyes* are highly complex, paired organs of special sense that, when stimulated by light, produce afferent *optic nerve impulses* encoding visual information. These nerve impulses are interpreted in the visual cortex of the cerebral hemispheres as a three-dimensional color representation of objects that lie in the direct line of vision.

Because the eyes are exposed at the body surface, they are vulnerable to injuries and infections. Ocular inflammation is therefore quite common. Degenerative changes can also occur, resulting, for example, in the inability to attain focus, partial loss of visual acuity, or increasing opacification of the lens. To some extent, these changes are age-related. Lost vision (ie, blindness) is an irreparable and devastating sensory loss that needs to be avoided as far as is possible.

An understanding of ophthalmologic disorders depends on a thorough and detailed knowledge of ocular structure. It is fortunate that many key structural components of the eye are directly observable, eg, by means of a headband loupe (magnifying lens), ophthalmoscope, or slit-lamp (biomicroscope). They are normally clearly visible through the cornea, the "transparent window of the eye." Furthermore, the eyes are readily accessible to ultrasonic examination. Availability of noninvasive investigative methods compensates for the extreme hazard of obtaining tissue biopsies from the eyeball.

The Wall of the Eye Is Made Up of Three Coats

It is important to be aware that in descriptions of the eye and its component parts, *outer* and *inner* refer to the *eye as a whole*. The three concentric coats that constitute the wall of the eye are shown, both separately and combined, in Fig. 10-5. The outermost, *fibrous coat* has a supporting function. Over most of the surface of the eye, the external coat constitutes the white, opaque *sclera* (Gk. *scleros,* hard). Anteriorly, it is represented by the transparent *cornea.* The optic nerve sheath and the lamina cribrosa are also parts of this fibrous coat, which is continuous with the dura mater. The middle, *vascular coat* is also known as the *uvea* (L. *uva,* grape) because it is darkly pigmented and encloses the jelly-like vitreous body like the skin of a grape. This middle coat is represented by the *choroid* (the vascular layer in the posterior part of the eye), the *ciliary body* (a ring-shaped structure, situated at the corneoscleral junction, ie, the *limbus,* that contains the *ciliary muscle* that maintains tension on the ciliary zonule of the lens), and the *iris* (the circular diaphragm that regulates the size of the pupil). The innermost, *retinal coat* is a double layer. The outer layer is a darkly pigmented, simple cuboidal epithelium called the *retinal pigment epithelium* (RPE) that, like the uvea, absorbs light that has undergone scattering or reflection. The inner layer, known as the *neural retina,* contains the *rods* and *cones* (ie, photoreceptors) and other retinal neurons. Optic nerve fibers from the neural retina join the *optic nerve.* Concentric superimposition of these three coats, with the addition of the transparent *lens,* essentially reconstructs the main anatomical parts of the eyeball (Fig. 10-5, *right panel*). The iris and the lens together separate the comparatively small *anterior* and *posterior chambers* of the eye, which both contain a transparent, protein-containing fluid known as *aqueous humor.* The main ocular cavity, commonly referred to as the *vitreous cavity* (*space* or *chamber*), contains a transparent semisolid gel called the *vitreous body* (Fig. 10-6).

Cornea

The *cornea* is an avascular transparent window made of dense connective tissue, with a layer of epithelium on each side (Fig. 10-7). Its anterior covering, *stratified squamous non-keratinizing epithelium,* is resistant to wear and tear. If the

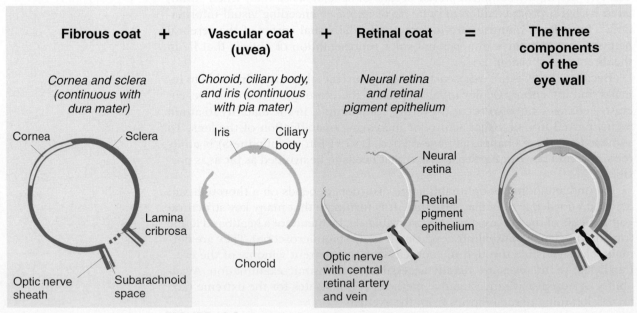

FIGURE 10-5 The three coats constituting the wall of the eye.

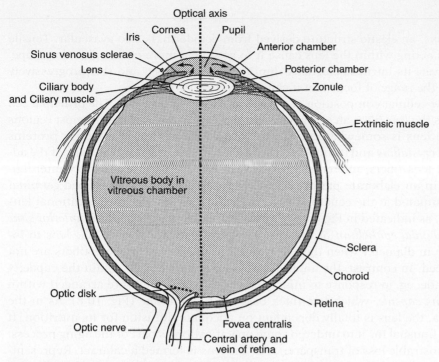

FIGURE 10-6 Main parts of the eye (right eye, in horizontal section).

normal protective film of tears is not present, this epithelium, which is provided with pain receptors, may ulcerate. The basement membrane of the epithelium binds it to an anterior acellular layer of interstitial matrix known as *Bowman's membrane.* The thick central region of the cornea, termed the *substantia propria,* is a proteoglycan-containing matrix that contains embedded type I collagen fibrils and fibrocytes. Posteriorly, the cornea has a simple squamous epithelium and thick basement membrane, known as *Descemet's endothelium* and *membrane,* respectively. This epithelium is responsible for keeping the substantia propria in a state of partial hydration. The cornea becomes cloudy if Descemet's endothelium fails to withdraw enough water. Another cause of corneal opacification is intense scarring of the cornea following injury.

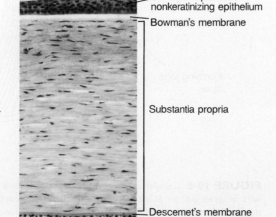

FIGURE 10-7 Cornea (horizontal section, with anterior border at top).

Lens

The *lens,* an elastic structure derived from ectoderm, is also avascular. Tensile forces acting within the lens cause it to assume a more or less globular shape. However, its intrinsic elasticity diminishes with aging, and this progressively limits the range of focus that it can achieve.

The cellular composition of the lens is shown in Fig. 10-8. The principal cell type is the *lens fiber,* an elongated columnar epithelial cell that in most regions of the lens is somewhat curved. Its cytoplasm contains distinctive proteins called *crystallins* and its nucleus has degenerated. The lateral margins of the adjacent lens fibers, interconnected by cell junctions, are extensively interdigitated in an elaborate pattern of knobs and recesses. A ring-shaped *germinal zone* situated at the equatorial border of the lens can produce additional lens fibers, as indicated in Fig. 10-8. Representing the periphery of the *anterior simple cuboidal epithelium* of the lens, the germinal zone enables the lens to increase in diameter when the eye grows, but the preexisting lens fibers are not replaced. In contrast, the anterior cuboidal epithelial cells retain the capacity to divide, eg, in response to injury. The two layers of cells are arranged within the *lens capsule,* which is a thick basement membrane (Fig. 10-8). As in the cornea, the lens is totally dependent on adequate diffusion for its nutrition. It is not unusual for it to undergo some opacification as part of the aging process. Demonstrable loss of transparency of the lens is termed a cataract. Representing one of the most common causes of visual impairment worldwide, cataracts lead to gradual painless loss of vision. Where available, lens extraction with accompanying implantation of a prosthetic intraocular lens is the most satisfactory remedy.

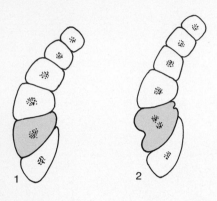

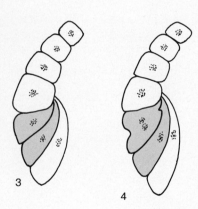

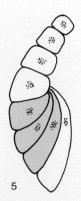

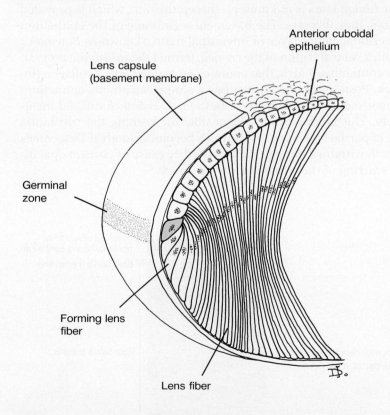

FIGURE 10-8 Cellular arrangement in the ocular lens (horizontal section, with anterior border at top). The series 1 through 5 (on the left) depicts production of additional lens fibers in the equatorial germinal zone of the lens.

Accommodation

The equatorial border of the lens is held under a certain degree of tension by the ciliary body, which is attached to the lens by a circular suspensory ligament known as the *ciliary zonule* (see Fig. 10-6). When the eyes are focused on distant objects, this tension opposes the elastic forces in the lens that makes it assume its globular shape. When bringing closer objects into focus, the *ciliary muscle*, a smooth muscle lying in the ciliary body (see Fig. 10-6), contracts. The zonular attachment to the ciliary body is moved *forward*, ie, closer to the equatorial border of the lens, by this action. Since the zonular attachment to the lens lies slightly anterior to the zonular attachment to the ciliary body, contraction of the ciliary muscle *eases the tension in the zonule*. Decreased tension allows the lens to bulge to a larger extent, an action described as *accommodation* for near objects. Since the thicker lens has a shorter focal length, it brings near objects into focus. Relaxation of the ciliary muscle leaves sufficient tension in the zonule to pull the lens into a flatter shape that brings distant objects into focus. Hence, reading "tires" the eyes, whereas gazing into the distance does not. As people approach middle age, they generally find that they need to move printed text farther away to bring it into focus. This is because the ocular lens is losing its elastic properties and does not return to a globular shape when the ciliary muscle contracts. *Presbyopia* (Gk. *presbys*, old man; *ōps*, eye) is diagnosed when the near point of vision recedes beyond 22 cm.

Iris and Iridocorneal Angle

The *iris* is the circular diaphragm surrounding the pupil that regulates the pupillary aperture and, hence, the amount of light reaching the retina. Its anterior surface is covered by a discontinuous layer of stromal cells. Posteriorly, it is covered by a double layer of pigmented cuboidal epithelial cells. In between lie the constrictor pupillae and the dilator pupillae muscles, which have antagonistic actions. Sympathetic noradrenergic nerve impulses and sympathomimetic drugs dilate the pupil (ie, cause *mydriasis*), whereas parasympathetic cholinergic nerve impulses and parasympathomimetic drugs constrict it (ie, cause *miosis*). Thus, phenylephrine (an adrenergic agonist) may be topically applied to dilate the pupil for ophthalmoscopic examination of the eye. Cocaine and amphetamines (which, of course, are not used for this purpose) have a similar sympathomimetic action on the iris. The *constrictor pupillae* is a circular band of smooth muscle fibers. The *dilator pupillae* is a thin sheet of myoepithelial cells that lie in a radial arrangement near the posterior border of the iris (Fig. 10-9). Eye color is determined by the distribution and concentration of light-blocking melanin-containing cells in the iris. The melanin in the posterior epithelium, seen through the stroma, looks blue. Additional melanized cells in the stroma make the eyes look brown.

The *iridocorneal angle*, which is also known as the *angle of the anterior chamber*, lies immediately posterior to the limbus. As may be seen on the right in Fig. 10-9, it is an acute angle. Associated with this angle is a ring-shaped band of scleral trabeculae, loosely arranged as a series of *trabecular sheets*, with a meshwork of *trabecular spaces* (spaces of Fontana) between them. Immediately peripheral to this loosely filled internal scleral sulcus is a ring-shaped scleral venous channel called the *sinus venosus sclerae* (*Schlemm's canal*). The posterior simple squamous (Descemet's) endothelium of the cornea extends as a lining layer into the trabecular spaces and sinus venosus sclerae.

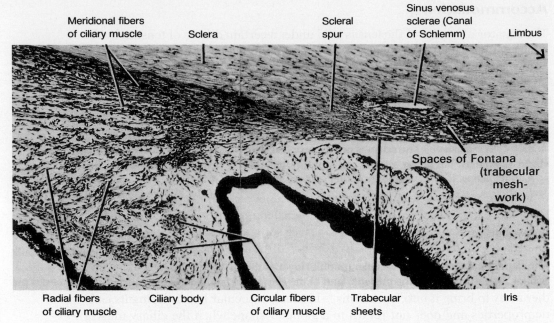

FIGURE 10-9 Iridocorneal angle (angle of anterior chamber). The sinus venosus sclerae (Schlemm's canal) lying in this angle provides the main exit route by which aqueous humor leaves the anterior chamber.

Pathway of Aqueous Humor

The *aqueous humor* that fills the anterior chamber of the eye is produced from small blood vessels in processes of the ciliary body. These processes border on the *posterior chamber,* which is the small intraocular space interposed between the posterior border of the iris and the anterior border of the vitreous body (see Fig. 10-6). Aqueous humor enters the *anterior chamber* from the posterior chamber by passing around the pupillary margin, as indicated by arrows in Fig. 10-6. Here, the posterior surface of the iris is gently pressed against the anterior surface of the lens, an arrangement that acts as a one-way flap valve. Whenever the hydrostatic pressure in the posterior chamber exceeds that in the anterior chamber, more aqueous humor is admitted to the anterior chamber. Aqueous humor cannot return to the posterior chamber.

The exit route for aqueous humor has clinical significance, since drainage of this fluid becomes markedly impaired if access to the sinus venosus sclerae (Schlemm's canal) is restricted. In *narrow-angle glaucoma* (a form of primary glaucoma), the anterior surface of the peripheral region of the iris lies very close to the drainage meshwork of trabeculae in the internal scleral sulcus. When the pupil is dilated, the unusually acute iridocorneal angle restricts access to the trabecular spaces and their venous drainage channel. Such obstruction to the outflow of aqueous humor from the anterior chamber causes painful episodes of elevated intraocular pressure. The normal rate of outflow of aqueous humor maintains an intraocular pressure of 10–20 mm Hg. Persistent elevation of the intraocular pressure >25 mm Hg impairs retinal nourishment and may cause visual field defects. It may also result in progressive opacification of the cornea. Progressive atrophy of the optic nerve head in the glaucomatous eye eventually leads to blindness.

Vitreous Body

The *vitreous body* is a highly hydrated, viscoelastic colloidal gel containing proteins and hyaluronic acid. It is supported internally by a loose meshwork of type

II collagen fibrils that are randomly arranged. The interstices of the gel, and internal pools of the sol phase, contain the lower molecular weight constituents present in aqueous humor. The vitreous body exhibits a fibrillar internal structure only after fixation for microscopy. Occasional small cells (*hyalocytes*) believed to produce hyaluronic acid and collagen are peripherally distributed in the vitreous body. Macrophages also are present. This avascular, transparent gelatinous mass provides support for the posterior border of the lens and keeps the neural retina tightly apposed to the RPE and the remainder of the eye wall.

If the vitreous body becomes damaged, eg, during surgical procedures such as lens extraction, there is an increased risk that these two layers of the retina may separate. The vitreous body is normally strongly adherent to the optic disk (nerve head of optic nerve), the posterior border of the lens capsule, the basement membrane of the ciliary epithelium covering the ciliary body, and the internal limiting membrane of the neural retina, which is the basement membrane of its tall columnar supporting cells (Müller cells).

Retina

The *outer layer* of the retinal coat is the *RPE*. The substantial melanin content of this heavily pigmented, simple cuboidal epithelium absorbs the light passing through the neural retina, minimizing glare due to reflection back into the eye. Continuous tight junctions between the lateral margins of these contiguous cells constitute an important part of the blood–retina barrier, a functional extension of the *blood–brain barrier*. A supplementary diffusion barrier exists between the endothelial cells of the retinal capillaries that supply the surface layers of the retina. The RPE cells also play a key role in restoring photosensitivity to the visual pigments that become dissociated by light, and they dispose of shed membranous disks from the adjacent photoreceptors (see Fig. 10-13, right side).

The *inner layer* of the retinal coat is the *neural retina*. This much thicker, more elaborate layer is brain-derived *nervous tissue* composed of two types of light-sensitive *photoreceptors* (*rods* and *cones*) and several other kinds of neurons (*bipolar, horizontal, amacrine,* and *ganglion cells*), together with supporting Müller cells and other glial cells such as fibrous astrocytes.

As outlined in Figs. 10-10, 10-11, and 10-12, the photosensitive *outer segments* of the photoreceptors lie in the deepest layer of the neural retina, adjacent to the RPE. Immediately internal to this is a layer made up of the inner segments of these cells. The photoreceptor *nuclei* lie in the *outer nuclear layer*. The *outer plexiform layer* contains synapses between (1) photoreceptors and (2) bipolar cells and horizontal cells. The *inner nuclear layer* contains the nuclei of bipolar cells and amacrine cells. *Amacrine cells* (Gk. *a*, without; *makros*, long; *inos*, fiber) are neurons with no recognizable axon. Some of their dendrites are presynaptic and others are postsynaptic. The nuclei of Müller cells can also be found in this layer. The *inner plexiform layer* contains synapses between bipolar cells and ganglion cells as well as synapses between amacrine cells and (1) bipolar cells and (2) ganglion cells. The *ganglion cell layer* contains the cell bodies and nuclei of ganglion cells, and also small retinal blood vessels. The innermost layer of the neural retina is made up of *optic nerve fibers,* along with long microvillous processes of Müller cells and medium-sized retinal blood vessels. At the inner surface of the retina, optic nerve fibers are unmyelinated, but where they extend centrally from the lamina cribrosa, they are myelinated. Müller cells are tall columnar cells that extend across almost the entire thickness of the neural retina. Their basement membrane is represented by the *internal limiting membrane* of the retina, and their nuclei lie in the inner nuclear layer.

Situated slightly lateral to the posterior pole of the eye, near the point of intersection between the optical axis and the plane of curvature of the retina (see Fig. 10-6), lies a shallow depression known as the *fovea centralis* (L. for central

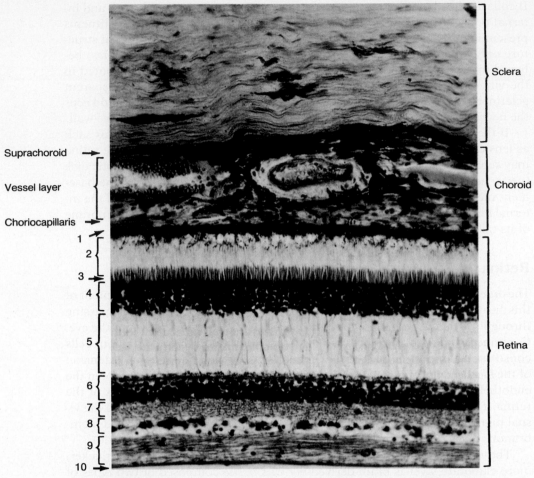

Sclera

Choroid

Suprachoroid →

Vessel layer

Choriocapillaris →

1
2
3 →
4

5

6
7
8

9

10 →

Retina

FIGURE 10-10 Retina, choroid, and adjacent region of sclera (medium power). For names of numbered layers, see Fig. 10-11.

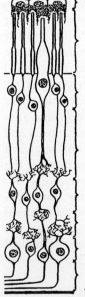

1. Retinal pigment epithelium

2. Outer and inner segments of photoreceptors

3. External limiting membrane
4. Outer nuclear layer

5. Outer plexiform layer

6. Inner nuclear layer (bipolar cells)

7. Inner plexiform layer

8. Ganglion cell layer

9. Retinal (optic) nerve fiber layer
10. Internal limiting membrane

FIGURE 10-11 Constituent layers of the retina.

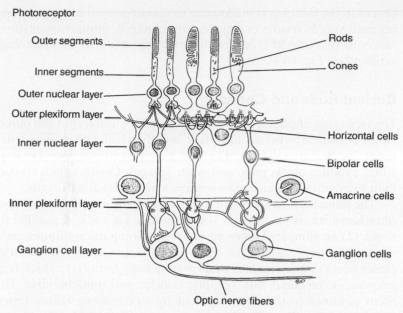

Photoreceptor
Outer segments — Rods
Inner segments — Cones
Outer nuclear layer
Outer plexiform layer
Inner nuclear layer — Horizontal cells
— Bipolar cells
Inner plexiform layer — Amacrine cells
Ganglion cell layer — Ganglion cells
Optic nerve fibers

FIGURE 10-12 Chief synapses and cellular organization in the neural retina.

pit). Approximately 1.5 mm in diameter, this part of the retina provides maximal visual acuity, because its photoreceptors are very closely packed and their outer segments are less thickly covered by overlying constituents of the retina. The fovea lies in a yellow pigmented area called the *macula lutea* (L. for yellow spot). In the central area (foveola) of the fovea, the tightly packed photoreceptors are all *cones* (cells providing color vision). This central area lacks retinal blood vessels. Macular (foveal) visual acuity is required for extremely fine visual resolution (eg, for reading important information printed in diminutive text). Loss of macular acuity as a consequence of degenerative changes is permanent. In contrast to the macula, the nerve head of the optic nerve (ie, the *optic disk* or *papilla*) is devoid of photoreceptors and, therefore, constitutes a "blind spot." It is the site of access of the central retinal artery and vein (see Figs. 10-4B, 10-6).

The columnar supporting and nutritive glial cells of the retina, Müller cells, are joined to the photoreceptors by band-shaped adhering (anchoring) junctions and are interconnected with each other, but not with the photoreceptors, by continuous tight junctions. Hence, there is strong intercellular attachment and an incomplete (ie, partial) permeability barrier at the level of the external limiting membrane.

Retinal Detachment

When the eye develops, the inner cellular layer of the optic cup gives rise to the neural retina, and outer cellular layer becomes the RPE. Although the two retinal layers adhere to each other, the strength of adhesion between the RPE and the neural retina is considerably less than that between the RPE and its underlying choroid. If one or more areas of neural retina become detached from the RPE, the condition is called a *detached retina*. Any separation may cause substantial damage, because the oxygen and nutrients reaching the cells in the outer third of the neural retina diffuse there from the capillaries in the choriocapillaris, a plexus of associated fenestrated wide capillaries situated in the vascular middle coat of the eye wall. The photoreceptors lie in this diffusion-dependent zone. Unless a reattachment procedure is performed, the restricted supply of oxygen and nutrients reaching retinal cells from capillaries supplied by the central retinal artery, which are confined to the inner third of the neural retina (but

KEY CONCEPT

Macular nutrition, and therefore visual acuity, is dependent on diffusion from the choriocapillaris.

absent in the foveola), is inadequate to sustain retinal function. Loss of the main nutrient supply results in degenerative changes. Similar separation of the neural retina from the RPE occurs on a much greater scale as a histological fixation artifact (see Fig. 10-4C,E).

Retinal Rods and Cones

The two types of photoreceptors are basically similar, but the outer segment of cones is conical, whereas in rods it is cylindrical. Other ultrastructural differences are shown in detail in Fig. 10-13. *Rods*, which respond to low light intensities, produce black, gray, and white images. *Cones*, which respond to higher light intensities, produce color images and resolve finer details.

The main parts of each type of photoreceptor are (1) a rod-shaped or conical photosensitive *outer segment*, which contains a stack of parallel membranous disks, (2) an elongated *inner segment* containing microtubules and most of the other cytoplasmic organelles, (3) a *nuclear region*, and (4) a wide axonic process (*inner fiber*) that terminates as a *synaptic body* (*process*), which is an expanded presynaptic terminal with synaptic vesicles and mitochondria. The outer segment is joined to the inner segment by a *connecting cilium* representing the basal part of a cilium. Particularly in cones (Fig. 10-13, left side), the outer region of the inner segment (often described as the *ellipsoid*) contains the majority of mitochondria, whereas the inner region (known as the *myoid*) contains most of the organelles concerned with the synthesis of cytoplasmic and membrane proteins (polysomes, rER, and Golgi stacks). *Calycal processes* lie at the base of the outer segment. A distinctive type of synapse known as the *ribbon synapse* is found in the synaptic body. A similarly specialized type of synapse is present in hair cells of the inner ear. Its *synaptic lamella* (*ribbon* or *bar*) is believed to serve as a guide for synaptic vesicles, making simultaneous neurotransmission to more than one postsynaptic terminal possible.

Visual Pigments of Membranous Disks

The photosensitive *visual pigments* are made up of (1) a transmembrane disk membrane glycoprotein known as an *opsin* and (2) a light-sensitive 11-*cis*-retinal prosthetic group (*retinene$_1$*) that is the aldehyde of vitamin A$_1$. The visual pigment in retinal rods is *rhodopsin* (*visual purple*). In rods, the opsin is scotopsin, whereas in cones there are other opsins, collectively known as *photopsins*. All the opsins are multipass integral membrane glycoproteins that span the lipid bilayer of the disk membrane seven times. The cone opsins confer maximal photosensitivities, in three different populations of cones, to red, green, and blue light, respectively.

Photons convert the *cis* form of the retinal in rhodopsin to the all-*trans* isomer. Isomerization initiates a cascade reaction, one of the effects of which is the closing of some of the Na$^+$ channels in the cell membrane of the outer segment, which in turn leads to *hyperpolarization* of the cell. Hyperpolarization inhibits release of the synaptic neurotransmitter. Following a short delay, the retinal dissociates from the opsin, resulting in photopigment bleaching. Both the Müller cells and the RPE are believed to participate in the retinol–retinal interconversions and isomerization required to regenerate 11-*cis*-retinal for rhodopsin resynthesis.

The retinal photoreceptors are highly differentiated, and possess no proliferative capacity or mechanism for cell renewal. The necessary turnover of their visual pigment is facilitated by its integral incorporation into *membranous disks*, a stack of which forms through invagination of many double layers of cell membrane. In the rods, approximately 30 to 100 new disks are produced each day, and each disk becomes essentially separate and unattached. In the cones,

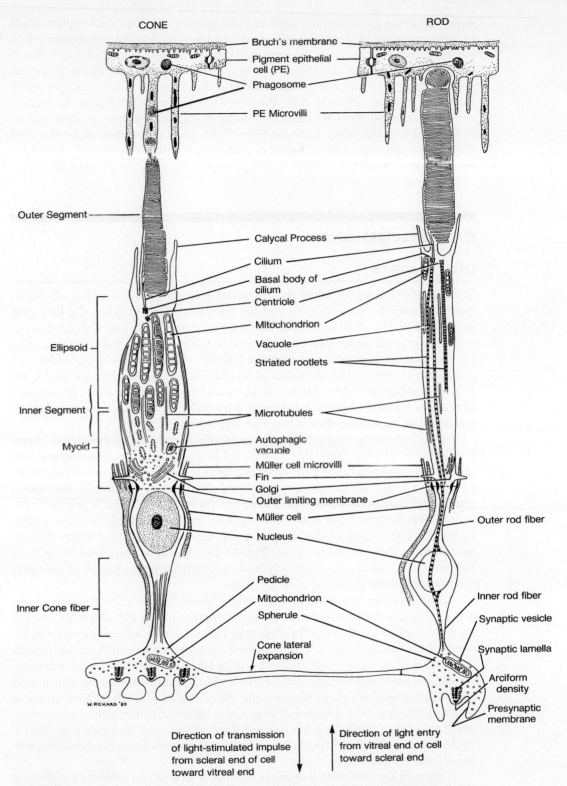

CONE

ROD

- Bruch's membrane
- Pigment epithelial cell (PE)
- Phagosome
- PE Microvilli

Outer Segment

- Calycal Process
- Cilium
- Basal body of cilium
- Centriole
- Mitochondrion
- Vacuole
- Striated rootlets

Ellipsoid

Inner Segment

Myoid

- Microtubules
- Autophagic vacuole
- Müller cell microvilli
- Fin
- Golgi
- Outer limiting membrane
- Müller cell
- Nucleus

Outer rod fiber

Inner Cone fiber

- Pedicle
- Mitochondrion
- Spherule
- Cone lateral expansion

Inner rod fiber
Synaptic vesicle
Synaptic lamella
Arciform density
Presynaptic membrane

W. RICKARD '80

Direction of transmission of light-stimulated impulse from scleral end of cell toward vitreal end

Direction of light entry from vitreal end of cell toward scleral end

FIGURE 10-13 Fine structure of retinal cones and rods, showing their relation to the RPE (Bruch's membrane is the adjacent region of the choroid).

many disks retain continuity with the cell membrane. The rods replace their membranous disks continuously, with a turnover time of approximately 2 weeks. Rhodopsin becomes incorporated into each disk while it is being formed. The cones evidently renew the visual pigment in their disk membrane at a comparable rate. However, the turnover time for disk renewal in cones is very much slower (9 to 12 months). In rods, the new disks formed each day at the base of the outer segment replace a number of older disks that are shed, as short stacks, from the tip of the outer segment (Fig. 10-13, right side). Rod disks are shed chiefly just after the normal hours of darkness. Comparable disk shedding occurs in cones. Stacks of shed disks are promptly phagocytosed by the RPE.

CASE DISCUSSIONS

D10-1 (CASE 10-1)

The essential reason for Marcella's impaired eyesight is extensive loss of attachment between the neural retina and the normally adjacent layer, the RPE that maintains it. The dark spots that she sees indicate that a hemorrhage has occurred from torn superficial blood vessels of the retina into the vitreous cavity. Careful examination of the superficial (vitreal) surface of the sectioned retina discloses the presence of additional new small blood vessels (see Figs. 10-1A, 10-2C), a pathological change known as *neovascularization of the retina*. Formation of these new *preretinal vessels* is largely a retinal response to angiogenic factors produced in the retina when it becomes hypoxic.

Newly formed preretinal vessels are extremely fragile. Diabetics are therefore likely to develop preretinal intravitreal hemorrhages that may impair their vision. Extravasated blood cells enter the narrow intraocular space between the posterior surface of the vitreous body and the anterior surface of the neural retina, and may then begin to penetrate the vitreous body. This is primarily because the iron liberated by hemolysis degrades hyaluronic acid, the main macromolecular constituent of the vitreous body. Ensuing shrinkage of the vitreous gel produces forward traction (see Fig. 10-1A). Multiple preretinal intravitreal hemorrhages, therefore, commonly lead to progressive separation of the vitreous body from the posterior pole of the eye.

Accompanying fibrovascular and glial (fibrous astrocytic) invasion of the preexisting interface between the posterior surface of the vitreous body and the anterior surface of the neural retina may cause fibrous adhesions to form between these two structures. The damaging consequences of such an occurrence are described as *proliferative diabetic retinopathy*. The newly formed preretinal vessels become increasingly invested by collagen and other interstitial matrix constituents as a result of fibrosis and gliosis (glial scarring). New collagen fibers also amass into substantial sheets and bands of fibrovascular connective tissue that extend radially from the periphery of the optic disk (see Figs. 10-1A, 10-2A). These abnormal fibrous structures adhere tightly to the posterior surface of the vitreous body.

If the proliferative retinal changes that occur in diabetic patients are allowed to progress, they may result in blindness, ie, reduce visual acuity to 20/200 (6/60) or below. Repeated resolution of multiple preretinal intravitreal hemorrhages causes progressive shrinkage of the vitreous body, which can lead to tractional detachment of the retina. The progressive forward traction exerted on adhering portions of the retina causes an increasing area of the neural retina to peel away from the adjacent RPE anchored to the choroid (see Figs. 10-1A, 10-2A). Even partial detachment of the neural retina is deleterious because it displaces the photoreceptors from their nearest source of nourishment, the capillaries in the choroid. Such separation results in visual deterioration and may lead to permanent visual field defects. Visual acuity becomes markedly impaired if the macular photoreceptors deteriorate as a result of tractional detachment. Peripheral vision becomes restricted under conditions of peripheral proliferative retinopathy.

D10-2 (CASE 10-2)

In Case 10-2, the patient's primary problem is a massive brain tumor known as a *meningioma*. This relatively slow-growing type of malignant tumor, mesenchymal in origin, is believed to arise from a constituent cell of arachnoid villi. Because a tumor with these dimensions substantially increases the brain volume inside the cranial cavity, it chronically elevates the intracranial pressure.

Increased intracranial pressure causes distinctive changes in both the ophthalmoscopic and the histological appearance of the retina. Seen with an ophthalmoscope through the dilated pupil, this patient's optic disks appear raised, with an indistinct margin (see Fig. 10-4A). A normal optic disk has a central depression, known as a physiological cup, and a fairly distinct margin (see Fig. 10-4B). Perceptible blurring of this margin or filling in of the *physiological cup*, especially if accompanied by congestion of the central retinal vein, are considered signs of *papilledema* (meaning edema of the optic disk). In contrast to a normal optic disk, the optic disk shown in Fig. 10-4A has an indistinct margin and its middle appears slightly out of focus because it is raised above the plane of the surrounding area of the retina. Also as a result of edema, the central retinal vessels appear somewhat indistinct at the site where they penetrate the center of the optic disk.

The cause of this patient's papilledema is elevated intracranial pressure. Increased hydrostatic pressure within the cranial cavity is transmitted to the subarachnoid space and, as a result, the optic nerves are compressed (see Fig. 10-5). Similar compression of the thin-walled central retinal vein, which follows a course within the optic nerve, causes this vein and its associated tributaries to become congested. Their pulsatile filling during the cardiac cycle becomes so reduced that it is barely detectable. Venous drainage from the retina is markedly impaired by severe compression of the central retinal vein. The resulting backpressure augments production of tissue fluid by the retinal capillaries, with the result that excess tissue fluid collects in the interstitial spaces of the retina. Edema of the optic nerve head can be recognized ophthalmoscopically as swelling and protrusion of the optic disk (*papilledema*).

If papilledema persists, the resulting compression may impair function of the optic nerve fibers (axons of ganglion cells) converging on the optic nerve head. Compared with normal optic nerve fibers, chronically compressed optic nerve fibers have a somewhat dilated and more widely separated appearance (compare parts D and E in Fig. 10-4). Some shrinkage artifact is to be expected in histological sections (see Fig. 10-4E), but there is no evidence of edema in a normal optic disk.

BIBLIOGRAPHY

Benson WE, Brown GC, Tasman W. Diabetes and Its Ocular Complications. Philadelphia, W.B. Saunders, 1988.

Bok D. Retinal photoreceptor-pigment epithelium interactions. Invest Ophthalmol Vis Sci 26:1659, 1985.

Jakobiec FA, ed. Ocular Anatomy, Embryology, and Teratology. Hagerstown, Md., Harper & Row, 1982.

Kuszak JR. The ultrastructure of epithelial and fiber cells in the crystalline lens. Int Rev Cytol 163:305, 1995.

Kuszak JR, Peterson KL, Brown HG. Electron microscopic observations of the crystalline lens. Microsc Res Tech 33:441, 1996.

L'Esperance FA, James WA. Diabetic Retinopathy: Clinical Evaluation and Management. St. Louis, C.V. Mosby, 1981.

Marshall J, ed. The Susceptible Visual Apparatus. Vision and Visual Dysfunction, vol. 16. Boca Raton, Fla., CRC Press, 1991.

Masland RH. The functional architecture of the retina. Sci Am 255(6):102, 1986.

Okano T, Fukada Y, Yoshizawa T. Molecular basis for tetrachromatic color vision. Comp Biochem Physiol [B] 112B:405, 1995.

Scuderi G, Morone G, Brancato R. Atlas of Clinical Ophthalmoscopy. Milano, Masson S.p.A., 1987.

Spalton DJ, Hitchings RA, Hunter PA, eds. Atlas of Clinical Ophthalmology, ed 2. London, Mosby-Year Book, 1994.

Urrets-Zavalia A. Diabetic Retinopathy. New York, Masson Publishing Inc., 1977.

Yau K-W. Phototransduction mechanism in retinal rods and cones: The Friedenwald lecture. Invest Ophthalmol Vis Sci 35:9, 1994.

Subject Index

Subject Index

Page numbers in bold face indicate major discussions; f following a page number indicates a figure; t following a page number indicates a table.

A

A bands, 101f, 102
Absorption, of drugs, 5
Accommodation, 293
A (α) cells, 248, 248f, 249f
Acetaminophen
   nephrotoxicity of, 179
   and toxic hepatitis, 214
Acetycholine, 148
Acid phosphatase, prostatic, 273
Acidophils, of anterior pituitary, 245t
Acinus
   of liver, 206–207, 206f
   of lung, 150, 153
Acne vulgaris, 26
Acquired immunodeficiency syndrome, 53
Acrosome and acrosome vesicle, 266, 266f
ACTH. See Adrenocorticotrophic hormone
Actin, 101–102, 102f
α Actinin, 102, 131
Acute inflammation, 22f, 47t, **48**
Acute myelomonocytic leukemia, 34, 64
Addison's disease, 24t
Adenohypophysis, 243
Adenoma
   corticotroph, 278
   prolactin cell, 277
Adhering (anchoring) junctions, **19t**, 20f, 123, 123f, 125f
Adhesion belt, 19t, 20f
Adhesion plaque, 19t
Adrenal(s), 240, 240f, 241f
   cortex and medulla, 240f–242f, 241
Adrenaline. See Epinephrine
Adrenocorticotrophic hormone, 241, 246, 247, 278
Afferent and efferent arterioles, of renal corpuscle, 171f, 172
AIDS. See Acquired immunodeficiency syndrome
Albinism, 24t
Alcohol
   effects on pancreas, 216
   effects on liver, 209f, 210, 214
   metabolism and elimination, 209f, 210, 214
Alcoholic cirrhosis, 214
Alcoholic hepatitis, 214, 215

Alcoholic hyaline, 214, 216
Alcoholic pancreatitis, 216
Aldosterone, 180t, 240f, 241
Alkaline phosphatase, 82, 83, 87
Allergic inflammation, 47t, 64
Allergic reactions, 49–51
Alopecia, male pattern, 26
Alveolar-capillary barrier, 154, 154f
Alveolar ducts, 154, 154f
Alveolar edema, 138, 158
Alveolar sacs, 154, 154f
Alveolar walls. See Interalveolar walls
Alveoli
   of breast, 263
   pulmonary, 153
Amacrine cells, 295, 297f
Amiodarone chlorhydrate, effect on nerve function, 77, 115
Analgesic nephropathy, 179
Anaphylaxis, systemic, 50
Anasarca, 181
Anastomoses, portal-systemic, 210–212, 211f
Anchoring filaments, 136, 137f
Anchoring junctions. See Adhering junctions
Androgen-binding protein, 269
Androgens, 240f, 241
   effects on hair follicles, 26
   ovarian, 256, 257t
Anemia
   aplastic, 62
   in chronic renal failure, 181
   megaloblastic, 62
   microcytic hypochromic, 62
   pernicious, 62
Anisocytosis, 62
Aneurysm, 131
Angiotensin, 148, 179, 180t
   actions of, 180t
   and vascular tonus, 134t
Angiotensin-converting enzyme, 148, 180t
Angiotensinogen, 179, 180t
Anisocytosis, 62
Anterior chamber
   angle of, 293, 294f
   of eye, 291f, 294

Anterior pituitary, 243f–245f, 244, 245t, 246f, 247t
  acidophils and basophils, 245t
  hormones secreted by, 245t
    regulation of release of, 245t
Antidiuretic hormone, 178, 180t
  and vascular tonus, 134t
Antigen-presenting cells, 55, 59
α_1-Antitrypsin, 143, **158–159, 160f**
Anulus fibrosus, 99, 100f
Aortic valve, 138
Aplastic anemia, 62
Apoptosis, 10, 55
Appendectomy specimens, 189f
Appendicitis, 201, 216
Appendix, 200, 201f
Appositional growth, of bone, 84
Aqueous humor, 294
Arcuate arteries, 169, 170f
Artery(ies)
  arcuate, 169, 170f
  bronchial, 150
  coronary, 121f, 122f, 139
  distributing. See Arteries, muscular
  elastic, 133t
  of kidney, 169–170, 170f
  muscular, 132, 133t
  nutrient, of bones, 94
  posterior interventricular, 121f, 139
Arterioles, 132, 133, 133t, 134f
  afferent and efferent, of kidney, 171f, 172
Articular cartilages, 86, **98–99**, 114
Ascites, 215
Ascorbic acid, and collagen formation, 79
Astrocytes, 107
Astrocytomas, 107
Atheromatous plaques, 132
Atherosclerosis, stages of, 135t
Atherosclerotic (fibrous) plaques, 132, **135t**, 139
Atretic follicles, 251–252, 252f, 253f
Atrioventricular node, 129
Auerbach's plexus, 191f, 192
A-V bundle, 128f, 129
A-V node, 128f, 129
Axon, 105
Axonal transport, 105–106
Axoneme, 266, 267f
Axoplasmic flow, 106
Axoplasmic transport, 105–106
Azurophilic granules, of neutrophils, 49, 50t

B
Band neutrophils, 37f, **39t**, 43f
Barrier
  alveolar-capillary, 154, 154f
  blood-brain, 108
  blood-retina, 295
  blood-testis, 270, 272f
  blood-thymus, 56
Basement membranes, 5–6, 80, 81f
  epidermal, 18t, 21f

glomerular, 6
Basophilic erythroblast, 43f
Basophils
  of anterior pituitary, 245t
  of blood, 37f, **39t**, 47t
    granule contents, 50t
B cell(s), 53
  activation of, 55
  antigen receptor, 53
B (β) cells, of pancreas, 248, 248f, 249f
Benign prostatic hyperplasia, 271, 281
Bertin, columns of, 169
Bile canaliculi, 205f, 207
Bile pigments, recirculation of, 208f
Bilirubin
  conjugated and unconjugated, 207, 208f, 213t
  direct and indirect, 212, 213t
  excretion, 207, 208f
  recirculation, 207, 208f
Blisters, 23
Blood, peripheral, normal values, 36t
Blood-brain barrier, 108
Blood cell counts, 36t, 38t
Blood count, complete, 36
Blood pressure regulation, renal involvement, 179
Blood-retina barrier, 295
Blood-testis barrier, 270, 272f
Blood-thymus barrier, 56
Blood vessels, 131, 132f, **133t**, 134f
B lymphocytes, 53
Body(ies)
  ciliary, 290, 290f, 291f, 293
  Herring, 247
  lamellar, 155, 156f
  Mallory, 214, 216
  polar, 254, 254t
  psammoma, 275
  vitreous, 291f, 294
Bombesin, 148
Bone
  blood supply, 94, 95f
  calcification, 82–83
  cancellous, 83–84, 83f
  compact (dense), 83–85, 84f, 85f
  contact healing of, 97
  fracture repair, 96–97
  growth of, 91–93
  immature, 85
  lamellar, 84
  matrix
    composition, 82, 82t
    coupling proteins of, 94
  mature, 84
  mineralization, 82–83
  modeling and remodeling, 93
  morphogenetic (osteoinductive) proteins, 94
  parathyroid hormone effects on, 90
  reactive, 236
  remodeling unit, 94
  resorption, 88–89, 89f
  scans, for metastatic cancer, 74f, 75f, **114**, 236

trabecular (spongy), 83–84, 83f
types of, 83–85
woven (woven-fibered), 85
Bone marrow, 38, 41
cellular composition of, 42f
evaluation of, 40f
transplants of, 31, 33, 63
Border, ruffled, of osteoclasts, 88, 89f
Bowman's capsule, 171
Bowman's membrane, 291, 291f
Breast
carcinoma, 280–281
lactating, 263, 263f
resting (inactive), 262, 262f
Bronchi, 149f, 151, 151f
Bronchi
support of, 151f
tonus regulation in, 153
Bronchial arteries, 150
Bronchial carcinoma, 161
Bronchiectasis, 161
Bronchioles, 152–153, 151f, 153f
respiratory, 154, 154f
support of, 151f
tonus regulation in, 153
Bronchitis, 149f
Bronchopneumonia, 159
Bronchospasm, 153
Brunner's glands, 198, 198f
Brush border enzymes, 197
Bullae, 23
Bullous pemphigoid, 16
Bullous pemphigoid antigen, 16, 21f
Bundle of His, 129
Burns, 23–24

C

Cadherin, 19t, 20f
Calcification, ectopic, dystrophic, and metastatic, 83
Calcitonin, 148, 251
receptor for, on osteoclasts, 90
Calcium channel, and calcium release, 103, 124f
Calcium handling, in cardiac muscle, 123–125, **124f**
Calcium release channel, in skeletal muscle, 103
Calculi, renal, 177–178, 183
Caldesmon, 131
Callus, 96
Calmodulin, 130
Canal
cervical, 259, 260f
haversian, 84, 85f
Schlemm's, 293–294, 294f
Canaliculi, 84
bile, 205f, 207
Cancellous bone, 83–84, 83f
Cancer
bone scan detection of metastases, 114
of breast, 281
chemotherapy, 8
metastases in bone scans, 236

prostatic, markers, 273
Capillaries
blood, 133, 133t, 134f
glomerular, 171f, 173f
lymphatic, 133t, 136, 137f, 197
Capsular space, 176, 178f
Capsule
Bowman's, 171
lens, 292, 292f
Caput medusae, 211f, 212
Carcinoid tumors, 148
Carcinoma
of breast, 280–281
bronchial, 161
cervical, 280
ductal and intraductal, 280
large cell keratinizing, 280
prostatic, 271, 281
in situ, 279
squamous cell, 161
Cardiac glands, 192, 193
Cardiac muscle, 122–126, 123f, 124f, 125f, 126f, 127t
calcium handling in, 123–125, **124f**
Cartilage, 85–86
articular, 86, **98–99**, 114
elastic, 86
hyaline, 85–86
matrix composition, 82, 82t
physical properties of, 86
Casts
fatty, 176, 181
granular, 181
hyaline, 176, 181
waxy, 176
Cataract, 292
Caveolae, of smooth muscle, 131
C cells, 237, 251
Cecum, 200
Cell, organization of, 1–2
Cell cycle, 7–8
Cell death, programmed, 10, 55
Cell nests, 85
Cell proliferation, regulation of, 7
Cells. *See also under individual names*
hematopoietic, 41, 43f, 63
myeloid, 43f
stem, 8
Central vein, of liver lobules, 205, 206f
Centroacinar cell, 201, 202f
Cervical canal, 259, 260f
Cervical glands, 260f, 261
Cervical intraepithelial neoplasia, 279
Cervical mucus, 261
Cervix, uterine, 258–261
Chief cells
of fundic glands, 193, 194f, 195f
of parathyroid glands, 250, 250f
Chloasma, 24t
Chondrocalcin, 82
Chondrosarcoma, 113
Chromaffin cells, 241

Chromophils, 244, 245f
Chromophobes, 244
Chronic inflammation, 46, 47t
Chylomicrons, 197
Ciliary body, 290, 290f, 291f, 293
Ciliary muscle, 291f, 293, 294f
Ciliary zonule, 291f, 293
Circumferential lamellae, 93
Cirrhosis, alcoholic, 214
Collagen, 79–80, 80f
    types of, 79t, 80
Collecting ducts and tubules, renal, 175
    resorption and secretion in, 177f
Colon, 200
Colostrum, 263, 264f
Compact bone, 83–85, 84f, 85f
Complete blood count, 36
Cones, retinal, 297, 297f, 298, 299f
Constrictor pupillae, 293
Convoluted tubule
    distal, 171f, 174, 175f, 176f, 177f
    proximal, 171f, 173, 174f, 176f, 177f
Corbular sarcoplasmic reticulum, 125, 125f
Cornea, 290–291, 291f
Coronary artery, 121f, 122f, 139
Corpus albicans, 252f, 255
Corpus luteum, 254–255, 256f
Corpuscles
    Hassal's, 56
    renal, 164f, 171–172, 171f
    thymic, 56
Corticogonadotrophs, 245t
Corticothyrotrophs, 245t
Corticotroph adenoma, 278
Corticotrophs, 245, 245f, 246f
Corticotropin. *See* Adrenocorticotrophic hormone
Corticotropin-releasing hormone, 241, 245t
Cortisol, 240f, 241, 278
Cortisone, 241
Coupling proteins, of bone matrix, 94
Crypt base columnar cells, 198
CT scan, abdominal, 223f, 225f
Cushing's disease, 278
Cycle, menstrual, phases of, 257–258, 259f, 260f
Cystic fibrosis, 152
Cystinuria, 178
Cysts, subchondral, in osteoarthritis, 74f, 114
Cytochrome P-450 enzymes, 3, 209f, 210, 214
Cytokines, 46
Cytolysin, 55
Cytolytic (cytotoxic) T cells, 52t
Cytomegalovirus, 145, 159
Cytoplasmic dynein, 106

D

D (δ) cells, 248, 249f
Defensins, 49
Degenerative joint disease, 99
Delayed hypersensitivity T cells, 52t
Dendrites, 105

Dendritic cells, 21f
Dense bodies, 131, 131f
Dense bone, 83–85, 84f, 85f
Dermatitis, allergic, 22f, 51
Dermis, 16, 18t
Descemet's endothelium and membrane, 291, 291f
Desmoplastic reaction, 280
Desmosome, 19t, 20f, 26
Diabetes mellitus, 249
Diabetic retinopathy, proliferative, 300
Dictyotene, 253
Dihydropyridine receptor, 103
Dihydrotestosterone, 269
Dilator pupillae, 293
Dipalmitoylphosphatidylcholine, 155
Disaccharidases, 197
Disk(s)
    herniation, 99
    membranous, 298
    optic, 288f, 289f, 291f, 297, 301
Disse, space of, 205, 205f
Distal convoluted tubule, 171f, 174, 175f, 176f, 177f
Distributing arteries. *See* Muscular arteries
Dopamine, 245t, 264
Down syndrome, 278
Drug absorption, 5
Duchenne muscular dystrophy, 104
Duct(s)
    alveolar, 154, 154f
    collecting, renal, 175, 177f
        resorption and secretion in, 177f
    lactiferous, 262
    pancreatic, 202–203
    papillary, 169, 169f
    thoracic, 136
Ductus deferens, 273, 274f
Ductus epididymis, 273, 274f
Duodenum, 198, 198f
Dynein, 4, 106
Dyshesive disorders, of skin, 16
Dysphagia, 190t
Dysplasia, cervical, 279
Dysplastic nevus, 26
Dystrophin, 104

E

Ectropion, endocervical, 280
Edema, 78, 129, 138, 151
    alveolar, 138, 158
    interstitial, pulmonary, 158
    of optic disk, 301
    osmotic, 163, 181
    pulmonary, 138, 157f, **158**
Ehlers-Danlos syndrome, type VII, 80
Elastic artery, 133t
Elastic cartilage, 86
Elastic fibers and laminae, 81
Elastin, 81, 151f, 153, 160f
Embolism, 139–140

Emesis, causes and mechanism of, 196, 196f, 197f
Emphysema, 158, 160f
Encephalitis, 106
Endocardium, 126
Endochondral ossification, 92f
Endometrium, 257–258, 260f
   bleeding of, 258
   spiral (coiled) arterial supply, 258
Endomysium, 78
Endoneurium, 78, 108f
Endoplasmic reticulum, smooth-surfaced, 3
Endoreduplication, 45
Endosteum, 84
Endothelial cells
   adhesion molecules of, 48–49, 48f
   inflammatory mediators from, 47t
Endothelin, 134t
Endothelium, Descemet's, 291, 291f
Endothelium-derived relaxing factor, 134t
Endotoxin, 63, 161
Enteric nervous system, 192
Enteroendocrine cells, 193, 194–196, 195f, 198
Enterohepatic circulation, 207, 208f
Enterokinase, 197
Eosinophils, 37f, **39t**, 47t, 51, 64
   granule contents, 50t
   in nasal polyposis, 35f, 64
Ependymal cells, 107
Epicardium, 126
Epidermis, 14, 18t
Epimysium, 78
Epinephrine, 240f, 241, 242f, 276
   and vascular tonus, 134t
Epineurium, 78, 108f
Epiphyseal plates, 90f, 91, 91f, 116
Epiphyseal separation, 95
Erythroblast
   basophilic, 43f
   polychromatophilic, 43f
Erythrocytes, 37f, 38, **39t**
   polychromatophilic, 41, 43f
Erythropoietin, 42f
   cellular sources of, 180
   recombinant, and anemia, 181
Esophageal sphincters, 192, 196f
Esophageal varices, 211f, 212, 212f, 215
Esophagitis, reflux, 192
Esophagus, 190t, 191f, 192
Estrogen, 254, 255f, 256, 257f, 262, 263
   and osteoporosis, 113
Estrogen receptor assay, and breast cancer, 280–281
Estrogenic phase, 257
Ethanol (ethyl alchohol), metabolism and oxidative
     elimination of, 209f, 210
Ethylene glycol, nephrotoxic effect of, 182
Excitation-contraction coupling, in skeletal and cardiac
     muscle, 124f
Exocervix, 261, 279
Exotoxins, 159
Eye, 289–290, 291f

F
Fallopian tubes, 256
Fat-storing cells of Ito. *See* Lipocytes
Fatty casts, 176, 181
Fatty streak, 135t, 140
F cells, 248, 249f
Ferritin, 207, 208f
Fever, 159–160
   anti-inflammatory drugs and, 161
Fibers, coarse (outer dense), 266, 267f
Fibrillin, 81
Fibrocartilage, 86, 87f
Fibrosis, cystic, 152
Fibrous plaque, 135t
Fibrous sheath, 266, 267f
Filaments
   anchoring, 136, 137f
   intermediate (IF), 19t, 20f
   thick and thin, of skeletal muscle, 101, 101f, 102f
Filtration slit diaphragm, 176, 178f
Flagellum, 266, 266f
Fluid
   ascitic, 215
   testicular, 269
Foam cells, 135t
Focal contact, 19t, 20f
Folate, and anemia, 62
Follicle-stimulating hormone, 247t, 255f, 257f, 269
Follicles
   atretic, 251–252, 252f, 253f
   lymphoid, primary and secondary, 59
   mature (Graafian), 252, 252f
   ovarian, primary and secondary, 251, 252f, 253f
   primordial, 251, 252f, 253f
Follicular dendritic cells, 55, 59
Follicular epithelial cells, of thyroid, 237, 238f
Follicular granulosa cells, 256, 257f
Follicular lutein cells, 254
Follicular phase, 257, 257f
Fovea centralis, 291f, 295
Fracture repair, 96–97
Fundic glands, 192, **193**, 194f, 195f
Fundus
   of eye, 288f
   of stomach, 192, 193f

G
G$_0$, 8
Galactorrhea, 277
Gallbladder, 203f, 207
Ganglia, 108
Ganglion cells, of retina, 295, 297f
Gastrin, 196
Gastrointestinal endocrine cells, 193, 194, 198
Gastrointestinal tract, organization of, 189, 191f
G cells, 196
Germ cells, 252, 254t, 265, 265t
Gland(s)
   adrenal, 240, 240f, 241f
   Brunner's, 198, 198f

Gland(s) *(contd.)*
  cardiac, 192, 193
  cervical, 260f, 261
  fundic, 192, **193**, 194f, 195f
  interstitial, 256
  mammary, 262
  parathyroid, 250, 250f
  pituitary, 243–248, 243f–246f, 245t, 247t
  prostatic, 271, 272f, 281
  pyloric, 194
  sebaceous, 17f, 18t, 26
  sweat, 16, 17f
Glaucoma, narrow-angle, 294
Glial cells, 106–107
Glial fibrillary acidic protein, 107
Glioblastomas, 107
Gliomas, malignant, 107
Gliosis, 107
Glomerular basement membrane, 6, 171f, 173f, 176, 178f
Glomerulonephritis, 172, 181
Glomerulus, 171f, 172
Glucagon, 248–249, 249f
Glucocorticoids, 241
Glucose transporters, 249
Glycosuria, 249
Goiter, 239–240, 239f, 277
Golgi apparatus, 2
Gonadotrophs, 245, 245f
Gonadotropin-releasing hormone, 245t, 257f, 259f, 277
Granular casts, 181
Granulation tissue, 139
Granules
  azurophilic, of neutrophils, 49, 50t
  neutrophil, 49, 50t
  specific,
    leukocytic and mast cell, composition of, 50t
    of neutrophils, 49, 50t
Granulosa cells, 256, 257f
Graves disease, 239f, 240
Gray matter, 105
Ground substance, 78
Growth factors, 7
  hematopoietic, 41, **42f**, 63
  insulin-like, 246
Growth hormone, 246, 247t
  releasing and inhibiting hormones, 245t
Guillain-Barré syndrome, 111

H
Hashimoto's thyroiditis, 276
Hassal's corpuscles, 56
Haversian canal, 84, 85f
Haversian systems, 84, 85f
Head cap, 266, 266f, 267f
Heart, impulse-conducting pathways of, 127–129, 128f
Heart failure (left, right), 129, 140
Heart failure cells, 155
Heart rate, regulation of, 129
Helicobacter pylori, 213
Helper T cells, 52t

Hematopoiesis, 38, 40f
  extramedullary, 61
Hematopoietic cells, 41, 43f, 63
Hematopoietic growth factors, 41, **42f**, 63
Hematopoietic stem cells, transplantation of, 63
Hematuria, 176
Hemianopsia, bitemporal, 243
Hemidesmosome, 19t, 20f
Hemochromatosis, 208f
Hemodynamic (hydrostatic) edema, pulmonary, 138
Hemoglobin degradation, 207, 208f
Hemoglobin S, 64
Hemorrhoids, internal, 211f, 212
Hemosiderin and hemosiderosis, 207, 208f
Henle, loop of, 171f, 173–174, 176f, 177f
Hepatic sinusoids, 205, 205f
Hepatic venules, terminal, 206, 206f
Hepatitis
  alcoholic, 214, 215
  toxic, 214
Hepatocytes, 3, 210
  alcohol metabolism in, 209f, 210
  and α_1-antitrypsin deficiency, 158–159, 160f
  functions of, 203
Herring bodies, 247
High endothelial venules (HEVs), 57t, 58, 59–60
Histamine, 47t, 50t, 134t
Histiocyte, 55
HIV. *See* Human immunodeficiency virus
Hormone(s)
  adrenocorticotrophic, 241, 246, 247, 278
  antidiuretic, 178, 180t
  corticotropin-releasing, 241, 245t
  follicle-stimulating, 247t, 255f, 257f, 269
  gonadotropin-releasing, 245t, 257f, 259f, 277
  growth, 246, 247t
    regulation of release, 245t
  luteinizing, 247t, 255f, 257f, 269
  melanocyte-stimulating (MSH), 246, 246f, 247t
  ovarian steroid, 257f
  parathyroid
    actions of, 90, 250–251
    osteoblast receptor for, 87
  receptors for, 237
  thyroid, 237–238
  thyroid-stimulating, 238f, 239, 239f, 247t
  thyrotropin-releasing, 245t
Human immunodeficiency virus, 53
Hyaline, alcoholic (Mallory's), 214, 216
Hyaline cartilage, 85–86
Hyaline casts, 176, 181
Hyaline membrane disease, 157
Hydrochloric acid, production by parietal cells, 193–194
Hydrocortisone, 240f, 241
Hydropic swelling, 182
Hydroxyapatite, 82t, 83
Hyperbilirubinemia, 212, 213t, 214
Hypercalcemia, 251
Hyperkeratosis, 25
Hypermelanosis, 24t
Hypersensitivity, 49–51

Hypertension
  portal, 210, 215
  pulmonary, 129, **138–139**, 140
Hyperthermia, malignant, 103
Hypoalbuminemia, and edema, 215
Hypocalcemia, 251
Hypomelanosis, 24t
Hypophyseal portal circulation, 243, 244f
Hypophysis. *See* Pituitary

I

I bands, 101f, 102
Icterus. *See* Jaundice
Ileum, 199, 199f
Immature bone, 85
Immotile cilia syndromes, 152, 267
Immune responses, 51
Immunoglobulins, thyroid-stimulating, 238f, 239, 239f, 277
Inflammation, 46–47
  acute, 22f, 47t, **48**
    in psoriasis, 25
  allergic, 47t, 64
  chronic, 46, 47t
  subacute, 47t
Inflammatory mediators, cellular sources of, 47t
Inhibin, 269
Insulin, 248–250, 249f
Insulin-like growth factors, 246
Integrins, 19t, 20f, 49
Interaleolar walls, 154, 154f
Intercalated cells, 175, 175f
Intercalated disks, 122, 123, 123f, 125f, 126f
Interleukins, 42f
Intermediate filaments (IF), 19t, 20f
Internal hemorrhoids, 211f, 212
Internodal atrial pathways, 128f, 129
Interstitial cells, of testis, 268, 269, 270f, 271f
Interstitial edema, pulmonary, 138, 158
Interstitial gland, ovarian, 256
Interstitial growth, of cartilage, 86
Interstitial lamellae, 94
Intervertebral disks, 99
Intestine
  large, 190t, 199–200, 200f
  small, 190t, 196–199
Intramembranous ossification, 90
Intraocular pressure, 294
Intrinsic factor, 30, 62, 193
Iridocorneal angle, 293, 294f
Iris, 290f, 291f, 293
Ischemic attack, transient, 139
Ischemic phase, 258, 259f
Islets, of Langerhans (pancreatic), 248, 248f
Ito, cells of. *See* Lipocytes

J

Jaundice, 212, 213t, 214
Jejunum, 199

JG cells, 171f, 179, 180t
Joints
  anterior intervertebral, 99
  degenerative disease (osteoarthritis), 99, 114
  synovial, 97, 98f, 99
Junctional feet, 103
Junctional nevus, 26
Junctional sarcoplasmic reticulum, 125, 125f
Junctions
  adhering (anchoring), **19t**, 20f, 123, 123f, 125f
  tight, 4
Juxtaglomerular apparatus, 171f, 179
Juxtaglomerular cells, 171f, 179, 180t

K

Kartagener syndrome, 267
Karyotype, 229, 229f, 230f, 278
Keratinocytes, 21f
Kidney(s), 167–171
  blood supply, 169–171, 170f
  cortex, 165f, 167f, 168, 169f
  infarcts, 170
  lobes and lobules, 168–169, 169f
  medulla, 167f, 168, 169f
    interstitial gradient of, 178
  sites of regulated resorption, 177f
  tubules, 167
Kidney stones, 177–178, 183
Kinesin, 105
Kulchitsky cells, 148
Kupffer cells, 205, 205f
Kyphosis, 113

L

Lacis cells, 171f, 179, 180
Lactation, 264
Lactiferous duct, 262
Lactoferrin, 49
Lamellar bodies, 155, 156f
Lamellar bone, 84
Langerhans, islets of, 248, 248f
Langerhans cells, 21f, 22f, 51
Large intestine, 190t, 199–200, 200f
Left heart failure, 129, 140
Lens, 291f, 292, 292f
  capsule, 292, 292f
Lens fiber, 292, 292f
Lesion, aceto-white, 233, 280
Leukemia, acute myelomonocytic, 34, 64
Leukotrienes, and vascular tonus, 134t
Leydig cells, 269. *See also under* Interstitial cells
Ligaments, 78
Lipase, 193
Lipocytes, 205, 206
Liver, 190t, 203–207
Liver
  acinus, 206–207, 206f
  alcohol effects on, 209f, 210, 214
  fatty, 215

Liver (contd.)
  lobule, classic, 206, 206f
  pseudolobules, 214
  sinusoids, 205, 205f
Loop of Henle, 171f, 173–174, 176f, 177f
Low density lipoprotein, 135t
Lung, 144f, 148, 150
  acinus, 150, 153
  lobules, 150, 150f
  organization of, 150
Lutein cells, 254–255, 256f, 257f
Luteinizing hormone, 247t, 255f, 257f, 269
Lymph nodes, 57t, 58–60, 59f
Lymphatic capillaries, 133t, 136, 137f, 197
Lymphatics, 133t, 134f, 136
Lymphocytes, 37f, **39t** . See also under B cell(s), T cell(s)
  activated, 59
  lifespan of, 54
  small, large, and large granular, 54
Lymphoid follicles (nodules), 57t, 58, 59, 60
Lymphoid organs and tissues, distinctive features of, 57t
Lymphoid sheaths, of spleen, 60, 60f
Lymphoid tissue, mucosa-associated (MALT), 57t, 58
Lymphokines, 46, 47t
Lysozyme, 49

M
Macrocytes, 62
Macrophages, 135t, 155
  inflammatory mediators from, 47t
Macula adherens, 19t
Macula densa, 171f, 179
Macula lutea, 288f, 297
Macular acuity, 297
Malignant hyperthermia, 103
Mallory bodies, 214, 216
Mallory's hyaline, 214, 216
Mammary carcinoma, 281
Mammary glands, 262
Mammogram, 234f
Mammosomatotrophs, 245t
Mammotrophs, 245, 245f, 246f
Marginal zone, of spleen, 60
Mast cells, 47t, 50
  granule contents, 50t
Matrix, of bone and cartilage, composition, 82, 82t
Matrix vesicles, 83
Mature bone, 84
Mean corpuscular volume, 30, 62
Medullary rays, 168, 168f, 169f
Megakaryocyte, 43f, 45
Megaloblastic anemia, 62
Meiotic division, 253
Meissner's plexus, 191f, 192
Melanin, **23t**, 24, **24t**
Melanization, epidermal, 24, 24t
Melanocyte-stimulating hormone (MSH), 246, 246f, 247t
Melanocytes, 21f, 22f, 23t
Melanocytic nevus, 24t, 26
Melanoma, malignant, 25–26

Melanosomes, 23t
Melasma, 24t
Membrane
  basement, 5–6, 80, 81f
    epidermal, 18t, 21f
    glomerular, 6, 171f, 173f, 176, 178f
  Bowman's, 291, 291f
  cell, 3, 5
Membranous disks, 298
Memory B cells, 55
Memory T cells, 52t
Meningioma, 301
Menstrual cycle, phases of, 257–258, 259f, 260f
Menstrual phase, 258, 259f, 260f
Mesangial cells, 172, 172f, 173f, 176
Metamyelocyte, 43f, 44
Metarterioles, 133, 133t, 135f
MHC Class I and II surface glycoproteins, 52t, 53, 55
Microcirculation, 133, 135f, 136
Microfilaments (MF), 19t, 20f
Microglia, 107
Microsomal ethanol oxidizing system, 209f
Milk, 263, 264f
  ejection of, 264
Miosis, 293
Mitochondrial sheath, 266, 266f, 267f
Mitosis, incidence of, 10
Mitral stenosis, 137, 138–139
Mitral valve, 119, 119f, 120, 137–138
M line, 101f, 102, 125f
Moles, 14–15f, 24t, **26**
Mongolian spot, 25
Monocytes, 37f, **39t**, 48, 135t
Morphogenetic proteins, of bone matrix, 94
Motilin, 198
Motor end plate, 104
Motor unit, 100
MSH, 246, 246f, 247t
Mucosa, of gastrointestinal tract, 189
Mucosa-associated lymphoid tissue (MALT), 57t, 58
Mucous membrane, of gastrointestinal tract, 189
Mucous neck cells, 193, 194f, 195f
Müller cells, 295
Multiple sclerosis, 111
Muscle
  cardiac, 122–126, 123f, 124f, 125f, 126f, 127t
  ciliary, 291f, 293, 294f
  skeletal, 100–103, 101f, 102f, 103f, 127t
    calcium and excitation-contraction coupling in, 124f
  smooth, 127t, 129–131, 130f, 131f
  types, comparative features of, 127t
Muscular arteries, 132, 133t
Muscular dystrophy, 104
Myasthenia gravis, 104
Mydriasis, 293
Myelin, 111, 115
Myelin-associated glycoprotein, 111
Myelination, 110
Myeloblast, 43f, 44
Myelocyte(s), 43f, 44
Myeloid cells, 43f

Myeloid tissue, 38, 41
Myeloid:erythroid ratio, 41, 42f
Myeloperoxidase, 49
Myenteric plexus, 191f, 192
Myocardial infarction, 129, 139–140
Myocardium, 126, 128f, 129
Myofibril, 101f, 102, 103f, 123, 125f
Myoid cells, 269, 269f
Myometrium, 256
Myosatellite cells, 104
Myosin, 101–102, 102f
Myosin light-chain kinase, 131
Myositis ossificans, 112

N

Natural killer cells, 54
Nephritis
    interstitial, 183
    tubulointerstitial, 179
Nephrons, 167, 169f, 171, 171f
    resorption and secretion in, 177f
Nephrotic syndrome, 181
Nephrotoxicity, 179
Nerve cells, 105
Nerve endings, cutaneous, 18t
Nerves, peripheral, 76f, 108, 108f, 109f
    response to injury of, 109
Nervous system
    enteric, 192
    peripheral, 108
Neuroendocrine cells, 148
Neuroglia, 106–107
Neurolemma (neurilemma), 110
Neurons, 105
Neurophysin, 247
Neuropil, 105
Neutrophilia (neutrophilic leukocytosis), 63
Neutrophils, 37f, **39t**, 47t, 48
    band, 37f, **39t**, 43f
    granules, 49, 50t
    hypersegmented, 62
    maturation of, 46f
    microbial elimination by, 49
    primary granules. See under Azurophilic granules
    secondary granules. See under Specific granules
Nevus
    dysplastic, 26
    junctional, 26
    melanocytic, 24t, 26
Nitric oxide, 134t
Node(s)
    A-V and S-A, 128f, 129
    of nerve fibers, 110
Nodules, lymphoid, primary, and secondary. See under
        Follicles
Noradrenaline. See Norepinephrine
Norepinephrine, 148, 240f, 241, 242f, 276
    and vascular tonus, 134t
Normoblast, 41, 43f
Nucleoli, 1–2

Nucleus
    organization of, 1
    paraventricular and supraoptic, 247
Nucleus pulposus, 99, 100f
Nutrient arteries, of bones, 94

O

Oligodendrocytes, 107
Omeprazole, and acid secretion in the stomach, 194, 213
Oocytes
    primary, 253, 254t
    secondary, 254, 254t
Oogenesis, 252, 254t
Oogonia, 253, 254t
Opsins, 298
Opsonization, 49
Optic chiasma, 243, 277
Optic disk, 288f, 289f, 291f, 297, 301
Osmotic edema, 163, 181
Ossification
    endochondral, 92f
    heterotopic, 112
    intramembranous, 90
    primary and secondary centers of, 92f
Osteoarthritis, 99, 114
Osteoblasts, 87, 88f
Osteocalcin, 82
Osteoclasts, 88, 89f, 250, 251
    and bone calcium release, 88–90, 89f
Osteocytes, 88
Osteogenic cell sarcoma, 112
Osteogenic cells, 87
Osteoid tissue, 82
Osteoinductive proteins, of bone matrix, 94
Osteomalacia, 82
Osteomyelitis, 111
Osteons, 84
Osteophytes, 114
Osteoporosis, 94, 113
Osteoprogenitor cells, 87
Osteosarcoma, 112
Ovarian follicles, 251, 252f, 253f
Ovarian steroidogenesis, 256, 257f
Ovaries, 251, 252f
Ovum, 254, 254t
Oxyntic cells. See Parietal cells
Oxyphil cells, 250, 250f
Oxytocin, 247, 256, 264

P

P-450 enzymes, 3, 209f, 210, 214
Pacemaker cells, cardiac, 127, 129
Pain, referred, 110f, 111, 115
Pancreas, 190t, 201–203, 202f
Pancreatic ducts, 202–203
Pancreatic islets, 248, 248f
Pancreatic polypeptide, 249
Pancreatitis, and excessive alcohol consumption, 216
Pancytopenia, 62

Paneth cells, 198
Pap (Papanicolaou) smear, 231f, 279
Papanicolaou stain, 261
Papilla
  of eye, 297
  renal, 168, 169f, 179
Papillary duct, 169, 169f
Papillary necrosis, 179, 183
Papilledema, 301
Papillitis, necrotizing, 179, 183
Papillomaviruses, 280
Paracentesis, 215
Paracetamol, nephrotoxicity of, 179
Parafollicular cells, 237. *See also* C cells
Parakeratosis, 25
Parathyroid hormone
  actions of, 90, 250–251
  receptor for, on osteoblasts, 87
Parathyroids, 250, 250f
Paraventricular nucleus, 247
Parietal cells, 62, 193–194, 194f, 195f
Pars intermedia, 248
Pemphigus vulgaris, 16
Peptic ulcer, 213
Peptidases, 197
Perforin, 55
Pericardium, 126, 128f
Perichondrium, 85–86, 96, 96f
Pericytes, 78, 140
Perimysium, 78
Perineurium, 78, 108f
Periosteum, 84
Peripheral blood, normal values, 36t
Peripheral nerves, 76f, 108, 108f, 109f
  response to injury, 109
Perisinusoidal space, 205, 205f
Pernicious anemia, 62
Peyer's patches, 199, 199f
Phagocytosis, 49
Phenacetin, nephrotoxicity of, 179
Pheochromocytoma, 277
Photoreceptors, 298
Pitting edema, 78
Pituicytes, 247
Pituitary, 243–248, 243f–246f, 245t, 247t
  acidophils and basophils, 245t
  adenomas, 246
  anterior lobe, 243f–245f, 244, 245t, 246f, 247t. *See also*
    under Anterior pituitary
  posterior lobe, 243f–245f, 246
  tumors, 246
Plasma cell, 43f, 53, 54f
Platelets, 37f, 38, **39t**
  storage of, 61
Pleuritis, referred pain in, 115
Plexus
  myenteric (Auerbach's), 191f, 192
  submucosal (Meissner's), 191f, 192
Pneumocytes, types I and II, 154, 154f, 155f, 156f
Pneumonia (pneumonitis), 31, 115, 159
Podocytes, 172, 173f, 176

Polar bodies, 254, 254t
Polychromatophilic erythroblast, 43f
Polychromatophilic erythrocyte, 41, 43f
Polymorphs (polymorphonuclear leukocytes). *See*
    Neutrophils
Portal circulation, 210
Portal hypertension, 210, 215
Portal-systemic anastomoses, 210–212, 211f
Portal tracts (radicles), 204, 204f, 206f
Portal vein, 210, 211f
Postcapillary venules, 48, 140
Posterior chamber, of eye, 291f, 294
Prebone, 82
Presbyopia, 293
Pressure, intraocular, 294
Primary follicles, 251, 252f, 253f
Primary oocytes, 253, 254t
Primary spermatocytes, 265, 265t
Primordial follicles, 251, 252f, 253f
Pro-opiomelanocortin, 246, 246f
Procollagen, 79
Proerythroblast, 43f
Progestational phase, 257
Progesterone, 254, 255f, 256, 257f, 263
Progesterone receptor, and breast cancer, 281
Prolactin, 225, 245t, 247t, 263–264, 277
  releasing and inhibiting hormones, 245t
Prolactin cell adenoma, 277
Prolactinoma, 246, 277
Prolapsed disk, 100
Proliferative phase, 257, 258, 259f, 260f
Promyelocyte, 43f, 44
Prophase I, 253, 254t
Prostaglandins, and vascular tonus, 134t
Prostate, 271–273, 272f, 273f
  benign hyperplasia of, 271, 281
Prostate-specific antigen, 273
Prostatic acid phosphatase, 273
Prostatic adenocarcinoma, 281–282
Prostatic hyperplasia, benign, 271, 281
Protein synthesis, 2
Proteinuria, 181
Proximal convoluted tubule, 171f, 173, 174f, 176f, 177f
Psammoma bodies, 275
Psoriasis vulgaris, 25
Ptosis, 104
Pulmonary edema, 138, 157f, **158**
Pulmonary hypertension, 129, **138–139**, 140
Pulmonary interstitial edema, 158
Pulmonary surfactant, 148, 154, **155**, 157
Purkinje fibers, 128f, 129
Pyelonephritis, 183
Pyloric glands, 194
Pyloric sphincter, 196
Pyramid, renal, 168, 168f
Pyrosis, 192

R

Rabies virus, access route to CNS, 106
Reactive astrocytes, 107

Reactive bone, 236
Receptors
    adrenergic, of smooth muscle, 131
    cholinergic, of smooth muscle, 131
    dihydropyridine, 103
    hormone, 237
    ryanodine, 103
Red pulp, of spleen, 60
Referred pain, 110f, 111, 115
Reflux esophagitis, 192
Relaxin, 239
Remodeling, of bone, 93
Renal calculi, 177–178, 183
Renal columns, 168f, 169
Renal corpuscle, 164f, 171–172, 171f
Renal cortex, 165f, 167f, 168, 169f
Renal medulla, 167f, 168, 169f
Renin, 179–180, 180t
    and intravascular volume regulation, 180t
Rennin, 193
Respiratory bronchioles, 154, 154f
Respiratory distress syndrome, neonatal idiopathic, 157
Rete cutaneum, 21, 22f
Rete subpapillare, 21, 22f
Reticular cells, epithelial, of thymus, 56
Reticulocyte counts, 44
Reticulocytes, 37f, **39t**, 44, 45f
Retina, 286f, 291f, 295–297, 296f, 297f
    detached, 297, 300
    neovascularization of, 300
    neural, 295
Retinal pigment epithelium, 290, 290f, 296f, 299f, 300
Rheumatic fever, and heart disease, 119, 120, 138
Rheumatic heart disease, 138
Rhodopsin, 298
Ribbon synapse, 298
Rickets, 82
Right heart failure, 129
Rods, retinal, 297f, 298, 299f
Ruffled borders, 88, 89f
Ruptured disk, 100
Ryanodine receptor, 103

S
S-A node, 128f, 129
Sarcolemma, 101f, 103
Sarcomeres, 102
Sarcoplasmic reticulum, 101f, 102–103, 123–125, 125f
    corbular, 125, 125f
    junctional, 125, 125f
Satellite cells, of skeletal muscle, 104
Scans
    bone, 75f, 114, 236
    CT, abdominal, 223f, 225f
    thyroid, 220f, 275–276
    ultrasound, abdominal, 223f
Schiller's test, 280
Schilling test, 30, 62
Schlemm's canal, 293–294, 294f
Schwann, sheath of, 110

Schwann cells, 106, 108, 108f, 109f, 110
Sclera, 290, 290f, 291f
Scotopsin, 298
Scurvy, 79
Sebaceous gland, 17f, 18t, 26
Secondary follicles, 251
Secondary oocytes, 254, 254t
Secondary spermatocytes, 265, 265t
Secretory phase, 257, 258, 259f, 260f
Seminal vesicles, 274, 275f
Seminiferous tubules, 265, 265t, 268–269, 268f
Serosa, of gastrointestinal tract, 191f, 192
Serotonin, 193
    and vascular tonus, 134t
Sertoli cells, 268, 269, 269f, 272f
Sheath
    fibrous, 266, 267f
    mitochondrial, 266, 266f, 267f
    of Schwann, 110
Shift to the left, 63
Shock, hypovolemic, due to burns, 24
Sickle cell disease (anemia), 64
Sinoatrial node, 127
Sinus venosus sclerae, 293–294, 294f
Sinusoids
    of bone marrow, 41
    of liver, 205, 205f
    of spleen, 61
Skeletal muscle, 100–103, 101f, 102f, 103f, 127t
    calcium and excitation-contraction coupling in, 124f
Skin
    blood supply of, 20–21, 22f
    burns of, 23–24
    features and organization of, 14–16, 18t
    functions of, 19t
    key components of, 21f
    lesions, 16, 19t
    structure-function relationships of, 22f
Slow calcium channel, 103, 124f
Small intestine, 190t, 196–199
Smooth muscle, 127t, 129–131, 130f, 131f
    cells, 129–131, 135t
Smooth-surfaced endoplasmic reticulum, 3
Somatomedins, 246
Somatostatin, 148, 193, 245t, 248, 249f
Somatotrophs, 245, 245f, 246f
Space
    of Disse (perisinusoidal), 205, 205f
    urinary, 176, 178f
Specific granules
    leukocytic and mast cell, composition, 50t
    of neutrophils, 49, 50t
Sperm counts, 267
Spermatids, 265, 265t, 266
Spermatocytes, primary and secondary, 265, 265t
Spermatogenesis, 265–266, 265t
    duration of, 266, 268
Spermatogonia, types of, 265–266, 265t, 269f
Spermatozoon, 266, 267f
Spermiogenesis, 266, 266f
S phase, 8

Sphincter
esophageal, 192, 196f
pyloric, 196
Spleen, 60–61, 60f, 61f
circulation and vasculature of, 61, 61f
Splenectomy, 61
Spongy bone. *See* Cancellous bone
Squamous cell carcinoma, 161
Steatosis, 216
Stem cells, 8
Stercobilinogens, 207
Stereocilia, 273
Steroidogenesis, ovarian, 256, 257f
Stomach, 190t, 192–196, 193f–195f
Subacute inflammation, 47t
Subchondral cysts, in osteoarthritis, 74f, 114
Submucosal glands, of duodenum, 198, 198f
Submucosal plexus, 191f, 192
Substantia propria, 291, 291f
Sunburn, 24
Superoxide radicles, 49
Suppressor T cells, 52t
Supraoptic nucleus, 247
Suprarenals. *See* Adrenal(s)
Surface membrane immunoglobulin, of B lymphocytes, 53
Surfactant, pulmonary, 148, 154, **155**, 157
Sweat gland, 16, 17f
Synapses, 105, 116
ribbon, 298
Syndrome. *See under individual names*
Synovial fluid, 97
Synovial joints, 97, 98f, 99
Synovial membrane (synovium), 98, 111
Synovitis, 111
System, haversian, 84, 85f

T

T cell(s), 52t, 53. *See also under* T lymphocytes
activation of, 55
antigen receptor, 53
T lymphocytes, 52t, 53
inflammatory mediators from, 47t
subsets of, 52t
T tubules, 101f, 103, 123, 125f
T₃ and T₄, 238, 238f
Tamoxifen, 281
Tay-Sach's disease, 3
Tendons, 78
Teniae coli, 200
Terminal cisternae, of sarcoplasmic reticulum, 101f, 103
Terminal hepatic venules, 206, 206f
Testes, 264–265, 265f, 268f
Testosterone, 269
Tetany, 251
Tetraiodothyronine, 238
Theca interna and externa, 252, 256
Theca lutein cells, 255, 256f, 257f
Thick filaments, 101, 101f
Thin filaments, 101, 101f, 102f

Thoracic duct, 136
Thrombopoietin, 42f, 45
Thymic corpuscles, 56
Thymic hormones, 56
Thymus, 56, 57t, 58f
Thyroglobulin, 237–240, 238f
Thyroid, 237
adenomatous nodule, hyperplastic, 276
carcinoma, papillary, 275
cold nodule, 219, 220, 220f, 276
colloid, 238, 238f
scan, 220f, 275–276
Thyroid hormone, 237–238
Thyroid peroxidase, 237
Thyroid-stimulating hormone, 238f, 239, 239f, 247t
Thyroid-stimulating immunoglobulins, 238f, 239, 239f, 277
Thyroiditis
chronic, 276
Hashimoto's, 276
Thyroperoxidase, 237
Thyrotrophs, 245, 245f
Thyrotropin-releasing hormone, 245t
Tight junctions, 4
Tissue fluid, 78
Tonofilaments, 20f, 26
Tonus, 132
vascular, key regulators of, 134t
Trabecular bone, 83–84, 83f
Transcytosis, 5
Transformation zone, 280
Transient ischemic attack, 139
Transverse (T) tubules, 101f, 103, 123, 125f
Triad, 103
Trigonum fibrosum, 126
Triiodothyronine, 238
Trisomy 21, 278
Tropoelastin, 81
Tropomyosin, 101, 102f
Troponin, 101, 102f
Tubular necrosis, 182
Tubules
collecting, 175, 176f
kidney, 167
seminiferous, 265, 265f, 268–269, 268f
transverse (T), 101f, 103, 123, 125f
Tunica albuginea, of testis, 265, 265f
Type I pneumocytes, 154, 154f, 155f
Type II pneumocytes, 154, 154f, 155f, 156f

U

Ulcer, peptic, 213
Ultrasound scan, abdominal, 223f
Ultraviolet radiation, melanization response to, 24t
Urethra
male, 275
prostatic, 271, 272f, 275
Urinary calculi, 177–178
Urinary casts, 176, 181
Urinary crystals, 177

Urinary filtrate, production, 176, 177f
Urinary sediment, 176
Urinary space, 176, 178f
Urobilinogens, 207, 208f
Urolithiasis, 177–178
Uterine cervix, 258–261
Uterine tubes, 256, 258f
Uterus, 256
Uvea, 290, 290f

V

Vagina, 261, 261f
Valve
    aortic, 138
    mitral, 119, 119f, 120, 137–138
Varices, esophageal, 211f, 212, 212f, 215
Varicose veins, 132
Vasa recta, 170f, 174
Vasa vasorum, 131
Vascular tonus, key regulators of, 134t
Vasectomy, 273
Vasopressin, 247. *See also* Antidiuretic hormone
    and vascular tonus, 134t
Vein(s), 131, 133t
    central, of liver lobules, 205, 206f
    portal, 210, 211f
    varicose, 132
Vena cava, 132f
Venules, 133, 133t, 134f, 140
    terminal hepatic, 206, 206f

Vesicles
    matrix, 83
    seminal, 274, 275f
Vessels
    blood, 131, 132f, **133t**, 134f
    lymphatic. *See* Lymphatics
Villi, 197, 199f
Visual pigments, 298
Vitamin B_{12}, 30, 62
Vitamin C, and collagen formation, 79
Vitamin D_3, 251
Vitreous body, 291f, 294
Vomiting, causes and mechanism of, 196, 196f, 197f

W

Waxy casts, 176
White matter, 105
White pulp, of spleen, 60
Woven (woven-fibered) bone, 85

Z

Z lines, 101f, 102, 123, 125f
Zona fasciculata, glomerulosa, and reticularis, 240f, 241, 241f
Zonula adherens, 19t
Zonule, ciliary, 291f, 293
Zymogenic cells, of fundic glands, 193, 194f, 195f